DAVIS'S
Pharmacology Review
for the
NCLEX-RN

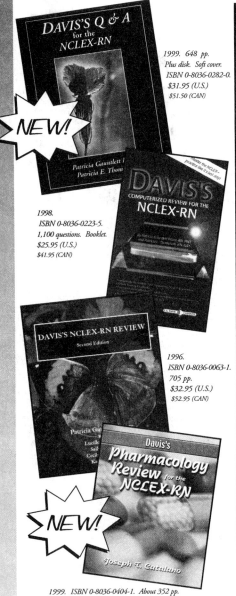
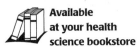
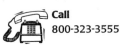

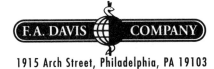

DAVIS'S
Pharmacology Review
for the
NCLEX-RN

JOSEPH T. CATALANO PhD, RN, CCRN
Professor of Nursing
East Central University
Ada, Oklahoma

F. A. DAVIS COMPANY ■ Philadelphia

F. A. Davis Company
1915 Arch Street
Philadelphia, PA 19103

Manufactured in Canada

Last digit indicates print number: 10 9 8 7 6 5 4 3 2 1

Acquisitions Editor: Alan Sorkowitz
Production Editor: Elena Coler
Designer: Maria Karkucinski
Cover Designer: Louis Forgione

As new scientific information becomes available through basic and clinical research, recommended treatments and drug therapies undergo changes. The author(s) and publisher have done everything possible to make this book accurate, up to date, and in accord with accepted standards at the time of publication. The authors, editors, and publisher are not responsible for errors or omissions or for consequences from application of the book, and make no warranty, expressed or implied, in regard to the contents of the book. Any practice described in this book should be applied by the reader in accordance with professional standards of care used in regard to the unique circumstances that may apply in each situation. The reader is advised always to check product information (package inserts) for changes and new information regarding dose and contraindications before administering any drug. Caution is especially urged when using new or infrequently ordered drugs.

Library of Congress Cataloging-in-Publication Data

Catalano, Joseph T.
    Davis's pharmacology review for the NCLEX-RN / Joseph T. Catalano.
      p.   cm.
    Includes bibliographical references and index.
    ISBN 0-8036-0404-1 (alk. paper)
    1. Pharmacology Outlines, syllabi. etc. 2. Pharmacology
Examinations, questions, etc. 3. Nursing Outlines, syllabi, etc.
4. Nursing Examinations, questions, etc.   I. Title. II. Title:
Pharmacology review for the NCLEX-RN.
    [DNLM: 1. Pharmaceutical Preparations—administration & dosage.
2. Drug Therapy—methods Examination Questions. 3. Pharmacology-
-methods Examination Questions.   QV 18.2 C357d 1999]
    RM301. 14.C38 1999
    615'.1'076—dc21
    DNLM/DLC
    for Library of Congress   99-17377
                                           CIP

To my parents, Thomas A. (deceased) and Kathryn V. Catalano
for the love of learning and knowledge
To my wife, Pamela M. Catalano and my daughters Sarah and Amanda
for their encouragement, devotion, and support
To my very anxious students,
who challenge my teaching skills daily

Education in nursing is generally considered to be a process through which an individual assimilates, analyzes, and finally internalizes information in a way that will increase the intellectual powers of the mind and provide a basis for giving safe client care. Although mastery of knowledge in all areas of nursing practice is important for the provision of safe client care, some areas seem to be more problematic for the student than others. Having taught the pharmacology course at our University for the past seven years, I have come to recognize that information about medications is one of these areas.

Davis's Pharmacology Review for the NCLEX-RN presents basic information about the most common medications a student or new graduate is likely to encounter in beginning practice. From experience, I have found that one of the best methods for mastering medication information is to learn the categories of the drugs. After the key information about the category, such as mode of action, uses, side effects, nursing implications, and so forth has been mastered, it becomes a process of associating the individual medication with the category. Although the students may not know all the details about a medication, if they know what category it belongs to, then they have a good idea of what the medication will do and what its side effects are.

In addition to the outline presentation of the general categories, the book presents approximately 155 of the most common, or prototypical, medications used in today's health care. These medications are presented in greater detail, including dosages, routes, and blood levels (if appropriate), and fetal risk category in a convenient chart form. These are also the medications that the graduate is most likely to encounter on the National Council Licensure Examination (NCLEX).

This book is directed primarily toward graduate nurses from all types of RN nursing programs (ADN, BSN, Diploma). Students who are currently enrolled in pharmacology classes may also find this book useful as a study guide. The only prerequisites for the use of the book are a basic knowledge of anatomy and physiology and perhaps a minimal knowledge of microbiology.

This NCLEX review book focuses exclusively on pharmacology in nursing, whereas most general review books include pharmacology only as a footnote. It is in an easy-to-read-and-learn outline format.

There are 550 questions about medications written at the higher cognitive level that require critical thinking, analysis and application rather than mere basic memory or recall about pharmacology. The correct answers and rationales for each of the distractors are also be included to enhance student learning. There is also a computer disk with an additional 150 questions included to simulate the NCLEX-RN computerized adaptive testing (CAT) that the graduate will be taking in the future.

Consultants

Renee I. L' Ecuyer, BSN, RN
Richland Memorial Hospital
Columbia, South Carolina

James Effinger
Student, BSN Program
University of New Mexico College of Nursing
Albuquerque, New Mexico

Karen S. Hair, RN
Atlantic Community College
Mays Landing, New Jersey

Kevin R. Kennedy
Student, Molloy College
Rockville Center, New York

Sheryl E. Radin
Student, Mount Carmel College of Nursing
Columbus, Ohio

Teresa Rogers
Student, University of Tennessee-Knoxville
Knoxville, Tennessee
President, Tennessee Association of Student Nurses

Heather M. Santa Barbara
Student, BSN Program
University of Delaware
Newark, Delaware

Kelly Sauer
Student, Salve Regina University
Newport, Rhode Island
President, Rhode Island Student Nurses Association

Laura Sherburne
Student, ADN Program
Mt. Hood Community College
Gresham, Oregon

Contents

Part Three
PRACTICE TESTS

Appendices

one

About the NCLEX-RN

1

Understanding the NCLEX-RN

The primary purpose of licensure examinations is to protect the public from unsafe or uneducated practitioners of the nursing profession. Passing the National Council Licensure Examination (NCLEX) examination indicates that graduates have attained the minimum level of competency deemed necessary by the state to practice nursing without injury to clients. Licensure is a legal requirement for all professions that deal with public health, welfare, or safety.

The NCLEX examination is a computerized test that is taken after the student is graduated from a school of nursing. With computerized adaptive tests (CAT), such as the NCLEX, the computer selects questions in accordance with the examination plan and, based on difficulty level, dependent on how the graduate answered previous questions.

The examination measures a wide range of basic nursing knowledge, including pharmacology. Pharmacology is a small (10%–15%) but important part of the NCLEX. It is also an area where graduates traditionally have difficulty, partially because of the large amount of seemingly unrelated information that needs to be mastered, and partially

because of the lack of direct experience with many of the medications. Although there is a relatively small number of questions about pharmacology on the NCLEX, theoretically, any medication in current use is fair game for a question. In reality, the majority of the medications asked about on the NCLEX are the more commonly used, or prototypical, medications that represent the whole group. There is also a minimal number of dosage and calculation questions on the NCLEX.

This book is designed to review the most commonly used or prototypical medications that appear frequently in questions on the NCLEX examination. It guides the graduate through a concise review of the pertinent information. The only really effective method of learning pharmacology is to master the groups or classes of medications and then relate specific medications to those classes. The outline and text portions of this book present the most common classes of medications and concise information about 150 of the most common or prototypical medications that the graduate is likely to encounter on the NCLEX or in practice after graduation.

The second section of the book consists of NCLEX-type questions about pharmacology. In all past NCLEX examinations, questions about medications have included the generic name followed by the brand name of the medication in parenthesis, for example, "digoxin (Lanoxin)." The questions in this book use this format for medication names. These questions are designed to help the graduate obtain a sense of what the actual NCLEX questions are like and reinforce key information about specific medications. All the sample questions in this first chapter overview of the NCLEX are also about medications, again to provide a taste of the type of questions the NCLEX might ask.

NCLEX TEST PLAN

Several substantive changes were made in the NCLEX-RN CAT test plan effective April 1998. The test plan consists of three components: (1) Client Health Needs, (2) Level of Cognitive Ability, and (3) Integrated Concepts and Processes.

COMPONENT 1: CLIENT HEALTH NEEDS

The NCLEX examination asks questions about four general groups of material called *client health needs*. These are Safe and Effective Care Environment, Physiological Integrity Needs, Psychosocial Integrity Needs, and Health Promotion and Maintenance Needs.

In general, all questions about medications might be placed in the Safe and Effective Care Environment category. Because nurses do not prescribe medications, their primary responsibilities are giving the right medication, to the right client, at the right time, in the right dose, and by the right route (five rights). These are primarily safety measures. Medication questions may also be categorized by the clinical area in which the medications are used, particularly if the medication is unique to that area. For example, ritodrine (Yutopar) is used only to control premature labor, and therefore it is given only in the obstetric unit. Questions about it may fall into the Health Promotion and Maintenance need category because that category includes obstetrics.

SAFE AND EFFECTIVE CARE ENVIRONMENT

   a. Management of Care 7% to 13%
   b. Safety, Infection Control 5% to 11%

Total questions in this category make up approximately 20% of the questions on the NCLEX examination. These questions deal with overt safety issues in client care, such as use of restraints, medication administration, safety measures to prevent injuries (e.g., putting up side rails), preventing infections, safety measures with pediatric clients, and special safety needs of clients with psychiatric problems.

This needs category also includes questions about laboratory tests, their results and any special nursing measures associated with them, legal and ethical issues in nursing, a small amount of nursing management, and quality assurance issues. Questions on these issues are intermingled with other questions throughout the examination.

PHYSIOLOGICAL INTEGRITY NEEDS

   a. Basic Care and Comfort 7% to 13%
   b. Pharmacological/Parenteral Therapies 5% to 11%
   c. Reduction of Risk Potential 12% to 18%
   d. Physiological Adaptation 12% to 18%

The Physiological Integrity Needs are concerned with adult medical and surgical nursing care as well as with pediatric clients. It makes up the largest groups of questions; about 50% to 55% of the total number of questions come from this category. It generally includes the more common health-care problems that the nurse deals with on a daily basis, such as diabetes, cardiovascular disorders, neurological and renal diseases. Questions about nursing care of the pediatric client, such as growth and development, congenital abnormalities, child abuse, burn injury, and fractures, are a few of the many potential topics that may be questioned.

PSYCHOSOCIAL INTEGRITY NEEDS

a. Coping and Adaptation 5% to 11%
b. Psychosocial Adaptation 5% to 11%

Psychosocial Integrity Needs are those health-care issues that revolve around the client with psychiatric problems. This category comprises about 15% of the examination and includes questions about the care of clients with anxiety disorders, depression, schizophrenia, and organic mental disease. Also included in the Psychosocial Integrity Needs section are questions about therapeutic communication, crisis intervention, and drug abuse.

HEALTH PROMOTION AND MAINTENANCE NEEDS

a. Life Span Growth and Development 7% to 13%
b. Prevention and Early Detection of Disease 5% to 11%

Health Promotion and Maintenance Needs deals with pregnancy, labor, and delivery; the care of the newborn infant; growth and development; and contagious diseases, particularly sexually transmitted diseases. This section comprises about 15% of the total examination. Teaching and counseling are important parts of nursing care during pregnancy, and knowledge of diet, signs and symptoms of complications, fetal development, and testing used during pregnancy is necessary.

COMPONENT 2: LEVELS OF COGNITIVE ABILITY

The levels of cognitive ability component of the NCLEX examination measures how knowledge has been learned and how it can be used by the nurse. For the NCLEX examination, knowledge is tested at three different levels.

Level 1 consists of knowledge and comprehension questions. Only about 15% of the questions are at this level. These questions involve memory of specific facts and the ability to understand those facts in relationship to a pathophysiological condition. Examples of these types of questions would include knowledge of specific anatomy and physiology, medication dosages and side effects, signs and symptoms of diseases, laboratory test results, and the elements of certain treatments and interventions. The ability to remember and to understand information is the most basic way of learning. Although this type of knowledge is important and underlies the other levels of knowledge, by itself it is not sufficient to ensure safe nursing care. An example of a level 1 question is:

An adult client is to be started on lanoxin (Digoxin) for congestive heart failure. Which of the following doses would the nurse consider appropriate for this medication?

a. 0.025 mg PO qid
b. 2 mg IV qd
c. 0.125 mg PO qd
d. 5 mg PO bid

The correct answer is c. The normal dosage range for this medication is 0.125 mg to 0.25 mg once a day. The graduate either does or does not know the correct dosage.

Level 2 consists of questions that ask the nurse to analyze and to apply the information learned by memory to specific client care situations. Analysis and application questions are more difficult to answer because they require the nurse to take the information learned through memory and do something with it. Analysis involves the ability to separate information into its basic parts and decide which of those parts is important. Application requires that the nurse be able to use that information in client care decisions. Examples of this type of question may include questions about the interpretation of electrocardiogram (ECG) strips, interpretation of blood gas values, making a nursing diagnosis based on a set of symptoms, or deciding on a course of treatment. These types of questions provide a better indication of the nurse's ability to care for clients. An example of a level 2 question is:

A client who has been receiving 200 mg of IV aminophylline every 6 hours IV is becoming restless and developing tachycardia. His theophylline level is 26.4 μg/mL. The nurse would suspect that the client:

a. Needs a higher dosage of medication to control the symptoms
b. Is theophylline-toxic
c. Should be started on a sedative to reduce his anxiety
d. Requires more ambulation to use up his excessive energy

The correct answer is *b*. The graduate needs to know not only the therapeutic range for theophylline (10–20 μg/mL) but also how to use that information to determine the developing condition based on the client's symptoms.

Level 3—synthesis and evaluation—takes the process one step further. Approximately 85% of the questions are at level 2 or level 3. Questions at the synthesis and evaluation level ask the nurse to make judgments about client care. One factor that adds to the difficulty of answering this type of question is that there is often more than one correct answer for the question. The nurse is asked to choose the best answer from among several correct answers. Questions at this level often ask about the priority of care to be given, the priority of nursing diagnosis formulated, how to best evaluate the effectiveness of care that has been given, and the most appropriate nursing action to be taken. It is felt that the ability of the nurse to make decisions about nursing care at these higher levels is the best indication of the thought processes expected of a nurse demonstrating safe nursing care. An example of a level 3 question is:

An adult client with type 1 diabetes is becoming lethargic and disoriented and having deep, blowing-type respirations. His blood glucose is 378, and his arterial blood gases (ABGs) are as follows: pH—7.13; Po_2—98; Pco_2—36; HCO_3—8. If all of the following medications are ordered for this client, which should the nurse give first?

  a. 25 U NPH insulin SC
  b. Oxygen by nasal prongs at 4 L/min
  c. Amitriptyline (Elavil) 30 mg PO
  d. Sodium bicarbonate 75 mEq IV push

The best answer to this question is answer *d*. Answers *a*, *b*, and *c* are for medications that should be given eventually, but at this particular time, correcting the acid-base balance of this client, who is in severe metabolic acidosis, must receive highest priority. This question requires not only that the graduate know the symptoms of diabetic ketoacidosis (DKA) and the normals for ABGs (recall) but also that the graduate interpret the ABGs (analysis) and select the medication to be given first from several correct options (judgment).

COMPONENT 3: INTEGRATED CONCEPTS AND PROCESSES

The Integrated Concepts and Processes component includes:

Nursing Process
Concepts of Caring
Therapeutic Communication
Cultural Awareness
Documentation
Self-Care
Teaching/Learning

These concepts will be integrated throughout the examination and included as elements in the four needs categories.

The Nursing Process has traditionally been a very important part of the NCLEX. The NCLEX-RN CAT uses the five-step nursing process: assessment, analysis, planning, implementation, and evaluation. Each of the questions that the graduate answers will fall into one of these five categories. It is important that the graduate keep in mind the phase of the Nursing Process when answering questions. Often questions that ask, "What should the nurse do first?" are looking for an assessment-type answer because that is the first phase in the Nursing Process. Questions on the Nursing Process are equally divided on the examination (about 20% in each category).

1. The assessment phase primarily establishes the data base on which the rest of the Nursing Process is built. Some of the components of the assessment phase include both subjective and objective data about the client, significant history, history of the present illness, signs and symptoms, environmental elements, laboratory values, vital signs, and so forth. Often the examination will ask the nurse to distinguish between appropriate and inappropriate assessment factors. An example of an assessment phase question is:

A type 1 diabetic client is receiving propranolol hydrochloride (Inderal) for a cardiac condition. Which of the following would be the most important assessment of this client made by the nurse?

a. Hyperglycemia
b. Hypoglycemia
c. Hypertension
d. Hyperthyroidism

The correct answer is *b*. Beta-blockers like Inderal mask or suppress some of the clinical signs of hypoglycemia, such as elevated blood pressure and tachycardia. Monitor the client for diaphoresis, fatigue, tremors, hunger, and disorientation.

2. The analysis phase of the Nursing Process involves developing and using nursing diagnosis

for the care of the client. The NCLEX examination uses the North American Nursing Diagnosis Association (NANDA) nursing diagnosis system. Also, questions concerning nursing diagnosis often ask the graduate to set priorities in regard to the diagnoses. An example of analysis phase question is:

A client is admitted with chronic bronchitis, superventricular tachycardia, and fever. The physician prescribes theophylline (Aminophylline) IV, propranolol (Inderal) PO, and acetaminophen (Tylenol) PO. The following nursing diagnoses are all appropriate; which one has the highest priority on the nurse's care plan?

a. Anxiety related to fear of hospitalization
b. Ineffective airway clearance related to retained secretions
c. Alterations in cardiac output (decreased) related to rapid heart rate
d. Ineffective thermoregulation related to fever

The correct answer is *b*. Nursing diagnoses that deal with airway always have highest priority. With this client, the respiratory complications may be compounded because betablockers like Inderal, which is being used to slow the heart rate, may worsen chronic obstructive respiratory disorders.

3. The planning phase of the Nursing Process primarily involves goal setting for the client. Included in the planning phase are such factors as determining expected outcomes, setting priorities for goals, anticipating client needs based on the assessment, and so forth. An example of a planning phase question is:

A client is determined to have been in respiratory failure and is started on IV aminophylline every 4 hours. Which of the following goals would have the highest priority for this client?

a. Ambulate twice a shift the length of the hall.
b. Complete the client's bath and A.M. care before breakfast.
c. Maintain an oxygen saturation of 90% throughout the shift.
d. Keep the head of the bed elevated to promote proper ventilation.

The correct answer is *c*. Answer *a* is unrealistic for this client. Answer *b* is not client centered, and answer *d* is a nursing intervention, not a goal. Maintaining an oxygen saturation of 90% is realistic, measurable, and client-centered.

4. The intervention/implementation phase of the Nursing Process involves identifying those nursing actions that are required to meet the goals stated in the planning phase. Some of the material that is included in the intervention/implementation phase are provision of nursing care based on the goals, prevention of injury or spread of disease, medications and medication administration, giving treatments, carrying out procedures, charting and keeping of records, teaching about health care, monitoring changes in condition, and so forth. An example of an intervention/implementation phase question is:

A postoperative client is given prochlorperazine (Compazine) IM for nausea. Which of the following actions by the nurse would be most appropriate after the administration of this medication?

a. Assess the client's skin color for cyanosis.
b. Give 60 mL of clear liquid to help settle the client's stomach.
c. Place the client in a right lateral position.
d. Assess the client's blood pressure for hypertension.

The correct answer to this question is *c*. Compazine depresses the cough reflex, making the client more vulnerable to aspiration. Positioning the client on the side or with the head elevated helps prevent aspiration.

5. The evaluation phase of the nursing process determines whether or not the goals stated in the planning phase were met through the interventions. The evaluation phase also ties the steps of the nursing process together and makes the process cyclical. If the goals were met, there is no problem. If they were not met, then the nurse has to go back and see where the difficulty lies. Was there inadequate assessment data? Were the goals defective, or was there a deficiency in the implementation? Material that is included in the evaluation phase includes comparison of actual outcomes to expected outcomes, verification of assessment data, evaluation of nursing actions and client responses, and evaluation of the client's level of knowledge and understanding. An example of an evaluation question is:

A client is being prepared for discharge. He is to take a theophylline medication by mouth at home for his lung disease. The nurse will know that the teaching concerning theophylline medications has been effective if the client states,

a. "I can stop taking this medication when I feel better."

b. "If I have difficulty swallowing the time-released capsules, I can crush them or chew them."

c. "If I have a lot of nausea and vomiting or become restless and can't sleep, I need to call my physician."

d. "I need to drink more coffee and Pepsi Cola while I am on these medications."

The correct answer to this question is *c*. Answer *c* lists some side effects of theophylline medications that may indicate the onset of toxicity. The physician needs to know about these so that the theophylline level can be determined and the dosage can be adjusted accordingly. Other factors that the client could be taught about theophylline medications include avoiding excessive amounts of caffeine, never suddenly stopping the medication, taking it with a full glass of water and a small amount of food, and watching for interactions with over-the-counter (OTC) medications.

EXAMINATION FORMAT

Knowledge of the material covered by the NCLEX examination is evaluated by a multiple-choice test given on a computer. The questions are all constructed similarly and usually include a client situation, a stem or stem question, and four answers or distractors. All the questions on the NCLEX examination stand alone, although a similar situation may be repeated. Occasionally a single question may be included without a case situation.

The graduate is asked to select the one best answer from among the four possible choices. No partial credit is given for a "close" answer, and there is only one correct answer for any particular question. The questions are totally integrated from the content areas listed above in the approximate percentages identified. Each question carries an equal weight or value toward the final score.

The graduate may take between a minimum of 75 and a maximum of 265 questions. There is a time limit of 5 hours for the entire examination, although there is no minimum time limit. The test is graded on a statistical model that compares the graduate's responses with a pre-established standard. If the graduate can demonstrate to the computer that he or she has a knowledge level consis-

tently above that standard, then he or she passes the examination.

Each question is assigned a difficulty value on a 7-point scale, ranging from the easiest (-3), which all graduates should answer correctly, to the most difficult ($+3$), which almost all graduates would be expected to miss.

The National Council Board of Directors has again revised the passing standard of the NCLEX-RN CAT for 1998. The new passing standard is -0.35 on the NCLEX-RN logistic scale, 0.07 logits (units) above the previous standard of -0.42. This increase is similar to past increases in the difficulty level that occurred in 1995 (0.06 logit increase) and in 1992 (0.04 logit increase).

Because the NCLEX-RN examination is given by CAT, the increase in the passing standard does not necessarily require a higher number of items to be answered correctly by the graduate. However, it does require that the graduate answer questions correctly at a slightly higher difficulty level than last year's graduates. Questions are rated on a 7-logit scale, called the NCLEX-RN logistic scale, ranging from a -3 to a $+3$ (see below). The difficulty level of the questions is determined by the question writers and question reviewers.

The new passing standard was established by a nine-member panel of nurses that included diverse representation (based on region, nursing specialty, minority group, position as educator, status as new RNs) in conjunction with the results of a survey of nursing professionals, such as nursing administrators of all types of facilities and directors of nursing. After consideration of all the data, including current trends in health care, the National Council Board of Directors determined that safe entry-level practice for RNs required higher levels of knowledge, skills, and abilities than those required in 1995. The passing standard and test content will again be evaluated in 2001 to maintain the current 3-year cycle of revision.

NCLEX-RN LOGISTIC SCALE

Logits		
	$+3$	most difficult
	$+2$	
	$+1$	
	0	Approximate pass level
	-1	
	-2	
	-3	least difficult

The first few questions that the graduate is given are at the lower end of the difficulty scale. As the graduate answers those questions correctly, the difficulty level is raised to a point where the graduate begins to answer questions incorrectly. Then the computer will lower the difficulty level. The computer has a pool of some 2000 questions to choose from. An example of a low-difficulty level question is:

A client is to receive his morning dose of digoxin (Lanoxin), 0.25 mg PO. Which is the most appropriate action for the nurse to take before giving this medication?

    a. Place the bed rails in the "up" position.
    b. Make sure the urinal or bed pan is within reach.
    c. Take the client's apical pulse for 1 full minute.
    d. Evaluate the client's level of orientation.

The correct answer is *c;* digoxin is a negative chronotropic medication, which tends to slow the heart rate. If the pulse were below 60, the nurse should hold the medication and call the physician. This is a basic nursing measure all nurses should know.

An example of a high-difficulty level question is:

A client with Wolf-Parkinson-White (WPW) syndrome develops PSVT while the nurse is giving him his morning bath. If all of the following medications were available for the nurse to give PRN, which should she give for this condition?

    a. Digoxin (Lanoxin) 0.25 mg IV
    b. Verapamil (Calan) 10 mg IV
    c. Propranolol (Inderal) 20 mg IV
    d. Nitroglycerin (NTG) 0.4 mg SL

The correct answer is *b;* WPW is a congenital disorder of the conduction system of the heart that produces very rapid tachycardias. The most effective medications to control these fast dysrhythmias are the calcium channel blockers, particularly verapamil. Although beta-blockers (Inderal) and cardiac glycosides (Lanoxin) can slow fast heart rates, they are not effective for this condition. Nitroglycerin (NTG) would tend to speed up the heart rate. Few new graduate nurses would be expected to know this information unless a critical care course was included in their curriculum.

SYLVAN LEARNING CENTERS

The NCLEX examination is given at Sylvan Learning Centers. After graduates have completed their nursing program, they apply to the State Board of Nursing. Appointments at the examination sites are made on a first-come, first-serve basis, but graduates are required to make the appointment within 30 days after application. There are both morning and afternoon sessions, which are scheduled for 5-hour periods. Depending on the size of the center, between 8 and 15 graduates may be in one session.

The required computer skills are minimal. After the graduate types in his or her name, address, and identification number, the only two keys that are used are the space bar and the enter key. All other keys are locked out. The computer screen is split with the situation and stem question on the left side. The answers are on the right side. The space bar highlights a different answer each time it

---

Example of a Computer Examination Question

A client is being prepared for discharge. He is to take a theophylline medication by mouth at home for his lung disease. The nurse will know that the teaching concerning theophylline medications has been effective if the patient states,

    a. "I can stop taking this medication when I feel better."
    b. "If I have difficulty swallowing the time-released capsules, I can crush them or chew them."
    c. "If I have a lot of nausea and vomiting or become restless and can't sleep, I need to call my physician."
    d. "I need to drink more coffee and Pepsi Cola while I am on these medications."

is pushed. When the graduate decides which answer is correct, he or she pushes the enter key. A message comes on the screen asking the graduate if that is the answer he or she wants. If the answer is yes, then the enter key is pushed again. The question is then replaced with new questions and answers. No question is ever repeated, nor is the graduate able to change the answer once it is selected.

The NCLEX examination is graded on a pass/fail basis. If the graduate fails the examination, he or she must retake the entire examination. The National League for Nursing (NLN) requires a 90-day waiting period for retaking the examination, although individual states may require a longer period. The results are sent to the graduate 7 to 10 days after the examination is completed.

STUDY STRATEGIES

There is a number of ways to prepare for the NCLEX examination. To attempt to take the NCLEX examination with an "If I don't know it by now, I never will" attitude is to court failure. Carefully directed study and preparation will considerably increase the chances of passing the examination.

1. Review books: The material review books cover is the key material found on the NCLEX examination. These books usually follow the NCLEX Test Plan very closely. But a review book is just that; it reviews the material that the graduate should already know. Reviewing is an important process in reinforcing learning and mentally refreshing old or unused information.

   Review books are not really designed to present new information about the key material. If the graduate is totally unfamiliar with the material in a particular section of the review book, then he or she most likely will need to read a more complete textbook on that particular subject area.

   Another important function that a review book serves is to point out areas of weakness. If the graduate finds sections that seem to contain new material, it would be important to investigate that particular section in more detail. If the graduate finds most of the material familiar and easy to grasp, then he or she is

probably prepared for the NCLEX examination.

2. Group study: Group study can be an effective method of preparation for an examination such as the NCLEX examination. To optimize the results of group study sessions, there are several rules that should be followed.

   - Rule 1: Be very selective in regard to the members of the study group. They should be of a similar mind frame and orientation toward studying as the graduate. They should be graduates who are also going to be taking the NCLEX examination. The ideal number for a study group is between four and six people. Groups larger than six become difficult to organize and handle. After the group has been formed and has begun its study sessions, it may be necessary to ask an individual to leave the group if he or she is not preparing the part assigned, is disruptive to the study process, or displays negative attitudes about the examination.

   - Rule 2: Assign each study group member a particular section to prepare for each group study session. Study groups generally meet once or twice a week. For example, if next week the group is going to study the endocrine system, assign one group member the anatomy and physiology of the system, another member the pathologic conditions, a third member the medications used for treatment, another person the key elements of nursing care, and so forth. When the group comes together, each individual should present his or her prepared section. This type of preparation prevents the "Well, what are we going to study tonight?" syndrome that often plagues group study sessions.

   By following this process, the study is organized and allows for more in-depth coverage of the topic. It also permits the members of the group to ask questions of the other members, thereby reinforcing the information being discussed.

   - Rule 3: Limit the length of the study session. No individual study session should be longer than 90 to 120 minutes. Sessions that go for longer than 2 hours tend to get off the topic and foster a negative attitude about the examination. Also, try to avoid making group study sessions a party time. A few snacks and refreshments may be helpful in maintaining the energy level of the group, but a major party atmosphere will detract significantly from the effectiveness of the study session.

3. Individual study: No matter what other study and preparation methods are used, individual preparation for the NCLEX examination is a must. This preparation can take several forms.

First, a review book is valuable for indicating areas of your knowledge that are deficient. Reading and studying the appropriate textbooks and study guides can be helpful if approached in the correct manner. It is important that the graduate mentally organize the information he or she is reading into a format that is similar to what is found on the NCLEX examination. After each page of reading in a textbook or study guide, the graduate should be able to ask three or four multiple-choice questions about that information. These questions can be asked "mentally" or actually written out. The questions should answer the question, "How might the NCLEX examination test my knowledge of this material?"

A second and extremely effective method of individual study is to practice answering questions similar to those found on the NCLEX examination. When practice questions are answered, several important mental processes occur. First, the graduate is becoming more familiar with, and therefore more comfortable with, the format of the examination. In research, this process is called the *practice effect*, and has to be accounted for when analyzing the results from Pretest/Posttest type research projects. Individuals will do better on a posttest even without any type of intervention if they have practiced answering questions on the pretest. Similarly, the score on the NCLEX examination may increase by as much as 10% through the answering of practice questions.

A second result of answering practice questions is that it reinforces the information already studied. Although it is unlikely that a question on the NCLEX examination will be identical to a practice question, there are many similarities in the questions. Realistically, there are only a limited number of ques-

tions that can be asked about any given subject. After a while, the questions begin to sound very similar.

A third advantage of answering practice questions is that it reveals subject areas that require more study. It is relatively easy to say, "I know the CNS medications pretty well." It is quite another to answer correctly 10 or 15 questions about those medications. If the questions are answered correctly, then the graduate can move on to the next topic. If the majority of the questions are missed, then further review is required.

To obtain the optimal benefit from working on practice questions, it is better to spend 30 to 45 minute each day working on 10 to 20 questions rather than to try to work on 100 questions on one day during the week.

After the questions are answered, review them and compare them with the answers the book provides. Also look at the rationales and the categories the questions fall into.

FORMAL NCLEX REVIEWS

The NLN does not endorse or sponsor any review courses for the NCLEX examination directly, but many companies offer reviews shortly after graduation. These reviews can range from 2 to 5 days in length and cover the basic information found in review books. They are rather expensive, and the quality of the NCLEX reviews varies. In general, they are only as good as the people who are presenting the material.

TEST-TAKING STRATEGIES

The multiple-choice question test format is one of the most commonly used methods of testing the knowledge of material. Some people always seem to do well on multiple-choice question tests, but others seem to have problems with that test format. The individuals who always do well are not necessarily more intelligent; rather, they most likely have intuitively mastered some of the strategies or "tricks" necessary to do well on multiple-choice tests. Fortunately, once graduates become aware of these strategies and master them, they should be able to improve their scores on this type of examination.

Knowing how to take a multiple-choice examination and optimizing selection of the correct answers is a skill that can be mastered. When mastery of this skill is combined with knowledge of the key material, the probability of passing the NCLEX examination increases greatly. The following section lists and describes these important test-taking strategies.

STRATEGY 1

Read the client situation, stem question, and answers carefully. Many mistakes are made on this type of examination because the test taker did not read all parts of the question carefully. Read the question and answers and try to understand what knowledge the question is asking for. Also, when reading the stem question, look for any key words, qualifiers, or statements that may help in the selection of the correct answer or to eliminate incorrect answers.

STRATEGY 2

Treat each question individually. Use only the information that is provided for that particular question in answering the question. Although there may have been client situations earlier in the examination that were similar to the one presently on the screen, avoid mentally returning to these previous items for help. Also, be careful about reading into a question information that is not actually provided. There is a tendency to think of exceptions or unusual clients that the graduate may have encountered. By and large, questions on the NCLEX examination ask for textbook-type knowledge of the material.

STRATEGY 3

Monitor the time. Although the examination is not strictly speaking a timed examination, the graduate is never sure how many questions will need to be answered. If the graduate plans on taking all 265 questions in 5 hours, he or she will have approximately 70 seconds per question. Ac-

tually, most individuals who take this type of test average approximately 45 seconds per question, so it is likely that the test will be completed well before the time limit is up. Take a watch along to the examination. If any question takes more than 2 minutes, put an answer down and move on. Theoretically, the graduate could sit in front of the computer screen for 5 hours with the same one question.

STRATEGY 4

An educated guess is better than no answer at all. There is no penalty for guessing on the NCLEX examination. If the graduate is unable to make any decision at all about the correct answer, he or she should just select one and move on. At least there is a one in four chance to hit the correct answer. Statistically, answer *b* has a slightly higher probability (approximately 30%) of being correct than any other answer. However, wild guessing for large numbers of questions will have a negative effect on the total score.

STRATEGY 5

Use the process of elimination in selecting the correct answer. Usually one or more of the answers can easily be identified as being incorrect. By eliminating these answers from the possible choices, the graduate will be able to better focus attention on the answers that have been identified as having some chance of being correct. Go back and read the stem question over again and try to determine exactly what type of information is being asked for. If still unable to make a decision on which of the remaining two answers is correct, select one and move on. This method increases the probability of choosing the correct answer to one in two.

STRATEGY 6

Look for the answer that has the broader focus. Another method that may be used when the choices have been narrowed down to two is to examine the answers and try to determine if one answer may include the other. The answer that is broader, that is, includes the other answer, is the correct one. An example of this type of question is:

A client is admitted to the emergency room with an overdose of acetaminophen (Tylenol). The most important action for the nurse to take is to:

a. Call a code blue and begin cardiopulmonary resuscitation (CPR)
b. Assess the client's blood pressure, pulse, and temperature
c. Place the client in a sitting position to facilitate breathing
d. Monitor vital signs and evaluate liver enzymes

The correct choice is answer *d*. Answer *b* is also correct, but answer *d* includes the information in answer *b* and adds additional information. Tylenol is lethal to the liver. Again, reading all the answers carefully is essential before making a choice. Just reading answer *b* and selecting it without reading the rest of the answers would have led to an incorrect choice.

STRATEGY 7

Trust intuition. When a question and the answers are read for the first time, an intuitive connection is made between the right and left lobes of the brain. The end result is that the first answer selection is usually the best choice. When a question is read too many times, the graduate may start to "read into" it elements that are really not there.

STRATEGY 8

Look for qualifying words in the question stem. There are some important words that help determine what type of information is called for in the answer. Some of these words are:

First   Initial
Best   Better
Most   Highest priority

When these words appear in the question stem, it is an indication that more than one of the choices is correct. The task then becomes to select the one answer that should be first or the answer to receive the highest priority. An example of a "first" type of question is:

A 62-year-old client has a history of coronary heart disease. He is brought into the ER complaining of chest pain. The initial action taken by the nurse is to:

a. Give the client NTG gr 1/150 SL now
b. Call the client's cardiologist about his admission
c. Place the client in a high-Fowler's position after loosening his shirt
d. Check the client's BP and note the location and degree of chest pain

The correct choice is answer *d*. It is important to remember that when asked for an "initial" or "first" action, think of the Nursing Process. The first step in the Nursing Process is always assessment. If there is no assessment choice, then look for a planning choice, and so forth. The other three answers provided for this question are also correct and should be done at some point, but in this particular situation, the first need is to assess the client's chest pain to determine if it is indeed cardiac in nature. Many other conditions also cause chest pain.

STRATEGY 9

Look for negatives in the question stem. Although there are very few negative questions on the NCLEX examination, negative words or prefixes in the question stem change how the correct answer is selected. Some common negatives include:

Not	False
Least	Except
Unlikely	Inconsistent
Inappropriate	Untoward
Unrealistic	All but
Lowest priority	Atypical
Contraindicated	Incorrect

In general, when a negative question is asked, it indicates that three of the choices are correct and one is incorrect. The incorrect choice is the answer. When a negative question appears, the test taker needs to ask, "What is it they don't want me to do in this situation?" An example of this type of question is:

A client is admitted to the Medical Unit. He is still having some mild chest pain. Which of the following medications would be inappropriate for relief of chest pain?

  a. Diltiazem (Cardizem)
  b. Propranolol (Inderal)
  c. Digoxin (Lanoxin)
  d. Meperidine (Demerol)

The correct answer is *c*. Digoxin is a positive inotropic medication and increases contractility and the oxygen demands of the heart. It is likely that it would actually increase chest pain in this client. The other three medications relieve chest pain by somewhat different mechanisms. But notice that if the question was not read carefully and the reader missed the *in-* prefix of "inappropriate," then certainly answer *c* would not have been selected.

STRATEGY 10

Avoid selecting answers that have absolutes in them. Answers that have absolutes in them are almost always incorrect choices. Some absolute words to be aware of include:

Always	All
Every	Never
Only	None

Health-care providers deal with very complex biochemical entities called human beings. Every person is different, and almost every rule will have an exception. An example of this type of question is:

In treating a client with cardiac chest pain with NTG 0.4 mg SL, the nurse realizes that:

  a. This pain is always caused by constriction or blockage of the coronary arteries by fat plaques or blood clots.
  b. True cardiac pain is never relieved without treatment.
  c. This type of pain is relieved only by NTG.
  d. Clients often attribute the pain to indigestion.

The correct answer is *d*. The answers to this question are very obvious in the demonstration of the "avoid the absolute" strategy. Coronary-type chest pain can also be caused by spasms of the coronary arteries as in variant angina (answer *a*). Chest pain sometimes can go away by itself, although it will probably return later (answer *b*). There are a number of medications that will also relieve chest pain besides NTG (e.g., morphine and

narcotics, calcium channel blockers and beta-blockers) (answer *c*).

STRATEGY 11

The answer that is presented differently is usually the incorrect answer. The NCLEX examination is difficult because the material is difficult. The examination is not designed to be "tricky" or difficult for the sake of confusing the test taker. On the other hand, the test question writers are not going to make the correct answer obvious. Therefore, if one answer is much longer or shorter than the other three, it is probably not the correct choice. Be wary of an answer that sounds as if it is trying to persuade the graduate that it is the correct choice by using explanation and rationalization. Again, it is probably incorrect. Also avoid answers that are different from the other three because of measurements or the way they are presented. An example of this type of question is:

A client has developed congestive heart failure. Which of the following would be a correct dosage for a loading dose of digoxin (Lanoxin) for an adult client?

  a. 0.75 mg divided into three doses q 8 hours
  b. 0.75 g divided into four doses q 8 hours
  c. 10 mg because the client is from an American Indian background and is a very large man, which causes slow absorption of the medication
  d. 0.25 mg

The correct answer for this question is *a*. The loading dose for digoxin is usually three times the maintenance dose (0.15 mg) divided over 24 hours. Answer *b* is in a different measurement form (grams instead of milligrams); answer *c* demonstrates the longer than average answer with rationale, and choice *d* is much shorter than any of the others. Look for the one of the "average length" answers as being the correct choice.

STRATEGY 12

Avoid selecting answers that refer the client to the physician. The NCLEX examination is for nurses and deals with conditions and problems that nurses should be able to act on independently. The answer that refers a client to the physician is usually incorrect and can be eliminated from the choice selection.

One exception to this rule is medication questions. Because the physician is the one who prescribes the medication, he or she is the only one who can legally change the dosage. If the nurse suspects that the dosage is incorrect, then there is a legal obligation to hold the medication and notify the physician.

STRATEGY 13

Avoid looking for a pattern in the selection of answers. The questions and answers on the NCLEX examination are arranged in a random fashion without any particular pattern to them. If something appears to be a pattern, ignore it. Any pattern is just coincidental. For example, if question 6 had answer *a,* question 7 had answer *b,* question 8 had answer *c,* question 9 had answer *d,* question 10 had answer *a,* and question 11 had answer *b,* you might expect that question 12 would have answer *c.* That is probably not the case. Another example of a pattern-type situation that sometimes occurs with answers on this type of test is that questions 22 to 29 have *c* as their answer. The answer to question 30 also seems to be *c,* but the tendency may be not to select it because of all the other *c* answers on the previous questions. The correct answer may very well be *c,* and if that is the best choice, go ahead and select it. It is important that each question is treated individually.

STRATEGY 14

Do not panic if you come across a totally unfamiliar question. Examinations such as the NCLEX examination are so designed that it is very difficult, if not impossible, for anyone to answer all of the questions correctly. As a result, there are questions that are very complex and deal with disease processes, medications, laboratory tests, and so forth that may be unfamiliar to the graduate. These questions may be encountered no matter how much review or study has been done.

Nobody knows everything! The important element to remember when encountering these types of questions is not to panic. It is just one question

out of many. Use some of the strategies already discussed in this book to select the best answer. Remember that nursing care is very similar in many situations, even though the disease processes may be quite different. Select the answer that seems logical and involves general nursing care. Common sense can go a long way on this type of examination. An example of this type of question is:

A 33-year-old black male client has been diagnosed as having a pheochromocytoma. Appropriate initial nursing care would involve:

   a. Administering large doses of xylometazoline to help control the symptoms of the disease
   b. Monitoring his vital signs closely, particularly the blood pressure
   c. Preparing the patient and family for imminent death
   d. Having the family discuss the condition with the doctor before informing the patient about the disease because of the protracted recovery period after treatment

The correct answer is *b.* Pheochromocytoma is a tumor of the adrenal medulla that causes an increase in the secretion of epinephrine and/or norepinephrine. One important result of having this type of tumor is that a hypertensive crisis may occur in some individuals. Monitoring the blood pressure would be an important nursing care measure. Also, assessment is the first step of the Nursing Process and would fit well with the qualifying word "initial," used in the question stem.

STRATEGY 15

When answers are grouped by similar concepts, activities, or situations, select the one that presents a different concept. If three of the four answers have some common element that makes them similar, and the fourth answer lacks this element, the different answer is probably the correct one. An example of this type of question is:

A female client has been treated for severe chronic emphysema for several years with bronchodilators and relatively high doses of prednisone (Deltasone). Which of the following activities would pose the least risk for this client in relationship to the side effects of prednisone therapy?

   a. Shopping at the mall on Saturday afternoon
   b. Spring-cleaning her two-story house

   c. Attending Sunday morning church services
   d. Serving refreshments at her 6-year-old son's school play

The correct answer is *b*. In answers *a, c,* and *d* there is the common element of contacting groups of strangers. Because of the suppression of the immune system, clients with this condition need to be protected from exposure to potential infections when they are taking steroid medications. Spring-cleaning her home, although strenuous, poses the least exposure to infection.

STRATEGY 16

Avoid selecting answers that make the client seem unworthy or ignorant. Nurses should not be making these types of judgments about clients. A question asked, for example, about why the client should not be told about her medications might include answers such as the following:

   She would not understand.
   Don't bother to explain.
   He's not intelligent enough.

These statements in answers make the answer incorrect.

STRATEGY 17

Look for the proper sequence of actions. Some things are always done before other things; for example, before any therapeutic communication can occur, a warm and trusting relationship must be established. Or, before doing a sterile procedure, the field must be cleaned and draped, or before giving a medication, the client should be assessed.

STRATEGY 18

If there is a lengthy nursing situation or case study, read the stem of the question *first*. This is not a real problem on the computerized NCLEX, because there is only limited room for long case studies. However, using this strategy ultimately saves some time by causing the graduate to focus attention on the information that needs to be obtained from case study rather than to read the case study, read the stem, then go back and reread the case study to obtain the information needed to answer the question. These types of questions are often found in psychiatric questions.

STRATEGY 19

Be positive about the examination! It is a generally accepted fact that people who have a positive attitude about an examination will score higher on the examination than people who are negative about it. Repeat the following phrases frequently: *I am an intelligent person! I will do well on the NCLEX examination! I have prepared for the examination and will receive a passing score! I deserve to pass this examination! If* (fill in the name of someone who passed the examination last year) *can pass the examination, so can I! I can't wait to show them what I know! I know I can do this!*

SUMMARY

Taking and passing the NCLEX-RN CAT examination is a necessary step in the process of becoming a professional registered nurse. Like all licensure examinations, its purpose is to protect the public from undereducated or unsafe practitioners. The examination is comprehensive and includes material from all areas of the graduate's nursing education. Although most graduates have some anxiety about taking this examination, knowledge about the examination format, its content, and strategies for taking the examination can lower the anxiety levels to an acceptable level.

In addition, many of these test-taking strategies can be applied to the student's course examinations taken while attending the nursing program. Although nothing is as effective for passing an examination as paying attention in class, good note taking, thorough study, and awareness of the important test-taking strategies may improve the student's overall score.

two

Pharmacology Content Outlines

2

Pharmacology in Nursing

CATEGORIES (CLASSIFICATIONS) OF MEDICATIONS

1. There are currently over 10,000 medications in use in the United States.
2. It is virtually impossible for anyone to memorize all the information about these medications.
3. All medications fall into one or more general categories or classifications.
4. Medications in a particular classification generally have the same use, similar modes of action, and similar side effects.
5. It is much easier to learn 12 or so major classifications.
6. Once the key information about a category is mastered, placing a medication with that category gives the graduate a great deal of information about the medication, even though he or she may not know the specific detailed information.
7. Illustrative situation: the nurse is to give bepridil (Bepadin) to a client for the first time but does not know anything about the medication except that it is a calcium channel blocker.

8. All medications in the classification of calcium channel blockers have similar uses, modes of action, and side effects.
   a. Common mode of action: inhibit or block the influx of calcium into the cells—particularly in the heart and vascular system—dilate blood vessels, and reduce the force of muscle contraction.
   b. Common uses: Various types of angina, hypertension, rapid dysrhythmias, post-myocardial infarction (MI), prevent vascular spasms.
   c. Common side effects: hypotension, A-V blocks, bradycardia, congestive heart failure (CHF), bleeding tendencies, dizziness.
9. Just from knowing the classification, the nurse will know a great deal about this medication and the client's condition.
   a. The client probably has some type of cardiovascular problem (bepridil is used primarily to control angina).
   b. The nurse should monitor the client for side effects such as hypotension, bradycardia, dizziness, and weakness.

10. Specific information unique to this medication is the dosage and administration (200 mg PO qd).
11. This book concentrates on the common classifications of medications but also includes specific information about the most commonly used or prototypical medications in each class.

DOSAGE CALCULATION REVIEW

1. There are few dosage calculation questions on the NCLEX.
2. The dosage calculation questions that are on the NCLEX are generally uncomplicated and straightforward because the graduate is not allowed to use a calculator during the exam.
3. It is important that the graduate master basic dosage calculations in order to ensure safe nursing practice.
4. The metric system is the primary system used for measuring and ordering medications, although in the United States some physicians may use a combination of systems, including the apothecary, household, or avoirdupois systems.
5. Some medications are measured in units.
6. The nurse must be able to make conversions from one system to another.
7. After verifying the order, the nurse should verify the medication dosage, particularly in pediatric clients, clients receiving chemotherapy, and elderly clients.
8. The nurse must also know how to calculate IV flow and drip rates.
9. Several different methods can be used for calculating dosages, including fractions, ratio and proportion, and desired/available methods.
10. The ratio and proportion method is used in this book.
11. System conversion/dosage calculation
    a. A physician orders acetaminophen (Tylenol) 600 mg for a client. Each tablet contains 5 grains. How many tablets should the nurse administer?
    b. First, convert milligrams to grains using the equivalency 60 mg = 1 gr.

    $$60 \text{ mg} : 1 \text{ gr} :: 600 \text{ mg} : x \text{ gr}$$
    $$60x = 600$$
    $$x = 10 \text{ gr}$$

    c. Second, calculate the number of tablets needed.

    $$5 \text{ gr} : 1 \text{ tab} :: 10 \text{ gr} : x \text{ tab}$$
    $$5x = 10$$
    $$x = 2 \text{ tab}$$

12. Dosage calculation
    a. A client is to receive heparin 5000 U IV. The medication comes in a vial labeled "10,000 units per mL." How many mL should the nurse give?
    b. Set up calculation:

    $$10,000 \text{ U} : 1 \text{ mL} :: 5000 \text{ U} : x \text{ mL}$$
    $$10,000x = 5000$$
    $$x = 0.5 \text{ mL}$$

    c. The client is to receive meperidine (Demerol) 50 mg IM. The medication is in a vial labeled "meperidine 75 mg/mL." How much should the nurse give?
    d. Set up calculation:

    $$75 \text{ mg} : 1 \text{ mL} :: 50 \text{ mg} : x \text{ mL}$$
    $$75x = 50$$
    $$x = 0.66 \text{ or } 0.7 \text{ mL}$$

13. IV calculation using drip factor
    a. A client is to receive 1000 mL lactated Ringer's solution in 8 hours. The administration set delivers 15 drops per milliliter. At what rate should the nurse regulate the IV?
    b. Use the formula for drip rate calculation:

    $$\frac{\text{Total number of mL}}{\text{Total number of min}} \times \text{drip factor} = \text{rate}$$

    $$\frac{1000 \text{ mL}}{8 \text{ h} \times 60 \text{ min}} \times 15 \text{ gtt/mL} = \text{gtt/min}$$

    $$\frac{1000 \text{ mL}}{480 \text{ min}} \times 15 \text{ gtt/mL} = \text{gtt/min}$$

    $$2.08 \text{ mL/min} \times 15 \text{ gtt/min} = 31.2 \text{ gtt/min (31)}$$

14. IV calculation for volumetric pumps using milliliters per minute.
    a. A client is to receive 1000 mL lactated Ringer's solution in 8 hours. At what rate should the nurse set the volumetric pump?
    b. Volumetric IV pumps or controllers are always set in mL per hour.
    c. Use formula for calculating volumetric pump rates:

$$\frac{\text{Total volume to infuse in mL}}{\text{Time to infuse in hours}} = \text{rate}$$

$$\frac{1000 \text{ mL}}{8 \text{ h}} = 125 \text{ mL/h}$$

    d. The client is to receive methicillin 1 g IVPB q 8 hours. The medication comes from the pharmacy mixed in 100 mL of fluid and is to run over 30 minutes. At what rate should the nurse set the volumetric controller?

    e. Calculate using the formula:

$$\frac{\text{Total volume in mL}}{\text{Time in hours}} = \text{rate}$$

$$\frac{100 \text{ mL}}{0.5 \text{ h}} = 200 \text{ mL/h}$$

REVIEW OF TERMINOLOGY RELATED TO MEDICATIONS

1. **Medication (drug)** is a pharmacological or chemical agent that is capable of interacting with a living organism to produce a biological effect.
2. Medication therapy or treatment is the use of a pharmacological agent to bring about a physiological change.
3. **Dispensing medications** is the act of distributing a supply of medications to a client (usually the role of a pharmacist).
4. **Prescribing medications** involves selecting an appropriate medication to treat a client's problem based on an assessment and diagnosis of the disease process (usually the role of physicians, dentists, nurse practitioners, veterinarians, physician's assistants).
5. **Administering medications** is any action that leads to the introduction of the medication into the client's body (usually the role of nurses, although most individuals who prescribe medications can also administer them).
6. **Medication potency** refers to the relative amount of medication required to produce the desired response.
   a. Medications with a high level of potency require only a small amount.
   b. Medications with a low level of potency require a much larger amount.

FACTORS THAT AFFECT CLIENT RESPONSE TO MEDICATION

1. Client compliance is the willingness of the client to follow the medication regimen as prescribed.
   a. Noncompliance or the client's voluntary refusal to follow the medication regimen is a major problem in the treatment of disease.
   b. Many factors contribute to noncompliance, including adverse effects of the medications, lack of knowledge concerning the medication or disease process, and complicated medication regimens.
2. Age affects how clients react to medications.
   a. Most medications are trial-tested with young to middle-age adults.
   b. Systemic metabolic differences in very young or very old clients may produce different responses to certain medications.
3. Gender affects how clients react to medications.
   a. Until recently, most medications were tested in young to middle-age men.
   b. Hormonal and metabolic differences in female clients can produce responses to medications that are different from male responses.
4. Body mass and build can affect how clients react to medications.
   a. Dosages for most medications are based on an adult man of average build who weighs 150 lb (75 kg).
   b. Clients who are markedly above the weight and build norms may require higher dosages of medications to achieve the same effects.
   c. Clients who are markedly below the weight and build norms may experience toxic reactions if given the standard dosage of some medications.

MEDICATION INTERACTIONS

1. When two medications are given at the same time, they often interact with each other in some way.
2. There are four different types of interactions that can occur:
   a. **Indifference** occurs when neither medication alters the effect of the other medication in any way.

(1) Each medication retains its effectiveness as if it were given alone.

(2) Example: Tylenol and Lanoxin.

b. **Additive interaction** occurs when the end effect is equivalent to the sum effect of each medication.

(1) It is possible to give lower doses of each medication.

(2) The interaction decreases the side effects of each medication.

(3) Example: Tylenol 3 (Tylenol plus codeine).

c. **Synergistic interaction** occurs when the two medications have an end effect greater than would be expected from the sum of the effects.

(1) Sometimes stated as "Medication X potentiates medication Y."

(2) The results of a synergistic interaction is often difficult to predict.

(3) Examples: Valium taken with alcohol; Phenergan given with Demerol.

(4) Some side effects may be increased because of this interaction.

d. **Antagonist interaction** occurs when the effects of two medications given at the same time cancel each other.

(1) The end result is that neither medication will produce its desired effect.

(2) Sometimes the medications' side effects may still persist even though the medications are not effective.

(3) Example: dicumarol (Coumadin) and vitamin K.

3. Certain foods taken with particular medications can produce any of the four interactions listed above. (These will be discussed when the medication is presented.)

4. **Incompatibility** is a type of interaction that can occur when IV medications are given together in the same solution.

a. The primary result of incompatibility is to cause the solution to produce solid particulates (precipitate).

b. Some medications that are particularly prone to incompatibility are sodium bicarbonate, phenytoin (Dilantin), diazepam (Valium), vitamins B and C solutions, glucagon, and nitroglycerin.

c. Although many incompatible medications are known and listed, use caution when mixing IV medications when the incompatibility is not known.

CONTROLLED (SCHEDULED) MEDICATIONS

1. Many central nervous system (CNS) medications have a potential for abuse and addiction.

2. In the *Controlled Substances Act* of 1971, the government developed a classification system to categorize medications according to their abuse potential.

3. In 1983, the Drug Enforcement Agency (DEA) in the Department of Justice became the nation's sole legal drug enforcement agency.

4. The five categories of potentially addictive medications are called *Schedules.*

a. *Schedule I* medications are very highly addictive.

(1) They can only be used for research purposes

(2) They require a special research/investigation clearance from the Food and Drug Administration (FDA) before use.

(3) Examples: heroin, cocaine, LSD, MDA, mescaline.

b. *Schedule II* medications have a high potential for addiction, and dependency always develops if taken for extended periods of time in large doses.

(1) These can be used medically.

(2) A new prescription must be written each time.

(3) There can be no telephone prescriptions.

(4) Examples: morphine, codeine, methadone, oxycodone (Percodan), pentobarbital, amphetamine.

c. *Schedule III* medications have a lower potential for addiction and abuse and may be combinations of medications.

(1) There is wide medical usage.

(2) A new prescription is required after 6 months or five refills.

(3) Examples: acetaminophen (Tylenol) with codeine, butabarbital (Butisol), benzphetamine (Didrex).

d. *Schedule IV* medications have some potential for abuse if used over long periods of time.

(1) A new prescription is required after 6 months or five refills.

(2) Penalties for illegal possession are less severe than for Schedule III medications

(3) These include many of the minor tranquilizers and antianxiety agents.

(4) Examples: pentazocine (Talwin), propoxyphene (Darvon), chlordiazepoxide (Librium), diazepam (Valium), flurazepam (Dalmane), phenobarbital.

e. *Schedule V* medications contain small amounts of controlled substances and have a low potential for abuse.

    (1) A new prescription is required after 6 months or five refills.

    (2) Some are dispensed without a prescription.

    (3) Examples: diphenoxylate (Lomotil), loperamide (Imodium), combination medications with less than 200 mg of codeine per 100 mL.

MEDICATION USE DURING PREGNANCY

1. A teratogen is any substance that can damage the rapidly growing cells in a fetus, often leading to birth defects.
2. Common teratogens include nicotine, x-rays, alcohol, viruses, and many medications.
3. Some medications have been tested for their safety during pregnancy, but many have not because of the potential dangers and ethical issues involved.
4. In general, when a woman is pregnant, the following rules should be followed:
   a. Use as few medications as possible.
   b. Use medications only when there is a clear need.
   c. If possible, delay all medications until after the first trimester.
   d. Use the smallest dose for the shortest time possible.
   e. Monitor the mother and fetus for adverse toxic effects.
   f. Avoid the use of combination medications.
5. Medications are categorized by the FDA based on their potential to produce injury to the fetus during pregnancy.
   a. Category A
       (1) Medications are generally considered safe during pregnancy.
       (2) Controlled human studies fail to demonstrate risk to the fetus.
       (3) Examples: folic acid (vitamin B_9), riboflavin (vitamin B_2), thiamine (vitamin B_1), thyroid (Thyrar).

   b. Category B
       (1) These medications are generally considered safe, but there may be some question about the safety.
       (2) Animal studies fail to demonstrate fetal risk, but no human studies have been conducted.
       (3) Animal studies show fetal harm, but controlled human studies fail to demonstrate fetal risk.
       (4) Examples: clozapine (Clozaril), dimenhydrinate (Dramamine), ampicillin, lidocaine.
   c. Category C
       (1) Evaluate benefits versus risks when using these medications.
       (2) Animal studies demonstrate fetal risk, but there are no human studies to rule out fetal risk.
       (3) No animal or human studies have ever been conducted to rule out risks.
       (4) Examples: clonidine (Catapress), codeine, digoxin (Lanoxin), atropine sulfate.
   d. Category D
       (1) Use only in life-threatening situations in which the benefits clearly outweigh the risks.
       (2) Controlled human studies show risk of abnormal fetal development.
       (3) Examples: diazepam (Valium), fluorouracil (5-FU), potassium iodide (Thyro-Block), lorazepam (Ativan).
   e. Category X
       (1) Use in pregnant women is always contraindicated.
       (2) Controlled human studies demonstrate clear fetal risk.
       (3) Examples: flurazepam (Dalmane), fluzastatin (Lescol), methotrexate (Rheumatrex), misoprostol (Cytotec), nicotine transdermal (Nicotrol).

TYPES OF CLIENT RESPONSES TO MEDICATIONS

1. **Predictable** reactions are one type of client response to medications.
   a. They are potential client reactions that are known from research and literature on that medication.
   b. These reactions are usually dose-related.

c. These reactions can be controlled and are not severe or life-threatening.

d. Predictable reactions include:

(1) Desired (expected) reaction (therapeutic effect)—the reason the medication is being used

(2) Adverse reaction (side effect)—any harmful, undesirable client response to a medication

(3) Secondary reaction—medications have more than one primary action and use

(4) Toxic reaction (effect)—a serious and potentially lethal type of adverse reaction that occurs when the blood level of the medication reaches toxic levels, producing permanent damage to organ systems

(5) Iatrogenic reaction (effect)—a condition produced by a medication that mimics a pathological disorder

2. **Unpredictable reactions** are less common, not dose-related, and caused by a unique or individual response by a client to a medication. They include:

a. **Hypersensitive (allergic) reaction,** sometimes called **anaphylactic reaction**

(1) It is an immune response (antigen-antibody) reaction to a medication the client has become sensitive to sometime in the past.

(2) It usually occurs in response to medications given by the IM, IV, or SC route, but it can occur with any route of administration.

(3) It is potentially lethal.

(4) Always obtain an allergy history before giving the first dose of IM, IV, or SC medications.

(5) It can occur with any medication at any time, even if the client has taken it before without problems.

(6) Symptoms include shortness of breath, dyspnea and cyanosis, wheezing and stridor, hives, rashes, and fever.

b. **Idiosyncratic responses** may be difficult to identify.

(1) The response is the opposite of what the expected response should be.

(2) The response may occur in the elderly or in clients who for some reason have an altered metabolism.

(3) For example, a client is given flurazepam (Dalmane) at bedtime for sleep but becomes anxious and agitated instead.

PHARMACOKINETICS

Pharmacokinetics is the study of the way medications are absorbed into the body, distributed to the tissues, metabolized and detoxified, and finally excreted from the body.

1. **Absorption** refers to the process whereby the medication enters the vascular system so that it can be distributed to the various tissue and organs in the body. The route of administration affects the absorption rate.

a. **The enteral route** involves administering the medication through the client's mouth.

(1) Oral route medications include pills, liquids, and suspensions and is relatively slow because absorption is dependent on the breakdown and absorption in the gastrointestinal (GI) tract.

(2) The oral mucosa (sublingual) route is very rapid because the medication is absorbed directly into the blood through the capillaries in the mucus membranes of the mouth. The medication needs to be water-soluble, and the client needs to be hydrated.

b. **The parenteral route** involves some method of introducing the medication below the skin layers.

(1) Intradermal (ID) injections place the medication between the layers of the skin. They have relatively slow absorption and are used primarily for diagnostic tests, such as purified protein derivative (PPD).

(2) Subcutaneous (SC) injections place the medication under the dermis layer of the skin where it is absorbed by the capillary system in the fat layer. It, too, has relatively slow absorption, but it is faster than ID.

(3) Intramuscular (IM) injections place the medication in the muscle layer of the body where it is rapidly absorbed into the large blood vessels found in the muscles.

(4) Intravenous (IV) injections place the medication directly into the bloodstream and provide for immediate absorption.

c. Topical route of administration involves applying the medication to a body surface and generally produces a very slow rate of absorption.

    (1) Topical creams and ointments are used to treat local irritations or infections and are not designed to be absorbed.

    (2) Transdermal drug delivery systems (TDDS) are gaining popularity and involve applying a medication-impregnated patch on a bare skin area to provide a slow but steady absorption rate of the medication.

    (3) Suppositories, either rectal or vaginal, allow the medication to absorb through either the rectal or vaginal mucosa. Absorption by this route is slow and erratic and depends on the hydration and condition of the mucus membranes.

d. **The inhalation route** involves introducing the medication into the lungs in a mist or gaseous form.

    (1) The medication is absorbed into the pulmonary capillaries from the alveoli.

    (2) It has the most rapid absorption of all the administration routes because of the large surface area and tremendous blood supply of the lungs.

    (3) It is used primarily for clients with respiratory conditions, although other medications can be administered by this route.

2. Distribution of medications to the target tissues or organs is accomplished through the cardiovascular system. Distribution is dependent upon cardiovascular function and general systemic hydration status.

a. Blood concentration levels are directly related to the effectiveness and side effects of a medication.

    (1) Peak concentration is the time when the level of the medication is the greatest in the blood. For IV medications, it is shortly after administration; other routes take longer.

    (2) **Minimum effective concentration** (MEC) is the lowest level of medication in the blood that will produce the desired effects.

    (3) **Minimum toxic concentration** (MTC) is the level in the blood at which the medication will begin to produce severe side effects or toxic effects.

    (4) **Therapeutic range** is the concentration of medication in the blood when the desired effects are produced without severe side effects; that is, the level between the MEC and the MTC (Fig. 2–1).

    (5) **Loading dose** is a larger-than-normal dose of medication given at the beginning of therapy to rapidly raise the blood level to the therapeutic range.

3. **Metabolism (detoxification)** of medications refers to the body's ability to change the medication from its basic chemical form into a more water-soluble substance that can be excreted by the renal system.

a. The liver is the organ that is responsible for most of the metabolism of medications in the body.

    (1) Clients with alterations in liver function (hepatitis, cirrhosis) may have difficulty metabolizing medications, causing the medication to reach toxic levels.

    (2) Some medications (e.g., calcium channel blockers) are converted from an inactive form to an active form in the liver.

    (3) Many medications have the potential to damage the liver (hepatotoxic) because of the liver's attempt to detoxify and metabolize them (e.g., acetaminophen [Tylenol], diazepam [Valium], calcium channel blockers, most anticancer medications).

b. Some medications are metabolized in the endocrine glands.

c. Because of their chemical structures, some medications are not altered chemically (metabolized) at all by the body and remain in their basic form until excreted.

d. In general, the body treats all medications as foreign substances that it will try to make less toxic and excrete as quickly as possible.

4. **Excretion** occurs when the medication is eliminated from the body.

a. The renal system is responsible for the majority of medication excretion in the body.

    (1) A well-functioning renal system is necessary for timely excretion of medications.

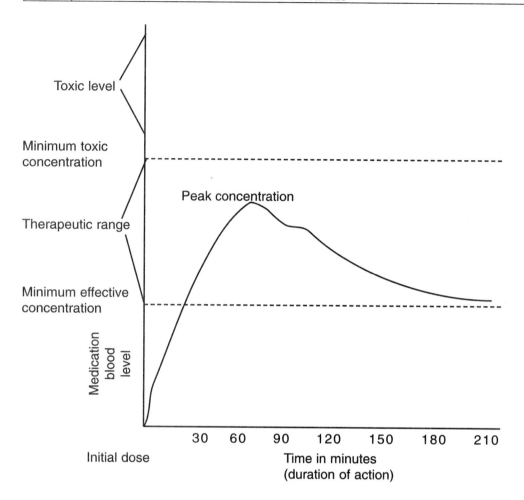

FIGURE 2–1. *Therapeutic range. This medication became effective in just under 30 minutes, reached its peak blood level at just over 1 hour (the time when side effects are most likely to develop), and has a duration of action of over 3½ hours.*

(2) Any disorder of the renal system (renal failure, renal disease, structural abnormalities) will prolong the excretion time and may lead to medication toxicity.

(3) Dehydration states may also prolong excretion times.

b. Some medications are also excreted by the following:
(1) Lungs
(2) Skin
(3) Salivary glands
(4) GI tract

c. Hemodialysis or peritoneal dialysis can be used to remove many medications from the circulatory system (artificial excretion).

d. **The half-life** of a medication is the amount of time required to lower the total medication level by one-half.

(1) Half-life is dependent on the rate of medication excretion in the body.

(2) Medication half-life predicts how long the medication remains in the body and is useful in determining administration frequency and elimination times in overdoses.

(3) The half-life of a medication remains the same despite increases or decreases in dose.

(4) After five half-lives, approximately 97% of the medication is eliminated from the body and is considered noneffective.

(5) The cumulative effect of some medications occurs because of the tendency to storage of the medication in certain tissues (e.g., fat) or organs (e.g., liver), extending the medication half-life.

PHARMACOLOGY FOR THE PEDIATRIC CLIENT

1. Developmental variations in infants and children indicate that they should not be treated simply as smaller versions of adults.
   a. There are pharmacokinetic differences in children of different age ranges, which determine the way children absorb, distribute, metabolize, and excrete medications.
   b. Children's responses to medications often occur more quickly and dramatically than in adults.
   c. Little research-based information exists related to the safety and effect of medications in children because most medications are tested on adults.
   d. Children's responses to medications vary dramatically between the neonatal, infant, young child, and adolescent stages.
   e. The circulatory and organ systems of children lack the reserve capacity found in adults, and even small overdoses of medications may be lethal.
2. Medication absorption in children is affected by several maturational factors.
   a. Emptying time of the stomach varies according to age group and may produce unpredictable medication results.
      (1) Oral medications given to infants leave the stomach in less than 3 hours.
      (2) Oral medications given to school-age or adolescent children may remain in the stomach up to 6 hours.
      (3) The nurse should anticipate diminished effect of medications absorbed in the stomach in infants but a more rapid and increased therapeutic response to intestinally absorbed medications.
      (4) Stomach acid pH is decreased in infants up to 9 months of age, which may affect medications that are either activated or deactivated by stomach secretions.
   b. The smaller muscle size of the infant and child reduces the volume capacity for IM injections and reduces the absorption rate.
   c. Topical medications tend to be more rapidly absorbed owing to the thinner stratum corneum (outer layer of skin), resulting in systemic rather than localized responses.
3. The distribution of medications to target organs is also altered in children because of their size and system immaturity.
   a. Children have a greater proportion of fluid per body weight (up to 85%) than adults (usually 60%).
   b. A greater proportion of the fluids in children are found in the extracellular spaces (up to 60%), whereas adults will have only 40% of fluid in extracellular spaces.
      (1) The larger proportion of fluid in children tends to dilute the medication and lower the serum levels of the medication.
      (2) The increased extracellular fluid in children leads to more rapid excretion of the medication than in adults.
   c. Infants and young children tend to have lower plasma protein and serum albumin levels than adults.
      (1) Many medications adhere to protein-binding sites, thus lowering the levels of the unbound or active medication.
      (2) In infants and young children, these lower-serum protein levels may lead to higher medication levels, toxicity, or increased excretion rate.
      (3) The effects of many medications given to infants and young children are often difficult to predict.
4. Metabolism and detoxification of medications in children is dependent on the maturity of the hepatic system and the body temperature.
   a. Hepatic function is very immature in newborn infants, leading to a slow metabolism of many medications.
      (1) Slow metabolismn of medications extends the half-life of the medication, requiring less frequent administration.
      (2) **The "gray baby" syndrome** is a type of cardiovascular collapse in infants producing cyanosis, hypotension, and circulatory failure caused by overly large doses of certain medications.

b. The temperature regulatory mechanism in infants and younger children is unstable and subject to fluctuations.
  (1) Increases in temperature increase the metabolism of most medications and shorten the half-life.
  (2) Subnormal temperatures decrease metabolism of medications and lengthen the half-life, leading to toxicity.
5. The excretion of medications in children is also affected by maturational differences from adults.
  a. Full-term neonates have only 30% of the glomerular filtration rate normally found in adults.
  b. Renal function increases until 12 months, when it is nearly equal to that of the adult.
    (1) The decreased renal function in young children reduces the amount of medication that can be excreted by the kidneys, increasing its half-life.
    (2) It is essential to monitor serum levels of medications closely in children.

DOSAGE CALCULATIONS IN PEDIATRICS

1. Because of the wide variations in pharmacokinetics for pediatric clients, many medication manuals do not give standard dosage ranges for children as they do for adults.
  a. Each medication prescribed for a pediatric client should have the dose calculated at the time the prescription is written, taking into consideration the child's age and physiological characteristics.
  b. Several formulas have been developed to give approximate dosages for pediatric clients.
    (1) Formulas based solely on the age of the child (Fried's rule, Young's rule) should be avoided because they do not take into consideration physiological variations.
    (2) Formulas based on weight (Clark's rule) are better and can provide a rough check of an ordered dosage as compared with standard adult dosages.
    (3) Clark's rule when the weight is in pounds:

$$\frac{\text{Child's weight in lb}}{150} \times \text{adult dose} = \text{pediatric dose}$$

    (4) Clark's rule when weight is in kilograms:

$$\frac{\text{Child's weight in kg}}{75} \times \text{adult dose} = \text{pediatric dose}$$

    (5) A more reliable method of dosage calculation for children uses the body surface area (BSA) of the child because BSA correlates more closely with the physiological function than weight or age alone.
    (6) A BSA nomogram must be used.
    (7) The formula for calculating dosage on BSA is:

$$\frac{\text{BSA}}{1.7} \times \text{adult dose} = \text{pediatric dose}$$

SPECIAL CONSIDERATIONS FOR PEDIATRIC PHARMACOLOGY

1. Client/parent education for pediatrics includes identifying to whom the teaching should be directed, the level of knowledge of the client, and the technical level of the information given.
  a. Teaching should be directed to the primary caregiver.
  b. It must be stressed that persons other than the primary caregiver (school staff, grandparents, baby-sitters) who may be responsible for giving medications understand the importance of maintaining the medication schedule.
  c. Client compliance is influenced by many factors.
    (1) Stress that the medication should be given for the full term of the prescription and not stopped because the child feels better.
    (2) Financial considerations may enter into the ability of the parents to purchase a particular medication.
    (3) Even simple directions should be repeated and reinforced to enhance learning.
    (4) Use of play therapy may be helpful in reducing a child's anxiety and fear of medications.

(5) Toddlers and preschoolers should be told about the administration procedures just before they are performed to lessen anxiety and fantasizing.

(6) Explanations and answers should be honest but reassuring.

(7) Teach parents the signs and symptoms of allergic reactions to medications and foods.

(8) Instruct parents not to threaten children with medications or injections; for example, "If you don't stop running around, the nurse will give you a shot."

2. Safe practices in medication storage and administration will help prevent accidental injections and overdoses.

a. Child-proof caps should always be replaced tightly on all medication bottles after use.

b. Even medications with child-proof caps should be stored out of reach or in locked storage areas when toddlers and young children are present in the home.

c. Be careful with medications left in a purse.

d. Parents should be taught about first aid for accidental ingestions.

(1) Know the poison control number, or keep it by the phone (1-800-392-8548).

(2) Most hospital ERs now have access to poison control information via Internet, or they have information in their own data bases.

(3) Syrup of ipecac, an emetic, should be kept in the home when there are young children present and used immediately by the parent if the child has ingested medication.

(4) Teach parents to always bring the container the ingested medication was in to the ER when they bring the child in.

PHARMACOLOGY FOR THE GERIATRIC CLIENT

1. Adults over 65 years of age are the fastest growing segment of our population.

a. Medication therapy is the most widely used form of treatment for diseases that affect the elderly.

b. Studies have found that up to 20% of the hospitalizations of adults over 65 years old are due to iatrogenic conditions produced by medications they are taking.

c. The elderly consume the largest amount of over-the-counter medications of our population.

2. Various anatomic and physiological changes occur as a person ages, which can alter both the therapeutic and adverse effects of medications.

a. These changes can be considered normal variations.

b. Changes in older adults are often slow and gradual.

c. Medication absorption is least affected by the aging process.

(1) Acid gastric secretions decrease, raising the pH of the stomach. This can affect the solubility of some medications, such as aspirin and barbiturates.

(2) Longer gastric emptying times and the presence of duodenal diverticula tend to delay or to reduce absorption.

(3) Decreased esophageal motility may make large capsules or tablets difficult to swallow, or they may have a tendency to lodge in the base of the esophagus, causing esophageal ulcers.

(4) The loss of subcutaneous fat and the increased fragility of veins often make IV administration of medications more difficult in the elderly.

(5) The loss of subcutaneous fat also increases the absorption rate of many topical ointments that are frequently used by the elderly.

d. Medication distribution to the tissues and target organs is altered by the aging process.

(1) Decreased cardiac output and changes in circulation may delay the onset or may extend the effect of medications.

(2) The decrease in lean body mass and the increase in the fatty tissue where medications are stored can result in prolongation of the medication's action, increased sensitivity, or toxic effects.

(3) Elderly clients generally have higher plasma levels of medications and more erratic distribution rates than young clients.

e. The metabolism of medications in elderly clients is difficult to predict and depends on several factors.

(1) A client's general health status, use of alcohol, health-care practices, nutritional status, medication use, and long-term exposure to environmental toxins or pollutants can affect the metabolism of medications.

(2) The aging process decreases total liver mass and hepatic blood flow, often resulting in delayed metabolism of medications and higher plasma levels of active medication.

(3) The lower-serum protein levels produce transient increases in the intensity of pharmacologic action of some medications because of the lack of protein-binding sites.

(4) Idiosyncratic reactions are more common in the elderly, because of unidentified alterations in metabolism.

  f. The excretion rate of medications is also affected by the aging process.

(1) The aging process causes a reduction in the number of functioning nephrons and decreased glomerular filtration rates.

(2) Reduced renal function leads to longer half-lives of medications, increased side effects, and potential for toxicity.

CLIENT TEACHING FOR THE ELDERLY CLIENT

1. Goals for teaching must be individualized for each client based on information from a thorough physical and mental assessment.

  a. Client instruction for clients who have sensory defects (vision, hearing, joint mobility) due to changes associated with the aging process need teaching plans that will allow them as much independence as possible while maintaining safety.

  b. The potential of injury caused by overdosing or underdosing of medications is increased in the elderly.

  c. Diminished memory capacity is especially problematic for the elderly client.

  d. Clients can learn at any age, even if the memory is not as acute or the attention span is shortened, if the nurse individualizes the teaching strategy.

(1) Begin teaching the client early in the hospitalization.

(2) Use effective adaptive devices if necessary (magnifying glasses, hearing aids).

(3) Avoid group teaching for the elderly; use individualized sessions whenever possible.

(4) Keep individual sessions to under 20 minutes maximum.

(5) Provide only essential information required for safe medication administration.

(6) Be concrete in explanations, using examples familiar to the client.

(7) Stress the unique colors, shapes, or sizes of medications in your explanations.

(8) Maintain a positive attitude even though the process may seem frustrating at times.

2. Frequent evaluation of the medication regimen is necessary in the elderly client.

  a. Elderly clients tend to see multiple physicians for various health-care problems and often are given prescriptions by one physician without the other physician's knowledge.

(1) They may be given the same medication by two different physicians, which can lead to accidental overdoses.

(2) Medication interactions are often not recognized unless the nurse evaluates all the medications the client is taking at the same time.

(3) Elderly clients often forget to include the many over-the-counter medications they frequently take.

  b. Evaluate the client's family and their ability to recognize adverse reactions to medications.

(1) Side effects of many medications mimic normal changes brought on by the aging process.

(2) Because of changes in metabolism in the elderly, side effects may be atypical or even suppressed.

  c. Careful and frequent monitoring of serum blood levels of medications is one of the best ways to ensure that the client's medications are not becoming toxic.

  d. Nutritional status should be evaluated frequently, because some medications may cause changes in the digestion of foods or in the use of nutrients by the body.

3

Medications Affecting the Nervous System

SUMMARY OF KEY ASPECTS OF THE ANATOMY AND PHYSIOLOGY OF THE NERVOUS SYSTEM

1. The nervous system is composed of two major parts:
   a. Central nervous system (CNS)
      (1) Brain
      (2) Spinal cord
   b. Peripheral nervous system
      (1) Autonomic (sympathetic, parasympathetic)
      (2) Somatic
2. The functional unit of the nervous system is the neuron, which is composed of three parts:
   a. Dendrites, which receive impulses through receptor sites.
   b. The cell body, which provides the vital functions that keep the neuron alive.
   c. The axon, which is the longest part of the neuron and which relays the impulses to the next neuron.
3. The axon from one neuron does not physically touch the dendrites from the next neuron.

4. **Synapses** are the "spaces" between the dendrites and axons.
   a. **Neurotransmitters** are chemical substances (hormones) that are released by the axon of one neuron and travel across the synapse to the receptor sites on the dendrites of the next neuron.
   b. This process promulgates the wave of electrical activity, which produces movement or sensation.
   c. There are many neurotransmitters, including:
      (1) Acetylcholine
      (2) Catecholamine (dopamine, epinephrine, norepinephrine)
      (3) Histamine (1 and 2)
      (4) Serotonin
      (5) Endorphins
      (6) Enkephalins
   d. Many of the medications affecting the nervous system work either by inhibiting or stimulating neurotransmitter production or by affecting receptor sites (Fig. 3–1).
5. Specialized terms are used when discussing medications affecting receptor sites:

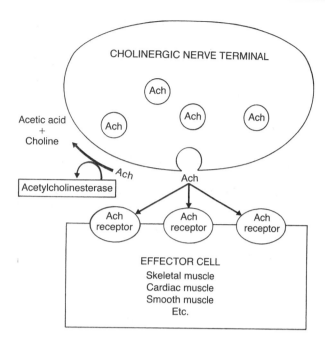

FIGURE 3–1. *Schematic of cholinergic axon terminal and effector cell. Acetylcholinesterase (Ach), located on the postsynaptic membrane, catalyzes the degradation of Ach to acetic acid and choline. (From Kuhn, M: Pharmacotherapeutics: A Nursing Process Approach, ed 4. FA Davis, Philadelphia, 1998, p 211, with permission.)*

a. **Affinity** is the tendency of a medication to attach or bind itself to a particular receptor site.

b. **Agonist** refers to a medication that binds with a receptor site to produce an effect.

c. **Antagonist** is a medication that inhibits or counteracts the effects of neurotransmitters or other medications at receptor sites.

d. **Specific binding medications** are medications that affect only one particular receptor site.

e. **Nonspecific binding medications** are medications that will affect several different receptor sites (most medications have this effect).

6. There are two major types of medication that have specific actions on receptor sites:

a. Medications with blocking effect, which are called blocker or antagonist medications.

b. Medications with stimulating effect, which are called stimulators or agonists and produce this effect by:

(1) Stimulating neurotransmitter production (directly—precursors that are converted to neurotransmitters)

(2) Mimicking the effect of the neurotransmitter (mimetic effect)

(3) Increasing the sensitivity of the receptor sites

7. The blood-brain barrier is a special property of the central nervous system.

a. The blood-brain barrier occurs because of the tightly compressed nature of the neurons of the brain.

b. The blood-brain barrier controls the exchange of substances between the circulatory system and the cells of the brain, protecting the brain from damage from toxins and infection.

c. Many substances, including medications, will not cross the blood-brain barrier.

PART A: GENERAL NEUROLOGICAL MEDICATIONS

MEDICATIONS THAT AFFECT THE AUTONOMIC NERVOUS SYSTEM

1. The autonomic nervous system (ANS) functions independently of conscious control and helps regulate most of the vital functions in the body.

2. The ANS carries impulses from the brain to:

a. Smooth (involuntary) muscles in the gastrointestinal (GI) system, blood vessels, and so forth

b. Glands in the endocrine system

c. Cardiac muscle tissue

d. Other organs such as the liver, pancreas, kidneys, and so forth

3. The ANS has two major divisions:

a. **The sympathetic branch,** also called the adrenergic or thoracolumbar branch, is responsive to activity and prepares the body to deal with stress or injury.

(1) It has a generalized, widespread body response.

(2) Epinephrine, norepinephrine, and dopamine are the primary neurotransmitters.

(3) Stimulation of the sympathetic branch produces increased heart rate, respiratory rate, pupil dilation, peripheral vasoconstriction, increased blood pressure, increased fat and glycogen breakdown, increased energy use, and suppression of the GI system.

b. **The parasympathetic branch,** also called the cholinergic or craniosacral branch, maintains normal functioning, or a homeostatic state, in the body.
   (1) It has a more discrete and localized effect on the body systems.
   (2) The primary neurotransmitter is acetylcholine.
   (3) Stimulation of the parasympathetic branch produces decreased heart rate, decreased respiratory rate, pupil constriction, peripheral vasodilation, sphincter tone relaxation, reduction of energy use, and stimulation of the GI system.
4. Both the sympathetic and parasympathetic branches send impulses to the same body organs and tissues.
5. The opposing effects of these two branches maintain a balanced state in the body.
6. Stimulating one branch or blocking the opposite branch will produce similar effects in the body.
   a. Stimulating the sympathetic branch or blocking the parasympathetic branch produces similar results.
   b. Stimulating the parasympathetic branch or blocking the sympathetic branch produces similar results.
7. Several key receptor sites have been identified for the neurotransmitters of the ANS:
   a. Alpha-adrenergic receptor sites (sympathetic branch) are located in the smooth muscles, blood vessels, and glands.
      (1) Alpha$_1$ sites respond to epinephrine, norepinephrine, and dopamine.
      (2) Alpha$_2$ sites respond to epinephrine, norepinephrine, and dopamine.
   b. Beta-adrenergic receptor sites (sympathetic system) are located in the heart, lungs, blood vessels, and uterus.
      (1) Beta$_1$ sites respond to epinephrine, norepinephrine, and dopamine and are located primarily in the heart.
      (2) Beta$_2$ sites respond primarily to epinephrine and are located primarily in the lungs, blood vessels, and uterus.
   c. Dopinergic receptor sites (sympathetic branch) respond primarily to dopamine.
   d. Muscarinic receptor sites (parasympathetic system) respond primarily to acetylcholine.
   e. Nicotinic receptor sites (parasympathetic system) respond primarily to acetylcholine.

8. Medications that affect the ANS are classified by what response they produce in either the sympathetic or the parasympathetic branches.

Medications that Stimulate the Sympathetic System (Adrenergic, Sympathomimetic)

1. Alpha-receptor stimulants (alphamimetics, alpha-agonists)
   a. Their primary effect is vasoconstriction, particularly in the skin arterioles, kidneys, and mesentery.
   b. Primary uses
      (1) Hemostasis
      (2) Pupil dilation
      (3) Nasal decongestion
      (4) Hypotension
      (5) Cardiac failure; cardiogenic shock
2. Beta-receptor stimulants (betamimetics, beta agonists)
   a. The primary effects are cardiac stimulation, smooth muscle relaxation, general vasodilation in key organs (brain, heart, muscles).
   b. Primary uses
      (1) Bronchodilation (asthma, anaphylaxis, chronic obstructive pulmonary disease [COPD])
      (2) Shock states
3. Dopamine receptor stimulants (dopaminergic, dopamine agonist)
   a. Their primary effects are CNS stimulation, cardiac stimulation, vasoconstriction, increased urinary output.
   b. Primary uses
      (1) Parkinson's disease
      (2) Cardiac failure, cardiogenic shock
      (3) Hypotension

Catecholamines

1. Modes of action
   a. Stimulation of both alpha- and beta-receptor sites
   b. Stimulation of dopamine receptor sites
2. Uses
   a. Nasal congestion
   b. Open-angle glaucoma
   c. Anaphylaxis
   d. Hypotension
   e. Bradycardia, heart blocks, asystole

f. Asthma, bronchitis
g. Cardiac arrest
h. Cardiogenic shock states, shock
3. Key medications (see Appendix D)
  a. dopamine (Intropin)
  b. epinephrine (Adrenalin)
  c. isoproterenol (Isuprel)
  d. norepinephrine (Levophed)
  e. dobutamine (Dobutrex)
4. Interactions: numerous, particularly mono-amine oxidase (MAO) inhibitors, antidepressants, digoxin, beta-blockers
5. General side effects:
  a. CNS (restlessness, anxiety, fear, headache)
  b. Cardiovascular (flushing, tachycardia, increased or decreased blood pressure, dysrhythmias—premature ventricular contractions [PVCs], ventricular tachycardia [VT])
  c. Musculoskeletal (weakness, tremors)
  d. GI (nausea, vomiting, diarrhea)
6. Nursing implications
  a. Catecholamines can be given only intravenously, subcutaneously, or by inhalation.
  b. Catecholamines are very potent; use carefully, double-check dosages.
  c. Monitor vital signs, heart rate, and blood pressure closely during and after administration.
  d. Monitor for the development of tolerance, edema, renal failure, and bleeding with long-term use.
  e. If giving intravenous injection, use large vein only.
  f. Monitor for infiltration (can cause tissue damage).

Medications that Reduce or Block the Effect of the Sympathetic Nervous System (Adrenergic Blockers, Antiadrenergics, Sympatholytics)

These are classified by their site of action:
1. Anatomic ganglionic blockers block transmission of the impulses through the synapses of the ganglia.
  a. They are not commonly used.
  b. There is low probability of these medications appearing on the NCLEX examination.
2. Alpha-blockers block alpha-receptor sites.

  a. These are used for hypertensive crisis, frostbite, and septic shock.
  b. There is low probability of these medications appearing on the NCLEX examination.
3. Beta-blockers block beta-receptor sites.
  a. They are the most commonly used of the adrenergic blockers for a variety of conditions, including:
    (1) Cardiovascular problems (hypertension, angina, supraventricular tachycardia (SVT), prevention of second myocardial infarction [MI])
    (2) Migraine headaches
    (3) Anxiety disorders
    (4) Wide-angle glaucoma
    (5) Pheochromocytoma
    (6) Hyperthyroidism
    (7) Reynold's disease
  b. Modes of action
    (1) These medications compete for the beta-adrenergic receptor sites.
    (2) They prevent the sympathetic response from the catecholamines.
    (3) They alter the function of the adrenal medulla, reducing the secretion of epinephrine and norepinephrine.
    (4) Most of these medications are nonselective and block both $beta_1$ and $beta_2$ receptor sites.
  c. Key medications (see Appendix D)
    (1) propranolol (Inderal)—prototype of this group
    (2) metoprolol (Lopressor)
    (3) nadolol (Corgard)
    (4) timolol maleate (Timoptic) (see Chapter 11)
  d. Interactions
    (1) With numerous medications.
    (2) Calcium channel blockers and digoxin potentiate the effect of beta-blockers.
  e. General side effects
    (1) Cardiovascular (hypotension, atrioventricular (A-V) blocks, congestive heart failure [CHF])
    (2) Respiratory (bronchoconstriction, bronchospasm)
    (3) Gastrointestinal (nausea, vomiting, diarrhea, abdominal cramping, flatus)
    (4) Central nervous system (dizziness, disorientation, memory loss)
    (5) Genitourinary (impotency in men)
    (6) Endocrine (hypoglycemia)

f. Nursing implications
   (1) Monitor blood sugar closely in diabetic patients for hypoglycemia.
   (2) Use with extreme caution in clients with asthma, bronchitis, or other respiratory disorders.
   (3) If giving intravenous injections, have atropine on hand as antidote.
   (4) Give on empty stomach for best results; food decreases absorption.
   (5) Instruct client to never stop taking this medication suddenly—rebound effect may cause chest pain or MI.
   (6) Teach client to monitor own blood pressure and pulse each day.
   (7) When used for hypertension, client must follow other health-care recommendations such as weight loss, low-sodium/low-fat diet, increase in exercise.

Medications that Directly or Indirectly Increase the Neurotransmitter Action of Acetylcholine (Cholinergic Agents, Parasympathomimetics)

There are two classes in this group:
1. Anticholinesterase agents
   a. These agents have very specific and limited uses.
   b. There is low probability of these medications appearing on the NCLEX examination.
2. Cholinergic agonists
   a. These are the most widely used of the cholinergic agents for:
      (1) Reduction of intraocular pressure in glaucoma
      (2) Stimulation of GI tract in postoperative clients
      (3) Stimulation of bladder and urinary tract function in postoperative clients
   b. Modes of action
      (1) Direct stimulation of cholinergic receptor sites
      (2) Ability to mimic the action of naturally occurring acetylcholine
      (3) Stimulation of the parasympathetic system
      (4) Usually given subcutaneously, orally, or intraocularly because of rapid breakdown when given intravenously or intramuscularly

c. Key medications (see Appendix D)
   (1) Pilocarpine HCL (Absorbocarpine; Ispotocarine; Pilocar)
   (2) Metoclopramide HCL (Reglan)
d. Interactions
   (1) There are few dangerous interactions.
   (2) Atropine is the antidote for overdose.
e. General side effects
   (1) Cardiovascular (vasodilation, tachycardia, postural hypotension)
   (2) Gastrointestinal (nausea, belching, vomiting, abdominal cramping, diarrhea)
   (3) Respiratory (dyspnea, wheezing, bronchospasms)
   (4) Genitourinary (urinary frequency, urgency, incontinence)
   (5) Central nervous system (tremors, muscular rigidity, anxiety, fear, seizures)
   (6) Sensory (blurred vision, constricted pupils [miotic], poor night vision, diaphoresis, salivation)
f. Nursing implications
   (1) Double-check route of administration.
   (2) Give oral medications on empty stomach.
   (3) Monitor for hypotension and tachycardia.
   (4) Instruct client to change positions slowly to prevent postural hypotension.
   (5) Assess bowel sounds and GI function in postoperative clients.
   (6) Monitor urinary output—keep bedpan or urinal within reach.
   (7) Promote good oral and general body hygiene because of diaphoresis.

Medications that Interrupt the Transmission of Impulses through the Parasympathetic Nervous System (Anticholinergic, Cholinergic Blocking Agents, Parasympatholytics)

These fall into two general classes.
1. Ganglionic blockers
   a. These are used only in surgery and in intensive care units.
   b. There is low probability of these medications appearing on the NCLEX examination.
2. Anticholinergic (antimuscarinic) medications
   a. These are commonly used for a variety of conditions, including:
      (1) GI conditions (spasms, diarrhea, ulcers)
      (2) Chronic asthma

    (3) Preoperative medications to reduce secretions

    (4) Motion sickness

    (5) Sinus bradycardia, heart blocks

    (6) Pupil dilatation (mydriatic)

  b. Modes of action

    (1) Suppression of the central nervous system

    (2) Relaxation of the smooth muscles of the bronchi

    (3) Blocking of the effects of the parasympathetic system and allowing the sympathetic system to take over

    (4) Similarity of end action to the sympathetic stimulants

  c. Key medications

    (1) atropine sulfate (prototype)

    (2) dicyclomine hydrochloride (HCL) (Bentyl)

  d. Interactions

    (1) Numerous and potentially dangerous

    (2) With all oral medications because delay in emptying time of stomach and because of decreased peristalsis

    (3) Most CNS medications (antihistamines, tranquilizers, analgesics, stimulants, etc.)

  e. General side effects (anticholinergic side effects)

    (1) Dry mouth

    (2) Decreased sweating—hyperthermia

    (3) Blurred vision, photophobia

    (4) Tachycardia

    (5) Urinary retention

    (6) CNS excitation (nervousness, irritability, disorientation, seizures)

    (7) Constipation

  f. Nursing implications

    (1) Instruct client to avoid alcohol, smoking, caffeine, and aspirin.

    (2) Instruct client to avoid milk before bed or between meals.

    (3) Give oral medications on empty stomach for best results.

    (4) Avoid giving medications with antacids.

    (5) Encourage good oral care for dry mouth (ice chips, hard candy).

    (6) Monitor older clients for urinary retention and constipation.

    (7) Instruct the client to avoid excessive exposure to heat, and monitor for heat stroke during summer.

    (8) Instruct the client to take the medication as prescribed, at the times indicated, and not to change dosage without physician's approval.

MEDICATIONS USED FOR THE RELIEF OF PAIN

Narcotic Analgesics

They are widely used for the relief of moderate to severe pain.

1. Modes of action

  a. These medications reduce the perception of pain by binding to the opioid receptor sites in the brain and block the transmission of pain to these receptor sites.

  b. They produce sedation by suppression of the CNS.

  c. They decrease the emotional response to pain.

2. Key medications:

  a. morphine sulfate (Prototype)

  b. meperidine HCL (Demerol)

3. Interactions

  a. With most other depressant CNS medications (tranquilizers, antihistamines, phenothiazines, etc.) potentiate the effect.

  b. CNS stimulants counteract the effect (amphetamines).

4. General side effects

  a. Respiratory (depression, respiratory arrest, decreased cough reflex)

  b. Cardiovascular (hypotension, bradycardia, diaphoresis, vasodilation, flushing, and diaphoresis)

  c. Gastrointestinal (nausea, vomiting, constipation)

  d. Pupil constriction

  e. Urinary retention

  f. CNS (drowsiness, disorientation, weakness, loss of coordination)

  g. Tolerance, addiction

5. Nursing implications

  a. Monitor rate and depth of respiration after giving intravenous or intramuscular medication.

  b. Put side-rails up after administration.

  c. Obtain baseline blood pressure prior to administering; hold if client is hypotensive.

d. Monitor for fluid retention and urinary retention.
e. Assess for response to medication (pain relief) and note on chart.
f. Avoid giving these medications to clients with head trauma or increased intracranial pressure (masks assessments).
g. These are Schedule II medications and must be signed for prior to administration.

MEDICATIONS THAT STIMULATE THE CENTRAL NERVOUS SYSTEM

1. CNS stimulants are very potent medications that are used on a limited basis for:
   a. Narcolepsy (sleep attacks)
   b. Attention deficit disorder (ADD), attention deficit hyperactivity disorder (ADHD)
   c. Extreme obesity
2. Modes of action:
   a. Stimulating the release or production of neurotransmitters in the CNS
   b. Increasing levels of norepinephrine, serotonin, and other neurotransmitters throughout the CNS
   c. Increasing the initiation and transmission of nerve impulses throughout the body
3. Key medications
   a. amphetamine (Dexedrine) (Prototype)
   b. methylphenidate HCL (Ritalin)
4. Interactions
   a. There are numerous interactions with most other CNS medications.
   b. Taken with other CNS stimulants, these medications may be fatal.
5. General side effects
   a. Cardiovascular (hypertension, tachycardia, ventricular tachycardia)
   b. CNS (restlessness, insomnia, hyperactivity, paranoia)
   c. Gastrointestinal (dry mouth, constipation, appetite suppression, weight loss)
   d. Genitourinary (urinary frequency, impotency)
   e. Endocrine (hyperthyroidism)
   f. Tolerance, high potential for addiction.
6. Nursing implications
   a. Assess clients for hypertension, dysrhythmias, and liver disorders prior to beginning administration.

b. Monitor blood pressure closely while on the medication.
c. Give the last dose 6 hours prior to bedtime.
d. Monitor for effectiveness and signs of addiction.
e. Most of these are schedule II medications and must be signed for prior to administration.

MEDICATIONS USED TO TREAT PARKINSON'S DISEASE

Parkinson's disease is a progressive neurologic disorder caused by depletion, degeneration, or destruction of dopamine in the basal ganglia of the brain.
1. Basal ganglia are a type of gray matter at the top of the brain stem that control muscular coordination.
2. There is usually a balance between the neurotransmitters dopamine and acetylcholine in the brain.
   a. Dopamine inhibits or decreases the activity of the involuntary neurons and muscles of the CNS.
   b. Acetylcholine increases the activity of the involuntary neurons and muscles of the CNS.
   c. With a decrease in dopamine, the involuntary activity of the CNS increases, leading to the classical symptoms of Parkinson's disease, including:
      (1) Involuntary muscular movements
      (2) Tremors at rest
      (3) Akinesia (loss of muscle control)
      (4) Muscular rigidity, drooling
      (5) Loss of postural reflexes (propulsive gate; toe walking)
      (6) Frustration
There are two groups of medications used.
1. Dopamine supplements
   a. Uses: controlling symptoms of Parkinson's disease
   b. Modes of action:
      (1) Increasing the dopamine levels directly with dopamine-like medications
      (2) Increasing the dopamine levels indirectly by administering a precursor to dopamine that the body can convert to dopamine

   c. Key medication
     (1) Levodopa (Dopar)—precursor of dopamine
   d. Interactions
     (1) Dopamine supplements interact with most central nervous system medications.
     (2) Clients should avoid over-the-counter cold and allergy medications.
   e. General side effects
     (1) Gastrointestinal (nausea, vomiting)
     (2) Cardiovascular (tachycardia, postural hypotension)
     (3) Genitourinary (dark-colored urine, urinary retention)
     (4) Neurological (visual difficulties, loss of effectiveness after 3–5 years)
   f. Nursing implications
     (1) Monitor blood pressure and pulse closely during early treatment.
     (2) Avoid using in clients with a history of glaucoma.
     (3) Give medications with meal or food to avoid GI irritation and upset.
     (4) Instruct the client to never stop taking the medication suddenly; there may be a rebound effect.
     (5) Monitor for effectiveness (control of symptoms), assess for tolerance.
2. Anticholinergic medications
   a. Uses
     (1) In the early stages of the disease
     (2) Help control symptoms such as drooling, muscle stiffness, and rigidity.
     (3) These medications may be used in conjunction with levodopa in the later stages of the disease.
   b. Mode of action
     (1) Blocking of some of the effects of acetylcholine
     (2) Blocking the effects of the parasympathetic system and allowing the sympathetic system to take over
   c. Key medications
     (1) benztropine (Cogentin)
     (2) trihexyphenidyl (Artane)
   d. Interactions
     (1) Numerous and potentially dangerous
     (2) With all oral medications because of delay in emptying time of stomach and because of decreased peristalsis

     (3) With most CNS medications (antihistamines, tranquilizers, analgesics, stimulants, etc.)
   e. General side effects (anticholinergic side effects)
     (1) Dry mouth
     (2) Decreased sweating—hyperthermia
     (3) Blurred vision, photophobia
     (4) Tachycardia
     (5) Urinary retention
     (6) CNS excitation (nervousness, irritability, disorientation, seizures)
     (7) Constipation
   f. Nursing implications
     (1) Instruct client to avoid alcohol, smoking, caffeine, and aspirin.
     (2) Instruct client to avoid milk before bed or between meals.
     (3) Give oral medications on empty stomach for best results.
     (4) Avoid giving medications with antacids.
     (5) Encourage good oral care for dry mouth (ice chips, hard candy).
     (6) Monitor older clients for urinary retention and constipation.
     (7) Instruct the client to avoid excessive exposure to heat, and monitor for heat stroke during summer.
     (8) Instruct the client to take the medication as prescribed, at the times indicated, and not to change dosage without physician's approval.

ANTICONVULSANTS

Key Terminology

1. Seizure is a physiological condition caused by abnormal electrical activity in the brain. This abnormal activity involves organized and repetitive discharges from some area in the brain and may or may not produce a convulsion.
2. Convulsion is the abnormal muscular activity that results from certain types of seizures.
3. Epilepsy, also called seizure disorder, is a class of disease that is caused by sudden abnormal electrical activity in the brain and may be manifested by a variety of types of convulsions.
   a. Idiopathic (essential, genetic) epilepsy
     (1) Most common type (90%).

(2) No direct physiological cause.

(3) Often genetic in origin.

(4) Seizures usually controlled with medication.

(5) Surgical oblation may be used in cases that do not respond to medications.

b. Acquired epilepsy

(1) Directly linked to brain pathology

(2) May be cured by removal of the pathology (e.g., brain tumor, hematoma, etc.)

4. Anticonvulsants

a. Uses

(1) For control of seizure activity

(2) Not for curing seizure disorders

b. Modes of action

(1) These medications decrease the abnormal electrical activity of the affected neurons in the brain.

(2) They prevent the spread of the abnormal impulses from one area to the brain to another.

(3) They inhibit the sodium and potassium ion movement across the cell membranes of affected neurons.

c. Key medications

(1) phenytoin (Dilantin) (prototype)

(2) carbamazepine (Tegretol)

(3) primidone (Mysoline)

(4) phenobarbital (Luminal)

d. General side effects

(1) Neurological (drowsiness, sedation)

(2) Cardiovascular (hypotension, bradycardia, dysrhythmias, cardiac arrest)

(3) Gastrointestinal (abdominal pain, cramping, nausea, vomiting, gingival hyperplasia [phenytoin])

(4) Endocrine (hyperglycemia)

(5) Respiratory (respiratory depression)

e. Nursing implications

(1) Obtain complete history prior to administration, noting liver and renal disease.

(2) Give medications with food or a full glass of water.

(3) Provide good oral care.

(4) Avoid over-the-counter medications with antihistamine, alcohol, or other CNS medications.

(5) Warn the client that some medications may turn the urine red or brown.

(6) Stress the need to take the medication exactly as ordered and not to change doses or times without physician's approval.

(7) Warn the client to never stop taking antiseizure medications suddenly because of possible rebound effect, leading to an increased number and severity of seizures.

(8) Instruct the client about the sedation effect, and warn against driving and other activities that require a high degree of coordination and alertness.

(9) Assess for effectiveness in the reduction of the number and severity of seizures.

ANALGESICS/ANTIPYRETICS/ANTI-INFLAMMATORY MEDICATIONS

1. Prostaglandins are chemical substances that are released whenever there is injury or damage to cells in the body, producing a variety of effects, including:

a. Pain—a subjective sensation of discomfort

b. Fever—elevation of body temperature that increases circulation and promotes healing process

c. Inflammation—redness, heat, swelling, and pain at the site of the injury

2. Medications

a. Uses

(1) For minor to moderate pain

(2) For fever associated with injury or infection

(3) For reduction of minor inflammation

b. Modes of action

(1) These medications block the transmission of impulses across the synapses of the pain receptor sites.

(2) They alter the function of the hypothalamus to set the body temperature lower.

(3) They inhibit the formation and release of prostaglandins to reduce inflammation.

c. Key medications

(1) acetylsalicylic acid (Aspirin)

(2) acetaminophen (Tylenol)

d. Interactions: few

e. General side effects

(1) Gastrointestinal (nausea, vomiting, GI bleeding [acetylsalicylic acid])

(2) Neurological (tinnitus [acetylsalicylic acid])

    (3) Endocrine (hypoglycemia [acetaminophen])
    (4) Renal failure, liver failure (acetaminophen)
  f. Nursing implications
    (1) Instruct client to take medications with full glass of water or food.
    (2) Monitor for GI complications (tarry stools, blood in stools [acetylsalicylic acid])
    (3) Avoid administering to children who have viral infection symptoms (acetylsalicylic acid)
    (4) Warn client not to exceed recommended dosages; increasing dose does not increase effectiveness.

SKELETAL MUSCLE RELAXANTS

1. Skeletal muscle pain may be caused by muscle strain from overexercise, traumatic injury, or unusual positioning.
2. Medications:
  a. Uses
    (1) Painful musculoskeletal conditions
    (2) Strains
    (3) Sprains and minor injuries
  b. Modes of action
    (1) These medications affect the CNS.
    (2) They decrease muscle spasms.
    (3) They block the effects of excitatory fibers in the CNS.
    (4) Their minor analgesic effect blocks pain receptor transmission.
  c. Key medication: orphenadrine citrate (Norflex, Norgesic) (prototype).
  d. Interactions: few, and only with a few CNS medications.
  e. General side effects
    (1) CNS (drowsiness, dizziness, dry mouth)
    (2) Genitourinary (urinary retention)
    (3) Cardiovascular (tachycardia, postural hypotension)
    (4) Anticholinergic side effects
  f. Nursing implications
    (1) Instruct client to avoid alcohol, smoking, caffeine, and aspirin.
    (2) Give oral medications only with food.
    (3) Encourage good oral care for dry mouth (ice chips, hard candy).
    (4) Monitor older clients for urinary retention and constipation.
    (5) Instruct the client to avoid excessive exposure to heat, and monitor for heat stroke during summer.
    (6) Instruct the client to take the medication as prescribed, at the times indicated, and not to change dosage without physician's approval.
    (7) Monitor for effectiveness; these medications are for short-term use only. Prolonged unrelieved muscle pain may indicate more severe disease process.

PART B: MEDICATIONS USED FOR PSYCHIATRIC CONDITIONS

SEDATIVES AND HYPNOTICS

1. Sedatives and hypnotics are commonly used for a wide range of conditions that may or may not have a psychiatric origin.
2. Medications: sedatives
  a. Uses
    (1) A sedative is a medication the primary purpose of which is to produce relaxation and to decrease levels of anxiety.
    (2) A hypnotic is a medication the primary purpose of which is to induce sleep (treat insomnia).
  b. Modes of action
    (1) Depression of the limbic system of the brain
    (2) Increase in the effectiveness of the inhibitory neurotransmitters
    (3) General suppression of the CNS
  c. Key medications
    (1) flurazepam (Dalmane)
    (2) temazepam (Restoril)
    (3) chloral hydrate (Noctec)
  d. Interactions
    (1) These medications interact with most CNS medications.
    (2) Alcohol potentiates effects markedly.
  e. General side effects
    (1) Neurological (drowsiness, dizziness, disorientation, weakness, "hangover" next day)
    (2) GI (nausea, vomiting, dry mouth)
    (3) Musculoskeletal (weakness, loss of coordination)
    (4) Respiratory (depression, arrest).
  f. Nursing implications
    (1) Avoid using in clients with glaucoma.

(2) Monitor respiratory status in clients with respiratory disorders.

(3) Instruct clients that these medications are to be used on a short-term basis only (2–4 weeks). If problems persist, symptoms may indicate a more severe condition.

(4) Warn client to avoid alcohol, over-the-counter cold and allergy medications, and other CNS medications.

(5) Clients should avoid driving and other activities that require concentration or coordination when taking these medications.

(6) Monitor for indications of abuse or addiction (increasing dosages, withdrawal symptoms).

(7) Warn clients that sudden withdrawal may cause seizures.

(8) Most of these are Schedule IV medications and must be signed for prior to administration.

MOOD-ALTERING MEDICATIONS

This is a broad class of medications that are used for a variety of psychiatric and nonpsychiatric conditions. The three major groups considered in this section are

1. Medications used to treat anxiety states
2. Medications used to treat major depression
3. Medications used to treat the manic phase of manic-depressive disorder

Medications Used to Treat Anxiety States

1. Anxiety is a normal response to a stressful situation that may manifest itself as:
   a. Apprehension
   b. Fear
   c. Nervousness
   d. Emotional and physical tension
   e. Generalized uneasy feeling
2. Prolonged, unresolved, severe anxiety may produce psychiatric conditions called *anxiety disorders*, which include:
   a. Phobia
   b. Panic and fugue state
   c. Obsessive-compulsive disorder
   d. Posttraumatic stress syndrome
   e. Psychosomatic disorders (conversion disorder, hypochondriasis, somatization)
   f. Eating disorders (bulimia, anorexia nervosa)
3. Antianxiety medications are one of the most frequently prescribed classes of medications in the United States.
4. Medications: the most commonly used class is the benzodiazepines.
   a. Uses
      (1) These medications can be used as hypnotics, sedatives, and relaxants.
      (2) They are sometimes used as anticonvulsants.
      (3) They are often used as preoperative sedatives or mild anesthetics.
      (4) They are used to treat moderate to severe anxiety and anxiety disorders.
   b. Modes of action
      (1) Suppression of the excitation centers in the cerebral cortex
      (2) Depression of the limbic system of the brain
      (3) Suppression of the thalamus and hypothalamus
   c. Key medications
      (1) chlordizephoxide (Librium)
      (2) diazepam (Valium)
      (3) oxazepam (Serax)
      (4) alprazolam (Xanax)
   d. Interactions
      (1) With most CNS medications.
      (2) Alcohol potentiates effects markedly.
   e. General side effects
      (1) Neurological (drowsiness, dizziness, disorientation, weakness, impaired motor coordination, decreased reaction time, partial amnesia)
      (2) GI (nausea, vomiting, dry mouth)
      (3) Respiratory (depression, arrest)
      (4) Withdrawal reaction after long-term, high-dose use.
   f. Nursing implications
      (1) These medications may cause birth defects; avoid using in pregnancy.
      (2) Monitor respiratory status in clients with respiratory disorders.
      (3) Instruct clients that these medications are to be used in conjunction with psychiatric treatment.

(4) Warn clients to avoid alcohol, over-the-counter cold and allergy medications, and other CNS medications.

(5) Clients should avoid driving and other activities that require concentration or coordination when taking these medications.

(6) Monitor for indications of abuse or addiction (increasing dosages, withdrawal symptoms).

(7) Warn clients that sudden withdrawal may cause seizures.

(8) Monitor for effectiveness. If client sleeps excessively, dose may need to be reduced or held.

(9) Most of these are Schedule IV medications and must be signed for prior to administration.

Medications Used to Treat Depressive States

1. Depression is a disorder of mood.
   a. There may be a single episode of depression caused by overwhelming loss, or
   b. There may be recurrent episodes or prolonged depression.
2. Depression is most commonly attributed to low levels of neurotransmitters in the brain, particularly serotonin and norepinephrine.
3. Symptoms will vary according to the severity of the illness, but they usually include:
   a. Psychologically depressed mood that is prolonged and severe and interferes with normal activities of daily living (ADLs).
   b. Lack of energy; client finds no joy in life events.
   c. Appetite disturbances—usually anorexia
   d. Sleep disturbances—difficulty falling asleep; alternatively, client may sleep at night but awaken after 2 to 4 hours of sleep and be unable to go back to sleep. Client may sleep fitfully or experience other disturbances in sleep patterns.
   e. Psychomotor retardation; slowing of movement and of mental and linguistic abilities.
   f. Feelings of low self-esteem or "worthlessness."
   g. Suicidal thoughts.
   h. Poor personal hygiene; poor posture; depressing, dark clothes.

4. Medications: three separate classes are used for the treatment of depression (tricyclics, bicyclics selective serotonin reuptake inhibitors [SSRI], and MAO inhibitors).
   a. Uses
      (1) Tricyclics are used for moderate to severe depression and are the most commonly used class.
      (2) Bicyclics are used for mild to moderate depression and are rapidly gaining popularity.
      (3) MAO inhibitors are used for severe depression that does not respond to other medications but are used only as a last resort because of the many dangerous side effects.
   b. Modes of action
      (1) Tricyclics inhibit the reuptake of neurotransmitters, increasing the norepinephrine and serotonin levels and enhancing sympathetic activity.
      (2) Bicyclics (SSRI) inhibit CNS neuron uptake of serotonin but not of norepinephrine, thereby increasing only the serotonin levels.
      (3) MAO inhibitors inhibit the monamine oxidase enzyme that destroys epinephrine, norepinephrine, serotonin, and dopamine in the synapses, thereby increasing the levels of these neurotransmitters.
   c. Key medications
      (1) doxepin (Sinequan) (tricyclic)
      (2) amitriptyline (Elavil) (tricyclic, prototype)
      (3) fluoxetine (Prozac) (bicyclic, prototype)
      (4) isocarboxazid (Marplan) (MAO inhibitor, prototype)
   d. Interactions
      (1) Tricyclics: most CNS medications, alcohol, MAO inhibitors.
      (2) Bicyclics: most CNS medications, alcohol, MAO inhibitors.
      (3) MAO inhibitors: tricyclics; bicyclics; foods containing tyramine (see Nursing implications); most CNS medications, particularly sympathetic stimulants (dopamine, levophed, isoproterenol)
   e. General side effects
      (1) Tricyclics incur anticholinergic side effects, including dry mouth, blurred vision, constipation, orthostatic hypotension, weight gain, nausea, urinary retention, and tachycardia.
      (2) Bicyclics incur only a few anticholinergic or cardiovascular side effects, weight loss

or gain, dizziness, drowsiness, low blood pressure, and sleep difficulties.

(3) MAO inhibitors incur anticholinergic side effects; hypertensive crisis (throbbing headaches, sweating, nausea, vomiting, stiff neck, restlessness, and cerebrovascular accident [CVA]) if taken with foods containing tyramine.

f. Nursing implications

(1) Monitor physical condition, including intake and output, fluids, sleep patterns, exercise. Give high-fiber, small-feeding diet.

(2) Assess thought processes for slow thinking, ruminating, blocking, restating. Allow time for client to respond to questions, limit choices, and use calm, matter-of-fact, nonjudgmental attitude.

(3) Continually monitor for signs of suicide; most dangerous time is 2 to 3 weeks after the initiation of antidepressant treatment.

(4) It takes 2 to 4 weeks before these medications become effective and show an improvement in mood.

(5) Give antidepressant medications late in the afternoon or early evening to maintain normal sleep patterns.

(6) Monitor for urinary retention.

(7) These medications may cause birth defects; avoid use in pregnancy.

(8) With MAO inhibitors, client needs to be oriented and compliant with instructions about diet.

(9) With MAO inhibitors, client must avoid foods containing tyramine (cheese, liver, beer, red wine, sour cream, citrus fruits, bananas, avocadoes, soy sauce, dried or aged foods, chocolate, pickled herring, chicken livers, yeast products, and yogurt).

(10) When changing from a MAO inhibitor to a tricyclic or bicyclic medication, or client must be drug free for 2 to 3 weeks.

Medications Used to Treat Manic Disorder

1. **Mania** is a disorder of mood, sometimes referred to as a bipolar disorder because it alternates with depression.
   a. Mania may be a mild and transient state.
   b. It may be severe and prolonged, requiring hospitalization.
2. Mania is probably due to unusually high levels of neurotransmitters in the brain, particularly dopamine, serotonin, and norepinephrine.
3. The symptoms of mania may vary based on the severity of the condition, but they include:
   a. Flight of ideas—thinking is speeded up, stream of thought is characterized by rapid association of ideas and there is use of "word salads."
   b. Elated, grandiose mood, in which the client appears self-satisfied, confident, and aggressive but may be covering up for feelings of inadequacy.
   c. Psychomotor excitement and continuous activity when the client sleeps infrequently.
4. Antimania medications
   a. Uses
      (1) Mild to severe manic disorder
      (2) Bipolar disorder
   b. Modes of action
      (1) These medications reduce concentrations of norepinephrine and serotonin by inhibiting their release and enhancing their reuptake by neurons.
      (2) Sodium is partially replaced by lithium in the cell membranes.
   c. Key medications
      (1) lithium carbonate (Eskalith) (prototype)
   d. Interactions
      (1) Thiazide diuretics increase lithium concentration by up to 50%.
      (2) Phenothiazines and nonsteroid anti-inflammatory drugs (NSAIDs) increase lithium levels.
      (3) Sodium increases lithium clearance and vice versa.
   e. General side effects
      (1) Mild toxicity (blurred vision, increased urination, diarrhea)
      (2) Moderate toxicity (irregularity, hypotension, slurred speech, syncope, vomiting, disorientation)
      (3) Severe toxicity (blackouts, seizures, hyperactive movements, shuffled gait, dysrhythmias, CHF, circulatory failure, coma, death)
   f. Nursing implications
      (1) Monitor physical condition closely because the manic state takes a tremendous toll on all the body systems.

(2) Provide small, high-caloric meals on a frequent basis that can be easily and quickly eaten.

(3) Encourage client to lie down and rest for short periods of time.

(4) Obtain a thorough nursing history—note any cardiovascular, renal, or liver disease.

(5) Monitor lithium blood level (therapeutic level = 0.5–1.5 mEq/L [may vary slightly]—toxicity is indicated when blood level is greater than 2.0 mEq/L).

(6) Regulate the dosages carefully, based on blood levels and effectiveness.

(7) Instruct the client that lithium is a drug used on a long-term basis.

(8) Take with food or snack to reduce GI irritation.

(9) Client should be encouraged to drink 2.5 to 3 L/d.

(10) Instruct client to maintain a normal sodium intake (3–4 g/d)

(11) Warn the client to avoid alcohol, sedatives, antihistamines, and other CNS medications without the physician's approval.

(12) If a dose is missed, it should be made up as soon as possible, but do not double up on doses.

(13) Stress the importance of avoiding dehydration and activities that may lead to dehydration, such as excessive sweating, saunas, hot weather, vomiting, or diarrhea (notify physician).

(14) Avoid driving and other activities requiring concentration or coordination.

(15) Instruct the client to avoid excessive intake of caffeine-containing liquids (coffee, tea, colas), inasmuch as these tend to increase diuresis.

(16) Stress the need for frequent follow-up visits to monitor blood levels.

Medications Used to Treat Psychotic States

1. **Psychosis** is an abnormal pattern of behavior characterized by a breakdown of integrated personality functioning, withdrawal from reality, emotional blunting, distorted and regressive behavior, poor communication, impaired interpersonal relationships, and disturbances in thoughts and behavior.

2. Although the exact cause for psychotic states is not known, there are several theories:

   a. *The biologic theory* claims that psychosis is a genetically linked disorder associated with insufficient levels of neurotransmitters, particularly dopamine and serotonin, in the brain.

   b. *The sociocultural theory* maintains that a stressful environmental or family situation produces the behavior changes that eventually manifest themselves as psychosis.

   c. Although there are several different types of psychotic states, schizophrenia is the most commonly seen.

3. The symptoms of schizophrenia may be varied, depending on the type and degree, but generally include:

   a. Associative looseness—verbalization of disturbed thought patterns. The client verbalizes successive ideas that appear to be unrelated to each other. These ideas may have meaning only to the client.

   b. Affect—flattened or inappropriate emotional response to a situation. Clients demonstrate apathy.

   c. Autism—substitution of reality by fantasy and daydreaming. Clients create their own "inner world" to live in.

   d. Ambivalence—coexistence of opposite feelings (e.g., feelings of love and hate for the same person (the "go-away-close" syndrome).

   e. Bizarre delusions or fixed ideas that may take the form of thought broadcasting or thought insertion

   f. Somatic, grandiose, religious delusions.

   g. Persecutory or jealous delusions.

   h. Disturbance of perception manifested as visual or auditory hallucinations.

4. Antipsychotic medications

   a. Uses

      (1) Effective in acute schizophrenia and psychosis

      (2) Modify thought disorders

      (3) Improve blunted effect and withdrawal

      (4) Not effective in controlling paranoid ideation and hostility

      (5) Decrease agitated, aggressive behavior

      (6) Antiemetic, antipyretic, sedation, hiccups (thorazine), potentiate narcotics

b. Modes of action
  (1) Dopamine receptor antagonist, which lowers the levels of dopamine in the brain.
  (2) Medication has anticholinergic and alpha-adrenergic blocking effect on the autonomic nervous system.
c. Key medications
  (1) chlorpromazine (Thorazine)
  (2) thiothinxene (Navane)
  (3) haloperidol (Haldol)
  (4) clozapine (Clozaril)
d. Interactions
  (1) These medications potentiate all CNS depressants.
  (2) They raise lithium levels.
  (3) They inhibit effect of anticonvulsants.
e. General side effects
  (1) Anticholinergic (orthostatic hypotension, tachycardia, dry mouth)
  (2) Photosensitivity
  (3) Sexual problems—cessation of menstruation, breast engorgement, impotency
  (4) Lower seizure threshold
  (5) Extrapyramidal effects (restlessness, pseudoparkinsonism [tremors, shuffling gait, muscle rigidity, salivation]); treatment (benztropine [Cogentin], trihexyphenidyl [Artane]).
  (6) Tardive dyskinesia (bizarre oral movements, tongue writhing, neck twisting, muscle spasms of back, trunk, pelvis)
  (7) Blood dyscrasia (agranulocytosis, white blood cell destruction, infection)
f. Nursing implications
  (1) Warn against overexposure to the sun, and encourage use of an appropriate sunscreen (SPF >15), and sunglasses.
  (2) Carefully monitor blood pressure, intake and output, infections, and constipation.
  (3) Monitor for poor temperature regulation (medication may depress thalamus, hypothalamus) during summer.
  (4) Assess liver function carefully prior to and during administration (medication may be contraindicated for liver disorders).
  (5) Teach the client not to discontinue drug without physician's order.
  (6) Administer smallest dose possible that will give the desired effect. Clients tend to become resistant over time, and they will be on these medications for life.
  (7) Encourage good oral care, and use hard candy and ice chips for dry mouth.
  (8) Stress the need to avoid other CNS drugs (alcohol, sedatives).
  (9) Instruct client to take missed dose as soon as possible; do not double up on missed dose.
  (10) Use with caution in epilepsy or seizure disorders.
  (11) Total detoxification is slow. After medication is stopped, it may take 2 to 3 weeks for client to become fully psychotic again.
  (12) Inform the client that these medications are not physically addictive but that they may cause a psychological dependency.

4

Cardiovascular System Medications

SUMMARY OF KEY ASPECTS OF THE ANATOMY AND PHYSIOLOGY OF THE CARDIOVASCULAR SYSTEM

1. The cardiovascular system is composed of the heart, the arteries, veins, and capillaries.
   a. The heart is a hollow, four-chambered muscular organ whose main function is to create a pressure gradient to keep blood circulating in the body.
      (1) The heart has its own internal circulatory system composed of the coronary arteries and their branches and subdivisions (Fig. 4–1).
      (2) The heart has its own internal conduction system of specialized cardiac tissue, composed of the synoatrial (S-A) node, intraatrial tracts, internodal pathways, atrioventricular (A-V) node, A-V junction, bundle of His, bundle branches, and purkinje fibers.
      (3) Although affected by various hormones, electrolytes, and the autonomic nervous system, the heart can function independently to maintain a normal rate and rhythm.
   b. Properties of cardiac muscle tissue
      (1) **Automaticity**—the heart can initiate impulses on its own without any external stimulation.
      (2) **Rhythmicity**—the heart initiates impulses at regular intervals.
      (3) **Conductivity**—because of the special structure of the muscle tissue in the heart, an impulse can spread throughout all the fibers, even without following the specialized conduction system.
      (4) **All-or-none response**—once a stimulating impulse is initiated, all the muscle tissues in the heart must depolarize.
      (5) **Nonregenerativity**—cardiac tissue that has been destroyed through infarction goes through a process in which it converts into scar tissue but will never regenerate into functioning cardiac muscle tissue.
      (6) **Contractility**—the heart increases the force of the pumping action and pressure of the ejected blood by shortening of the muscle fibers in the chambers.
      (7) **Irritability**—a general term that refers to muscle fibers' tendency to respond to

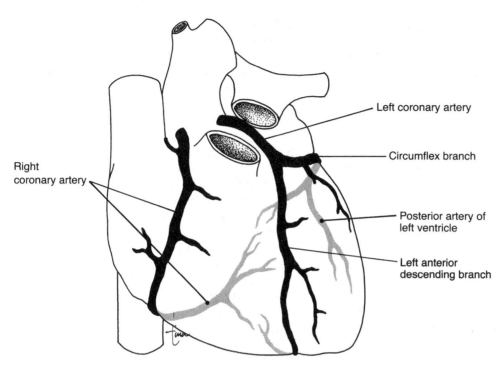

FIGURE 4–1. Coronary arteries. (From Kuhn, M: Pharmacotherapeutics: A Nursing Process Approach, ed 4. FA Davis, Philadelphia, 1998, p 403, with permission.)

external stimuli. Cardiac muscle fibers have increased irritability because of hypoxia, ischemia, abnormal electrolyte levels, certain hormones and medications, and physical trauma.

2. Key terms used in conjunction with cardiovascular medications

a. **Cardiac output** (CO) is the amount of blood measured in liters that is ejected from the left ventricle each minute.
   (1) CO = (HR)/(BPM) × SV (mL/beat) [HR = heart rate; BPM = beats per minute; SV = stroke volume; mL = ?]
   (2) CO is affected by both the rate of the heart and the force of contraction of the left ventricle.
   (3) Increasing the rate or force of contraction will increase the CO.
   (4) When cardiac output is increased, more oxygen is used by the heart, and the workload of the heart is increased.
   (5) Normal CO is 4 to 8 L/min.

b. **Afterload** is the resistance to the blood that is being ejected by the left ventricle.

   (1) Increasing the afterload increases the workload of the heart.
   (2) Constricting the blood vessels increases the afterload.
   (3) Decreasing the afterload decreases the workload of the heart.
   (4) Vasodilation decreases afterload.

c. **Preload** refers to the amount of blood that is in the heart just prior to contraction.
   (1) Vasoconstriction reduces preload.
   (2) Vasodilation increases preload.

d. **Refractory period** is that part of the cardiac cycle when the heart is in a recovery phase after depolarization.
   (1) **Absolute refractory period** refers to the period when the heart does not depolarize (contract) even under the influence of a very strong stimulus.
   (2) **Relative refractory period** refers to a part of the recovery phase at which a strong stimulus will cause partial and abnormal depolarization of the cardiac tissue.

e. **Titrate** is a term that refers to the adjustment of the dosage of a medication based on

CARDIOVASCULAR SYSTEM MEDICATIONS

a predetermined, specific physiological response.

   (1) A morphine drip may be increased or decreased, depending on how much pain the client is experiencing.

   (2) A dopamine drip may be increased or decreased, depending on heart rate and blood pressure.

f. **Inotropic medications** are medications that affect the force of contraction of the heart muscle fibers directly and the cardiac output indirectly.

   (1) Positive inotropic medications increase the force of contraction and increase the cardiac output.

   (2) Negative inotropic medications decrease the force of contraction and decrease the cardiac output.

g. **Chronotropic medications** are medications that affect the rate of the heart.

   (1) Positive chronotropic medications increase the heart rate.

   (2) Negative chronotropic medications decrease the heart rate.

h. **Dromatropic** medications are medications that affect the speed at which impulses pass through the conduction system of the heart.

   (1) Positive dromatropic medications increase the speed at which the impulses pass through the conduction system of the heart.

   (2) Negative dromatropic medications decrease the speed at which the impulses pass through the conduction system of the heart.

i. **Dysrhythmia** (arrhythmia) is a general term that refers to abnormalities in the electrocardiogram (ECG) pattern produced by the heart.

ANTIANGINAL/VASODILATORS

1. **Angina pectoris** is chest pain or pressure that is produced when the oxygen needs of the heart are greater than the oxygen being supplied to the heart muscle tissues. It is often produced by:

  a. Partial obstruction of the coronary arteries

  b. Spasms of the coronary arteries

2. There are three types of angina:

  a. Stable angina is:
   (1) Predictable
   (2) Associated with exercise
   (3) Usually relieved with nitroglycerin (NTG) or rest
   (4) Short-term (5 min)
   (5) Does not radiate
   (6) Shows no or minor ECG changes

  b. Unstable (crescendo, preinfarction) angina is:
   (1) Unpredictable
   (2) May or may not be associated with exercise or activity
   (3) Relieved only partially by NTG
   (4) Characterized by pain that often radiates
   (5) Shows nonspecific or ischemic changes on ECG

  c. Variant (Prinzmetal's) angina is caused by coronary artery spasms and is manifested by:
   (1) Severe, crushing, radiating pain
   (2) Pain that is unrelated to exercise/activity
   (3) ECG changes that show severe ischemia
   (4) Little or no relief with NTG and rest

3. Medications: nitrates as antianginal

  a. Historically, the first documented use of nitrates for the relief of chest pain was in the 1850s.

  b. Nitrates are available in a number of different forms and routes, including:
   (1) Sublingual (SL) tablets and sprays (rapid acting)
   (2) Intravenous (IV) liquids (rapid acting)
   (3) Topical ointments and extended-release patches
   (4) Oral tablets

  c. Uses
   (1) Immediate relief of chest pain during acute attacks
   (2) Prevention of anginal attacks long-term

  d. Mode of action
   (1) Direct dilation of coronary and systemic blood vessels increases the blood and oxygen supply to the heart muscle tissue.
   (2) Dilation of the blood vessels, particularly the systemic arteries, decreases the afterload and reduces the workload of the heart and the amount of oxygen required by the coronary tissues.
   (3) Dilation of the blood vessels tends to pool the blood in the peripheral vascular system, reducing the preload, further reducing the workload of the heart.

e. Key medications
  (1) NTG (Nitro-Bid) (Nitrostat)
  (2) Isorbide (Isordil)
f. Interactions
  (1) Potentiated by alcohol and antihypertensives
  (2) Inhibited by vasoconstricting medications
g. General side effects
  (1) Cardiovascular (tachycardia, hypotension, postural hypotension)
  (2) Central nervous system (CNS) (dizziness, weakness, syncope, flushing, severe headache)
  (3) Gastrointestinal (nausea, vomiting)
h. Nursing implications
  (1) Avoid using nitrates in clients with head trauma or increased intracranial pressure.
  (2) Instruct the client to be sitting or lying down when taking the medication and to change position gradually to prevent orthostatic hypotension.
  (3) Monitor clients closely after the initial dose for hypersensitive reactions (extreme hypotension).
  (4) If using sublingual tablets, the mucus membranes of the mouth should be moist.
  (5) IV NTG should be in a glass bottle and have special tubing to prevent leaching of the medication into the plastic.
  (6) Clients receiving IV NTG should have their blood pressures taken every 1 to 5 minutes.
  (7) SL tablets should be replaced every 3 to 6 months after opening and should be kept in a cool place protected from light.
  (8) Monitor clients for medication effectiveness.
  (9) Inform clients that long-term use of nitrates may lead to tolerance.
  (10) Teach clients that if they have no relief after 3 sublingual tablets, 5 minutes apart, they should call their physician.
  (11) Reinforce with the client the need to modify cardiac risk factors (stop smoking, lose weight, increase exercise, lower cholesterol and fat levels, avoid alcohol) in addition to taking medications for the control of angina.
  (12) Warn the client to continue the medication regimen as prescribed and to never stop taking the medication suddenly.
  (13) Instruct the client to follow the administration instructions exactly as found on the package inserts.

ANTIHYPERTENSIVES

1. **Hypertension** is a sustained blood pressure of 140/90 or higher (Fig. 4–2).
   a. The key word is "sustained," which refers to an elevated blood pressure that persists for a month or more.
   b. The diastolic pressure is more important, because that is the pressure that is in the vascular system at all times.
   c. Hypertension most often appears in adults between 25 and 55 years of age, although in children, it is a growing problem.
2. Types of hypertension
   a. **Essential (idiopathic—primary)** hypertension comprises 95% of all cases and has no direct physiological cause.
      (1) It is probably genetic in origin.
      (2) It may be related to stress (either anxiety or physiological) that increases renin release from the kidneys, producing chronic vasoconstriction.
      (3) It is often marked by prolonged elevation of the diastolic pressure above 95 mm Hg.
   b. **Secondary (acquired) hypertension** has a direct physiological cause. Causes include:
      (1) Pheochromocytoma—a tumor of the adrenal medulla that excretes norepinephrine or an epinephrine in large amounts
      (2) Renal failure
      (3) Hyperthyroidism
      (4) Coarctation of the aorta
   c. **Malignant hypertension** (hypertensive crisis) is a greatly elevated, sustained hypertension that causes necrosis of the small arteries in the organs (brain, heart, kidneys, liver).
      (1) Often leads to renal failure, CVAs, and heart failure
      (2) Diastolic blood pressure between 120 and 150
      (3) Should be treated as an emergency situation with vasodilating medications (IV nitrates)

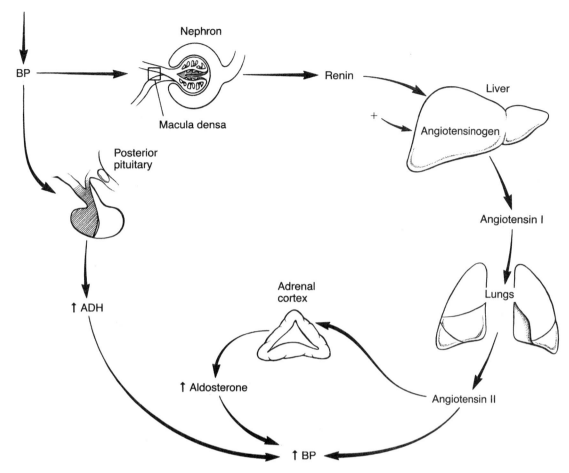

FIGURE 4–2. Blood pressure (BP) control. Several systems regulate blood pressure in the body. The renal system conserves volume and releases renin from the macular densa cells. Renin is eventually converted to angiotensin II, a powerful vasoconstrictor. The endocrine system releases antidiuretic hormone (ADH) from the posterior pituitary, which conserves volume, and aldosterone from the adrenal cortex, which conserves sodium. The nervous system, through the vasomotor center in the medulla, controls the size of the blood vessels. (From Kuhn, M: Pharmacotherapeutics: A Nursing Process Approach, ed 4. FA Davis, Philadelphia, 1998, p 425, with permission.)

3. Hypertension assessment
   a. Risk factors
      (1) Smoking
      (2) High-sodium/high-fat diets
      (3) Stressful life style/lack of exercise
      (4) Family history of hypertension
      (5) Ethnicity (African-American or Native-American)
      (6) Obesity
      (7) Renal disease
      (8) Insulin-dependent diabetes mellitus (IDDM)
   b. Symptoms of hypertension: few
      (1) Occipital headache in A.M.
      (2) Dizziness
      (3) Tinnitus
      (4) Pounding heart
4. Medications: five separate classes of medications are used in the treatment of hypertension (angiotensin-converting enzyme [ACE] inhibitors; diuretics; calcium channel blockers; adrenergic inhibitors; vasodilators).
   a. Uses
      (1) ACE inhibitors are used for mild hypertension.
      (2) Diuretics are used in conjunction with other antihypertensive medications for mild to moderate hypertension (see full discussion in Chapter 6).

(3) Calcium channel blockers are used to treat mild to moderate hypertension.

(4) Adrenergic inhibitors are used to treat moderate to severe hypertension resistant to other medications.

(5) Vasodilators are used to treat severe hypertension.

b. Modes of action

(1) ACE inhibitors block the conversion of angiotensin I into angiotensin II (a potent vasoconstrictor) in the renin-angiotensin mechanism of the kidneys.

(2) Diuretics reduce the total fluid volume of the body through excretion in the urinary system (see Chapter 6).

(3) Calcium channel blockers interfere with the influx of calcium ions into the cardiac muscle tissues and blood vessels, reducing the force of contraction (CO) and dilating blood vessels (reducing afterload).

(4) Adrenergic inhibitors block either alpha-receptors or beta-receptors or both along the sympathetic chain, both reducing the force of contraction of the heart (cardiac output) and dilating blood vessels (reducing afterload).

(5) Vasodilators directly dilate the blood vessels in the body by altering the cellular metabolism of calcium ions, reducing the afterload of the heart.

c. Key medications

(1) ACE inhibitors: captopril (Capoten)

(2) Diuretics: thiazide-(HCTX) (Diuril), loop-furosemide (Lasix) (see Chapter 6)

(3) Calcium channel blockers: diltiazem (Cardizem)

(4) Adrenergic inhibitors: methyldopa (Aldomet), propranolol (Inderal), nadolol (Corgard)

(5) Vasodilators: hydralazine (Apresoline), prazosin (Minipress)

d. Interactions

(1) ACE inhibitors: alcohol, other antihypertensives potentiate effect; psychiatric medications inhibit effect.

(2) Diuretics (see Chapter 6)

(3) Calcium channel blockers: beta-blockers and antidysrhythmics potentiate effect; H_2 inhibitors block metabolism.

(4) Adrenergic inhibitors: potentiate alcohol, antihistamines, antidepressants, lithium. Tricyclics and anti-inflammatory medications inhibit hypotensive action.

(5) Vasodilators: potentiate anticholinergics, inhibited by nonsteroid anti-inflammatory drugs (NSAIDs).

e. General side effects (similar for all groups)

(1) Cardiovascular: hypotension, orthostatic hypotension, bradycardia (adrenergic inhibitors), tachycardia (other groups), congestive heart failure, edema

(2) Central nervous system: headache, dizziness, weakness, syncope, depression

(3) Gastrointestinal: anorexia, nausea, vomiting, diarrhea, excessive flatus (beta blockers)

(4) Genitourinary: impotency, excessive urination and electrolyte imbalance (diuretics)

(5) Respiratory: chronic cough (ACE inhibitors), respiratory depression (adrenergic inhibitors)

f. Nursing implications (similar for all groups)

(1) Stress the need for taking the medication exactly as ordered and not skipping or changing dosages, even if client feels well.

(2) Instruct client on how to monitor blood pressure and pulse at home; notify physician if it is abnormal.

(3) Warn client to change positions slowly to prevent dizziness from orthostatic hypotension.

(4) Instruct client to avoid conditions that may produce dehydration (extreme heat, hot showers, saunas, and hot tubs).

(4) Caution client not to drive or operate hazardous equipment if client feels dizzy.

(5) Instruct client to avoid alcohol and other medications that may cause interactions.

(6) Stress the need to inform dentists and other health-care providers of condition and medications being taken.

(7) Reinforce the importance of altering hypertensive risk factors/lifestyle (control stress, increase exercise, low-sodium and low-fat diet, decrease caffeine intake, lose weight, stop smoking, decrease/stop alcohol intake) in addition to medications.

CARDIAC GLYCOSIDES

1. Cardiac glycosides are used primarily in the treatment of congestive heart failure (CHF).
2. CHF designates ineffective ventricular pumping due to enlargement and inefficient contractions of the heart.
   a. General symptoms: fatigue, anxiety, skin breakdown, tachycardia
   b. In right-sided failure the blood backs up into the venous circulation.
      (1) It often has pulmonary causes, such as chronic obstructive pulmonary disease (COPD [cor pulmonale]).
      (2) Specific right-sided failure symptoms include generalized peripheral edema, ascites, perhaps some liver engorgement.
   c. In left-sided failure the blood backs up into the lungs.
      (1) It often is caused by myocardial infarction (MI) or other cardiac pathology.
      (2) Specific left-sided symptoms: dyspnea, orthopnea, frothy blood-tinged sputum, paroxysmal nocturnal dyspnea (PND).
3. Medications: cardiac glycosides
   a. Uses:
      (1) Treatment of congestive heart failure
      (2) Treatment of atrial dysrhythmias
   b. Modes of action
      (1) Increases the concentration of calcium and sodium ions in the cardiac muscle cells by inhibiting ATPase
      (2) Positive inotropic effect (increases the force of contraction, oxygen use, and workload of the heart)
      (3) Negative chronotropic and dromotropic effects (slows the heart rate and decreases the rate of conduction)
      (4) Will shrink an enlarged heart
      (5) Affects all the cells in the body in some way
   c. Key medication: digoxin (Lanoxin)
   d. Interactions
      (1) Antibiotics may increase Lanoxin level to toxic
      (2) Antacids, antidiarrheals, and ion exchange resins reduce effectiveness
      (3) Diuretics increase the risk of toxicity and dysrhythmias
   e. General side effects

(1) Cardiovascular: bradycardia, pulse deficit, ventricular ectopic beats (premature ventricular contractions [PVCs], ventricular tochycardia [VT]), A-V blocks
(2) Gastrointestinal: early signs of toxicity—anorexia, nausea, vomiting, diarrhea
(3) Neurological: late signs of toxicity—headache, double vision, blurred or colored vision, restlessness or irritability, muscle weakness, fatigue
   f. Nursing implications
      (1) Assess client prior to administration for indications of renal or liver disorders.
      (2) Instruct client to take pulse for one full minute prior to taking medication. Hold if pulse is below 60 BPM in adult.
      (3) Instruct the client in the signs and symptoms of digoxin toxicity and stress the need to notify the physician if any appear.
      (4) Encourage the client to eat foods high in potassium, particularly if client is also taking a diuretic.
      (5) Warn client that the medication should be stored in a tightly closed container away from heat and light.
      (6) Stress the need for frequent follow-up visits with the physician to monitor digoxin blood levels (therapeutic level =0.5 to 1.5 mg/L; toxic levels >2.0 mg/L).

ANTIDYSRHYTHMIC AGENTS (ANTIARRHYTHMIC)

1. **Dysrhythmia (arrhythmia)** is generally defined as any deviation or abnormality in the ECG pattern.
2. The seriousness of a dysrhythmia is determined by:
   a. The part of the heart affected; most serious are:
      (1) Dysrhythmias that affect the ventricles
      (2) Conduction defects in the A-V node.
   b. The degree of reduced cardiac output that the dysrhythmia produces
   c. The symptoms that the dysrhythmia causes secondary to reduced cardiac output: common symptoms of dysrhythmias include:
      (1) Neurological (dizziness, weakness, syncope, unconsciousness)

(2) Cardiovascular (chest pressure and pain, shortness of breath, hypotension, tachycardia/bradycardia)

3. The treatment of cardiac dysrhythmias is extremely complex and is usually reserved for mastery in critical care or advanced dysrhythmia courses.

4. There are no ECG strips for interpretation on the NCLEX, although an occasional question may be asked concerning treatment of the most serious dysrhythmia, including:

a. Premature ventricular contractions (PVCs). These are early ectopic beats that arise from an irritable area in the ventricles often secondary to a myocardial infarction. They are most serious when they occur:
   (1) Frequently (more than 6 per minute)
   (2) In a bigeminal pattern (one normal beat followed by an ectopic beat in a repeating pattern)
   (3) In grouped patterns of two or three
   (4) Very early in the cardiac cycle so that the QRS complex of the PVC is near or on the T wave of the previous beat (R on T phenomenon)

b. Ventricular tachycardia. This occurs when an irritable area in the ventricles takes over all the pacemaker functions of the heart.
   (1) Cardiac output may be reduced to near zero.
   (2) It may cause death if not treated immediately.

c. Ventricular fibrillation. This occurs when there are multiple irritable areas in the ventricles, which cause a quivering of the ventricles without any organized, effective contraction.
   (1) It is a type of cardiac arrest.
   (2) All circulation stops.
   (3) The client is considered clinically dead.

d. Cardiac arrest. This occurs when there is no electrical activity in the heart.
   (1) All circulation stops.
   (2) Client is considered clinically dead.

e. High-grade A-V block (complete heart block). This occurs when no impulses can pass through the A-V node from the S-A node and atria.
   (1) A back-up pacemaker site must take over in order to maintain circulation (from A-V junction or ventricles).
   (2) Heart rate is usually much slower.
   (3) Back-up pacemaker sites are less reliable and may stop suddenly.

f. Paroxysmal supraventricular tachycardia (PSVT). This occurs when the atria become very irritable and begin to beat at rates in excess of 200 BPM.
   (1) The A-V node normally blocks some of the atrial beats from getting to the ventricles to keep the ventricular below 150 BPM.
   (2) Sustained episodes of PSVT place great demand on the heart.
   (3) This may lead to myocardial infarction, ventricular tachycardia, or cardiac arrest if not treated quickly.

5. Medications: antidysrhythmic agents are divided into several classes determined by their mode of action and dysrhythmia treated.

a. Uses
   (1) Class I-A: treat both atrial dysrhythmia (atrial fibrillation) and ventricular dysrhythmia
   (2) Class I-B: prevent or suppress ventricular dysrhythmia
   (3) Class II (beta-blockers): suppress or stop ventricular tachycardia and PVCs
   (4) Class III: back-up medications used to treat life-threatening ventricular dysrhythmias when Class I-A and I-B medications are not effective
   (5) Class IV (calcium channel blockers): used to stop and control PSVT and other atrial dysrhythmias
   (6) Unclassified: used to treat PSVT

b. Modes of action
   (1) Class I-A: depress myocardial contractility and excitability; prolong the refractory period
   (2) Class I-B: prolong repolarization time and stabilize cell membranes to sodium/potassium exchange
   (3) Class II (beta-blockers): negative inotropic and chronotropic effect (reduce workload of heart and oxygen demand), decrease atrial and ventricular irritability
   (4) Class III: slow automaticity and repolarization, block reentry through the A-V node
   (5) Class IV (calcium channel blockers): inhibit calcium entry into the myocardium by blocking slow channel entry sites of the cell membrane; negative inotropic,

CARDIOVASCULAR SYSTEM MEDICATIONS

negative chronotropic, and negative dromotropic effects

(6) Unclassified: inhibit reentry pathways through A-V node, produce vasodilation of coronary arteries; negative dromotropic effect

c. Key medications

(1) Class I-A: disopyramide phosphate (Norpace)

(2) Class I-B: lidocaine, (prototype) tocainide HCL (Tonocard)

(3) Class II (beta-blockers): propranolol (Inderal) (see above)

(4) Class III: amiodarone HCL (Cordarone)

(5) Class IV (calcium channel blockers): verapamil HCL (Calan, Isoptin) (see above)

(6) Unclassified: adenosine (Adenocard)

d. Interactions

(1) Class I-A: other antidysrythmics may cause cardiac arrest; alcohol potentiates effect

(2) Class I-B: used with beta-blockers; may cause toxicity

(3) Class II (beta-blockers): potentiate alcohol, antihistamines, antidepressants, lithium. Tricyclics and anti-inflammatory medications inhibit antidysrhythmic action.

(4) Class III: concurrent use of other antidysrhythmics and oral anticoagulants potentiate effects; digoxin toxicity may occur

(5) Class IV (calcium channel blockers): beta-blockers and antidysrhythmics potentiate effect; H_2 inhibitors block metabolism

(6) Unclassified: effects inhibited by caffeine and theophylline; nicotine increases risk of tachycardia; disyridmole potentiates effects

e. General side effects

(1) Class I-A: gastrointestinal (GI) irritation, thrombocytopenia, hypotension, heart block, tachycardia, dizziness, cardiac toxicity (widened QRS complex), urinary retention

(2) Class I-B: drowsiness, seizures (sign of toxicity), disorientation, slurred speech, somnolence, hypotension

(3) Class II (beta-blockers): bradycardia, hypotension, fatigue, weakness, impotency, heart block, fatigue, GI upset, flatulence

(4) Class III: orthostatic hypotension, dizziness, ventricular dysrhythmia, photosensitivity

(5) Class IV (calcium channel blockers): orthostatic hypotension, A-V blocks, CHF, edema, flushing, leg and muscle cramps

(6) Unclassified: shortness of breath, flushing, palpitations, chest pain, hypotension, nausea

f. Nursing implications

(1) Class I-A: Do not use in cardiogenic shock or high grade A-V block without pacemaker; hold if pulse below 60 or above 120 in adult; monitor blood pressure; watch for urinary retention.

(2) Class I-B: Monitor ECG continuously during lidocaine administration; monitor lidocaine blood levels (therapeutic 1.5 to 6 μg/mL; toxic >7); monitor for neurological side effects.

(3) Class II (beta-blockers): Avoid using in clients with COPD, CHF, and A-V block; hold if pulse <60 BPM; warn client to never stop taking suddenly—may precipitate MI.

(4) Class III: Monitor BP and pulse; reevaluate ECG for changes; use sunscreen.

(5) Class IV (calcium channel blockers): Monitor blood pressure closely during IV administration; administer IV slowly; assess for development of CHF; monitor BP and pulse.

(6) Unclassified: Monitor BP, pulse, and respiratory status closely; do not confuse with adenosine phosphate; check vial for crystals before administration.

MEDICATIONS USED TO TREAT SHOCK STATES

1. **Shock** is a general term used to describe an abnormal physiological state in which there is widespread, serious reduction of tissue perfusion.

a. If shock is prolonged, it will lead to:

(1) Generalized impairment of cellular function

(2) Inability of cells to use oxygen

(3) Inadequate microcirculatory perfusion of the vital organ

(4) Death

2. Organs that are particularly sensitive to poor perfusion include:
   a. Brain
   b. Kidneys
   c. Liver
   d. Heart
3. The "fight or flight" response is activated by shock states, and blood is shunted to the vital areas, especially the heart and brain.
4. General symptoms of shock include:
   a. Low blood pressure
   b. Cool, moist skin
   c. Low body temperature
   d. Tachycardia
   e. Stupor, coma
   f. Dilated, sluggish pupils
5. Types of shock
   a. Hemorrhagic: caused by excessive blood loss (surgery or trauma, GI bleeds, closed fractures, lacerated liver or spleen, intracranial hemorrhages)
   b. Hypovolemic: caused by fluid loss other than whole blood (burns, vomiting, heat stroke, diabetic ketoacidosis [DKA], excessive urination diabetes insipidus [DI])
   c. Neurogenic: caused by excessive systemic vasodilation secondary to paralysis of nerves that control the size of the blood vessels (medulla or spinal cord injury).
   d. Cardiogenic: caused by inability of the heart to produce adequate circulation secondary to ischemia, infarction, myocarditis, or cardiomyopathies; dissecting aortic aneurysm or pulmonary embolus
   e. Septic: type of neurogenic shock caused by bacterial toxins or necrotic tissues (septicemia, toxic shock syndrome [TSS], overwhelming infection)
   f. Anaphylactic: severe allergic antigen-antibody reaction to some foreign substance usually by injection, bee sting, or inhalation, producing severe bronchial spasms, wheezing, dyspnea, tachypnea, restlessness
6. A wide range of medications may be used for treatment of shock, depending on the cause, including:
   a. Antihistamines, bronchodilators, and epinephrine for anaphylactic shock (see Chapters 3 and 7)
   b. Antibiotics for septic shock (see Chapter 12)
   c. Sympathetic stimulants for cardiogenic shock (see Chapter 3)

5

Hematologic Medications

SUMMARY OF KEY ASPECTS OF THE ANATOMY AND PHYSIOLOGY OF THE CLOTTING MECHANISM

1. The coagulation process involves multiple steps and is complex (Fig. 5–1).
   a. The coagulation process or cascade is normally triggered by an injury that produces bleeding.
      (1) In response to the injury, the body begins to release the key clotting factors and substances necessary to produce a clot.
      (2) All the steps in the clotting process must be present for a clot to form.
   b. The body also produces its own anticlotting substances.
      (1) Anticlotting substances act in conjunction with the clotting process to allow for normal circulation in the vascular system.
      (2) Anticlotting substances are also normally released 7 to 14 days after a clot forms to help dissolve the clot and promote normal circulation.

2. Disruption of the balance between the clotting and anticlotting mechanisms in the body produces problems.
   a. Disruption of the clotting mechanism can cause uncontrollable bleeding.
   b. Disruption of the anticlotting mechanism can cause abnormal clot formation.
      (1) **Thrombus** is a blood clot that occurs in the vascular system.
      (2) **Embolus** refers to the obstruction of a blood vessel by some foreign substance, most commonly a blood clot.
      (3) **Thromboembolism** is a thrombus that breaks off and travels to another part of the body.
      (4) **Thrombophlebitis (venous thrombosis)** is a blood clot that forms on the wall of a vein and partially or completely blocks the flow of venous blood; it is often associated with an inflammation or infection of the blood vessel.

3. Symptoms of abnormal clot formation are dependent on the affected body part. Common areas include:

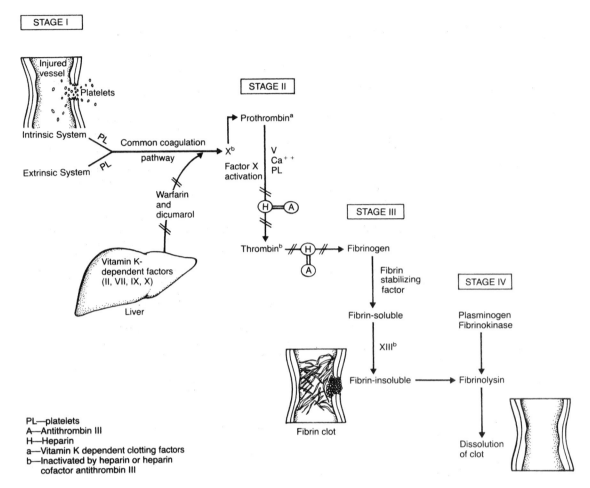

FIGURE 5–1. Schematic representation of the blood coagulation mechanism. The intrinsic system activates XII → XIIa, XI → XIa, IX → IXa, →X → Xa, which are all found in blood; the extrinsic system is activated by release of tissue thromboplastin, a factor not found in circulating blood, and then activates VII → VIIa and joins to activate IX → Xa and X → Xa. Activation of the intrinsic system takes several minutes to achieve a clot, whereas the extrinsic system takes only several seconds. From the activation of the extrinsic/intrinsic system the common pathway is entered. Stage II ultimately creates thrombin and stage III fibrin. Stage IV consists of clot resolution. (From Kuhn, M: Pharmacotherapeutics: A Nursing Process Approach, ed 4. FA Davis, Philadelphia, 1998, p 518, with permission.)

a. The lungs (pulmonary embolism). Symptoms include:
  (1) Localized chest pain
  (2) Tachypnea
  (3) Dyspnea
  (4) Blood-tinged sputum
  (5) Low-grade fever
  (6) Tachycardia
  (7) Pleural friction rub
b. Calf area of the legs. Symptoms include:
  (1) Localized tenderness and swelling

  (2) Sensation of warmth at clot site
  (3) Palpable cordlike structure
4. Some clients are at high risk for abnormal clot formation, including clients:
  a. On extended bed rest, or immobilized
  b. With IV catheters
  c. Who are obese
  d. Who develop atrial fibrillation
  e. With cancer
  f. Suffering from multiple sclerosis
  g. Who take oral contraceptives and smoke

h. Who are pregnant or postpartum
i. Over 40 years of age who must have surgery
j. Who are postfracture
5. Anticoagulant agents are used to treat abnormal clot formation.
   a. Anticoagulants are used to prevent the formation of new clots or prevent the enlargement of existing clots.
   b. Anticoagulants allow the body to use its own anticoagulation factors to dissolve the clot.
   c. Anticoagulants do *not* dissolve clots.
6. Medications: parenteral-only anticoagulants
   a. Uses
      (1) Short-term or emergency treatment of all types of blood clots
      (2) Postmyocardial infarction
      (3) Postbypass surgery and most vascular surgery
      (4) Hemodialysis
      (5) Early stages of disseminated intervascular coagulation (DIC)
      (6) Prolonged bed rest or immobilization states
   b. Modes of action
      (1) Found naturally in body tissues
      (2) Inactivates thrombin formation from prothrombin
      (3) Inactivates the activated parts of factors IX, X, XI, and XII
      (4) Combines with and increases the activity of antithrombin III
   c. Key medication: heparin sodium (Liquaemin, Lipo-Hepin)
   d. Interactions
      (1) Potentiated by acetylsalicylic acid (aspirin), ibuprophen, alcohol, some antibiotics
      (2) Inhibited by nitroglycerine products, digoxin (Lanoxin), antihistamines
   e. General side effects
      (1) Hematuria
      (2) Epistaxis
      (3) Ecchymosis; petechiae
      (4) Black, tarry stools
      (5) Bleeding from gums and mucus membranes
      (6) Heparin-induced thrombosis; white clot syndrome
      (7) Thrombocytopenia

(8) Rashes
(9) Hair loss
(10) Bone demineralization; osteoporosis
f. Nursing implications
   (1) Monitor partial prothromoplastin time (PTT) (normal = 30–45 seconds; therapeutic = 2–2½ times normal [60–80 seconds]).
   (2) Wait for daily PTT to come from laboratory before giving A.M. dose.
   (3) Always double-check dosage; use tuberculin (TB) syringe for small doses; medication is given in units.
   (4) Read package carefully; comes in different dosage strengths (1 mL = 1000 U; 1 mL = 5000 U; 1 mL = 10,000 U).
   (5) Monitor client closely for side effects, particularly signs and symptoms of bleeding.
   (6) Monitor IV site closely for signs of infiltration when administering IV push or drip.
   (7) Instruct the client to avoid over-the-counter medications that contain aspirin or ibuprophen.
   (8) Avoid giving the client IM injections if possible.
   (9) Maintain pressure on IM injection and venipuncture sites for 5 minutes.
   (10) Do not mix any other medications with IV heparin infusions.
   (11) Use an electric razor for shaving clients; soft toothbrush for oral care.
   (12) When giving medication subcutaneously, insert syringe into the abdomen above the iliac crest; do not rub injection site; do not aspirate.
   (13) Inform ancillary services (laboratory, x-ray, respiratory therapy, physical therapy) that the client is receiving anticoagulant therapy.
7. Medications: oral-only anticoagulants
   a. Uses
      (1) Long-term treatment or prevention of venous thromboembolic problems
      (2) Postmyocardial infarction or cardiac surgery
      (3) Postcerebral vascular accident (CVA)
      (4) Prophylactically for clients at risk
   b. Modes of action
      (1) Inhibit the formation and use of vitamin K in the liver

(2) Depress synthesis of factors VII, IX, and X

(3) Take 48 to 72 hours to reach therapeutic level in the bloodstream

c. Key medication: warfarin sodium (Coumadin) (prototype)

d. Interactions

(1) Potentiated by glucocorticoids, aspirin and ibuprofen, alcohol, some antibiotics

(2) Inhibited by barbiturates, estrogen, oral contraceptives, foods containing vitamin K (cabbage, cauliflower, broccoli, asparagus, tomatoes, fish, liver, cheese, egg yolks, red meat)

e. General side effects

(1) Bleeding and hemorrhage (see parenteral anticoagulants)

(2) Mouth ulcers

(3) Nausea, vomiting, diarrhea

(4) Red-orange color to urine

(5) Leukopenia, agranulocytosis

f. Nursing implications

(1) Avoid administering to clients with liver disorders.

(2) Monitor prothrombin time (PT): normal = 11 to 16 seconds; therapeutic 2 to 2½ times normal (25–35 seconds).

(3) Instruct the client to avoid over-the-counter medications that contain aspirin and ibuprofen.

(4) Instruct the client to avoid eating large amounts of foods that contain vitamin K (cabbage, cauliflower, broccoli, asparagus, tomatoes, fish, liver, cheese, egg yolks, red meat).

(5) Instruct the client that this medication is usually taken long-term at home, and stress the importance of taking it as prescribed.

(6) Instruct the client to wear a medical alert bracelet or band that identifies him or her as being anticoagulated.

(7) Instruct the client to avoid activities that may result in cuts or injury.

(8) Instruct the client to inform physicians, dentists, or other health-care providers prior to treatment that he or she is taking this medication.

(9) Reinforce the importance of frequent return visits to the physician for monitoring.

(10) Client may be on both heparin and coumadin for 2 to 3 days before discharge.

(11) Avoid giving the client IM injections, if possible.

(12) Maintain pressure on IM injection and venipuncture sites for 5 minutes.

(13) Use an electric razor for shaving clients; soft toothbrush for oral care.

8. Medications: thrombolytic agents

a. Uses

(1) Myocardial infarction

(2) Cerebral embolism (stroke)

(3) Pulmonary infarction due to embolism

(4) Large arterial or venous embolisms

(5) Clearing of clots in cannulae and catheters

b. Modes of action

(1) Dissolves blood clots

(2) Converts a plasminogen to plasmin, degrading fibrin in the clot

(3) Lyses protein fibers in clots

c. Key medications

(1) streptokinase (Streptase)

(2) alteplase (tissue plasminogen activator) (t-PA, Activase)

d. Interactions

(1) Potentiated by heparin, coumadin, aspirin, ibuprofen

(2) Inhibited by any medication or substance that inhibits bleeding

e. General side effects

(1) Excessive bleeding and hemorrhage

(2) Anaphylactic/allergic reactions with streptokinase

(3) Body temperature elevations

(4) Chest pressure, pain, or dysrhythmia

(5) Phlebitis at IV site

f. Nursing implications

(1) Monitor closely for bleeding, CVA, and dysrhythmia during IV administration.

(2) Mix carefully according to directions; use within 24 hours.

(3) Always use controller or pump for administration.

(4) Alert laboratory, x-ray, and other ancillary personnel that the client is receiving medications.

(5) Avoid giving aspirin and other anticoagulants without the physician's approval.

(6) Monitor PT, PTT, and complete blood count (CBC) closely.

(7) Hold pressure on all venipuncture sites for 5 minutes.

(8) Assess for previous reactions to streptokinase.

ANTIDOTES

1. Anticoagulant and thrombolytic medications are extremely potent and dangerous.
   a. Excessive dosages due to medication errors may lead to sudden and uncontrolled hemorrhage and death.
   b. Even individuals who receive the proper dosage may develop severe hemorrhagic conditions.
2. Each group of medications has its own particular antidote to counteract the unique effects of that medication.
   a. Protamine sulfate is the antidote for heparin.
      (1) It binds and inactivates heparin.
      (2) It must be given IV.
      (3) Dosage is based on amount of heparin received (1 mg per 100 units of heparin).
   b. Phytonadione (AquaMEPHYTON, vitamin K) is the antidote for oral anticoagulants (warfarin).
      (1) Promotes synthesis of coagulation factors II, VII, IX, and X
      (2) May be given PO, SC, or IM
      (3) Usual dose: 2.5–10 mg for adults; repeat q 6–8 h
   c. Aminocaproic acid (Amicar) is the antidote for antithrombolytic agents (streptokinase, t-PA).
      (1) Inhibits the activation of plasminogen and stabilizes clot formation
      (2) May be given PO or IV
      (3) Dosage based on amount of antithrombolytic medication used, but averages 4–6 g IV for adults
      (4) May also be used for heparin overdose

6

Urinary System Medications

SUMMARY OF KEY ASPECTS OF THE ANATOMY AND PHYSIOLOGY OF THE RENAL SYSTEM

1. There are normally two kidneys.
   a. They are located behind the parietal peritoneum.
      (1) Hilum is the concave notch in each kidney.
      (2) Cortex is the outer layer.
      (3) Medulla is the inner portion, divided up into 12 to 14 renal pyramids.
   b. Nephron is the functional unit of the kidney.
      (1) There are 1,000,000 to 1,250,000 nephrons; it is possible to lose 75% and do well.
   c. Nephron is composed of the following (Fig. 6–1):
      (1) Bowman's capsule
      (2) Proximal convoluted tubule
      (3) Descending and ascending loops of Henle
      (4) Distal tubule and collecting tubule
      (5) Glomerulus, which is impermeable to large protein molecules

   d. The blood is separated in the Bowman's capsules.
   e. Excretion and reabsorption of fluids, electrolytes, and wastes takes place in tubule system.
   f. Excretion and reabsorption occur because of diffusion, osmosis, and active transport.
      (1) As the filtrate moves through the nephron, a large portion of the water and ions is reabsorbed.
      (2) In the proximal tubule cells, carbon dioxide is converted into bicarbonate by the enzyme carbonic anhydrase.
      (3) Water and chloride ions are also reabsorbed in the proximal tubule.
      (4) Sodium ions are reabsorbed in the loop of Henle and the distal tubule in exchange for potassium ions.
      (5) Water passively follows sodium ions in either excretion or reabsorption.
      (6) Normal glomerular filtration rate (GFR) is 125 mL/min.
   g. Kidneys require a mean arterial pressure of 50 to 60 mm Hg to function.

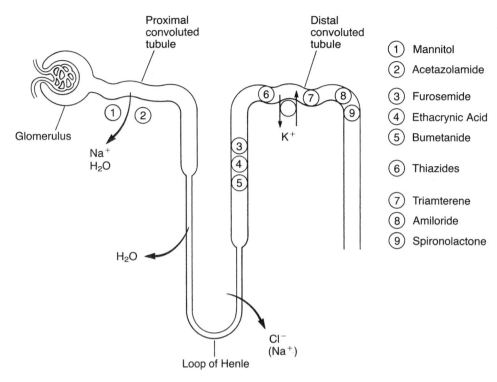

FIGURE 6–1. *Sites of action of diuretics. The primary site of action is presented. Many of these drugs have multiple sites of action. (From Kuhn, M: Pharmacotherapeutics: A Nursing Process Approach, ed 4. FA Davis, Philadelphia, 1998, p 546, with permission.)*

h. Normal adult produces 1 L of urine per 24 hours.
2. Functions of the kidney
  a. Regulation of volume and composition of body fluid
    (1) Fluid volume control
    (2) Electrolyte regulation
    (3) Excretion of metabolic waste, toxins, and drugs
  b. Regulation of acid-base balance: selectively controls
    (1) H ion secretion/retention (normal pH 7.35–7.45)
    (2) HCO_3 ion secretion/retention
  c. Regulation of body processes
    (1) Blood pressure regulation (renin-angiotensin mechanisms causing vasoconstriction)
    (2) Erythropoietin production (hormone necessary for the production of RBCs)
    (3) Calcium/phosphate balance

DIURETICS

1. Diuretics are medications that promote the excretion of sodium and water through the renal system.
2. Diuretics primarily function through the interference of reabsorption of sodium and chloride ions in the renal tubules.
  a. Diuretics are used in a number of disease processes in which reduction of excessive body fluid volume is important.
    (1) **Edema** is a condition in which there is build-up of fluid in extravascular tissues.
    (2) **Pitting edema** occurs most often in the extremities and is noted by the indentation left after pressure by a finger.
    (3) **Anasarca** is a generalized body edema often seen in renal disease or long-term right-sided congestive heart failure.
  b. Several hormones also affect the secretion of sodium and water in the renal system.

(1) Aldosterone is a hormone that causes sodium reabsorption.

(2) **Antidiuretic hormone (ADH)** is released by the pituitary gland during stress response and inhibits the secretion of sodium and water.

(3) Estrogen and corticosteroids increase sodium and water retention.

3. Medications: thiazide diuretics
  a. Uses
    (1) Hypertension
    (2) Congestive heart failure
    (3) Renal failure
    (4) Liver failure (controversial)
    (5) Decreased urine output states
    (6) Corticosteroid and estrogen therapy adjunct
  b. Modes of action
    (1) Lower peripheral vascular resistance (vasodilation)
    (2) Block sodium, chloride, and water reabsorption in the distal tubule system
  c. Key medications: chlorothiazide (Diuril); hydrochlorothiazide (HCTZ, Dyazide)
  d. Interactions
    (1) These medications potentiate effects of lithium, digoxin, and oral hypoglycemics.
    (2) Alcohol and antihypertensives potentiate effects of these medications.
  e. General side effects
    (1) Orthostatic hypotension
    (2) Hypokalemia; hyponatremia
    (3) Elevated/decreased glucose levels; may require increase insulin dose in diabetics
    (4) General dehydration (dry mouth, thirst, poor skin turgor)
    (5) Cardiac dysrhythmias
    (6) Nausea, vomiting, rashes
  f. Nursing implications (see general nursing implications at end of chapter)
    (1) Assess for allergies to sulfonamides prior to administration
    (2) Monitor blood sugar levels closely when used in clients with diabetes.
    (3) Monitor for the development of gout.
    (4) Administer with food to prevent gastrointestinal (GI) upset.
4. Medications: loop diuretics
  a. Uses
    (1) Marked edema states
    (2) Congestive heart failure
    (3) Renal dysfunction
    (4) Liver failure (controversial)
    (5) Moderate to severe hypertension
    (6) When less potent diuretics are not effective
  b. Modes of action
    (1) Block sodium and water reabsorption in the entire loop of Henle and ascending loop
    (2) Block sodium and water reabsorption in the proximal and distal tubules
    (3) Reduce preload and afterload
  c. Key medication: furosemide (Lasix)
  d. Interactions
    (1) Furosemide potentiates effects of lithium, anticoagulants, and digoxin.
    (2) Alcohol, nonsteroidal anti-inflammatory medications, and antihypertensives potentiate its effects.
  e. General side effects
    (1) Excessive urination and dehydration
    (2) Hypokalemia; hyponatremia
    (3) Transient deafness with rapidly administered IV doses
    (4) Decrease in white blood count (WBC) with long-term therapy
    (5) Circulatory collapse and hypovolemic shock
    (6) Orthostatic hypotension
    (7) Thrombocytopenia
    (8) Elevated blood urea nitrogen (BUN) (normal 10–20)
  f. Nursing implications (see general nursing implications at the end of chapter)
    (1) Give IM with Z-track method.
    (2) Give IV at 10 mg/min (1 mL/min)
5. Medications: osmotic diuretics
  a. Uses
    (1) Decrease intracranial pressure due to head trauma, surgery, stroke, and so forth.
    (2) Decrease pressure in cerebral spinal fluid following back trauma, surgery, or meningitis
    (3) Increase urine output in the oliguric phase of acute renal failure conditions
    (4) Correct edema states not caused by excessive sodium
    (5) Increase excretion of toxins and medication overdoses

b. Modes of action
   (1) Increase the osmotic pressure (hypertonic solution) in the vascular system
   (2) Draw fluid from the tissues into the vascular system, where it can be excreted
   (3) Inhibit renal tubular reabsorption of water
c. Key medication: mannitol (Osmitrol)
d. Interactions
   (1) Potentiates effects of digoxin
   (2) Decreases phosphate, potassium, and sodium levels
e. General side effects
   (1) Circulatory overload, congestive heart failure (CHF), or pulmonary edema caused by expansion of plasma volume
   (2) Rebound increased intracranial pressure after discontinuation (8–12 hours)
   (3) Sloughing of tissues around IV site if infiltrated
   (4) Cerebral dehydration, producing headache
   (5) Hypokalemia; hyponatremia
   (6) Excessive diuresis and dehydration
f. Nursing implications (see general nursing implications at the end of chapter)
   (1) Avoid using in clients with CHF, chronic renal failure, pulmonary edema, or pregnancy.
   (2) Assess IV site frequently during administration for signs of irritation or infiltration.
   (3) Check bottle prior to administration for presence of crystals; do not administer if crystals are present. Place bottle in hot-water bath, then reduce to room temperature and assess for crystals.
   (4) Always administer through a filter.
   (5) Bottle may be warmed to dissolve crystals prior to administration.
   (6) Never administer with other IV medications or blood products.
   (7) Monitor intake and output (I & O) every 1 hour during administration.
6. Medications: carbonic anhydrase inhibitors
a. Uses
   (1) Decrease intraocular pressure in glaucoma
   (2) Relieve symptoms of premenstrual syndrome (PMS)
b. Modes of action

   (1) Reduce the secretion of the enzyme carbonic anhydrase to decrease the secretion of hydrogen ions
   (2) Increase the alkalinity of the urine
   (3) Increase bicarbonate, sodium, and water excretion
   (4) Reduce the production of intraocular fluid
c. Key medication: acetazolamide (Diamox)
d. Interactions
   (1) Potentiated by other diuretics
   (2) Potentiates the effects of amphetamines and salicylates
   (3) Inhibits tricyclic antidepressants
   (4) Lowers lithium levels
e. General side effects
   (1) Anemia (hemolytic)
   (2) Headaches
   (3) Hypokalemia; hyponatremia
   (4) GI upset
   (5) Depression, anxiety, drowsiness
   (6) Hyperglycemia
f. Nursing implications (see general nursing implications at end of chapter)
   (1) Do not mix with fruit juices—these medications do not dissolve
   (2) Use honey or syrup to disguise bitter taste of liquid.
   (3) IM injections may cause severe pain and abscesses.
   (4) Administer with food or antacids to prevent GI upset.

GENERAL NURSING IMPLICATIONS FOR USE OF DIURETICS

a. Avoid sudden position changes to prevent orthostatic hypotension.
b. Monitor I & O during therapy.
c. Monitor blood pressure (BP) and pulse during therapy.
d. Encourage intake of foods high in potassium.
e. Stress need for return visits to physician for monitoring of sodium and potassium levels.
f. Administer early in the day and evening to prevent nocturia (last dose should be given before 5 P.M.).
g. Warn client about the signs and symptoms of decreased effectiveness (edema, weight gain, elevated BP).

h. When used for control of hypertension, stress the need for other measures (eat low-sodium diet, increase exercise, lose weight, stop smoking).

i. Instruct client to avoid the use of *all* alcohol products.

j. Warn diabetic clients that diuretic use may make glucose control difficult.

7

Respiratory System Medications

SUMMARY OF KEY ASPECTS OF THE ANATOMY AND PHYSIOLOGY OF THE RESPIRATORY SYSTEM

1. The respiratory system is composed of several different structures
   a. Upper air way (nose, mouth, sinuses)
   b. Larynx
   c. Trachea
   d. Bronchi
   e. Bronchioli
   f. Alveoli
      (1) The alveoli with their surrounding capillaries are the functional units of the lungs, where actual gas exchange takes place.
      (2) The average adult has between 1,000,000 to 1,500,000 alveoli.
   g. There are two lungs: the right lung has three lobes; the left lung has two.
   h. The lungs are lined with the visceral pleura; the chest cavity, with the parietal pleura.
      (1) These two layers of connective tissue provide a smooth surface for the normal movement of the lungs.

      (2) **The pleural space** is the potential space between the visceral and parietal plurae and contains a small amount of fluid that acts as a lubricant.
      (3) There is negative pressure in the pleural space to help keep the lungs expanded.

2. Control of ventilation
   a. The centers for respiratory control are located in the brain stem (pons).
   b. Pco_2 is the normal stimulant for respirations.
      (1) When the Pco_2 level increases, it triggers the breathing center in the brain (normal Pco_2 = 35–45)
      (2) Pco_2 is the most powerful stimulant for respirations.
   c. Po_2 (hypoxic drive) is a backup mechanism for the stimulation of respirations (normal Po_2 = 80–100)
      (1) Some clients, such as chronic obstructive pulmonary disease (COPD) clients, maintain high levels of Pco_2 in the 50 to 60 range.
      (2) Respirations are triggered by their low Po_2 levels in the 50 to 60 range.

d. Problems with the hypoxic drive
   (1) The client is hypoxic all the time.
   (2) It is less sensitive to body needs (it takes a greater fluctuation in the O_2 level).
   (3) Anything that interferes with respirations at all (such as an upper respiratory infection) can cause respiratory distress.
   (4) High levels of supplemental oxygen may cause respiratory arrest.
3. Pulmonary physiology
   a. In the lungs, oxygen is exchanged for carbon dioxide through diffusion and osmosis.
   b. Inspiration is an active process creating a negative pressure in the chest cavity owing to the contraction of the diaphragm and intercostal muscles.
   c. Expiration is a passive process that creates a positive pressure in the chest cavity owing to relaxation of the respiratory muscles.
4. Defense mechanisms of the respiratory system
   a. The upper airways filter and heat the air.
   b. The epiglottis prevents foreign objects from entering the lungs.
   c. The cough reflex helps rid the lungs of foreign substances and mucous.
   d. Ciliated mucus membranes line the bronchioles and help remove small particulate matter.
   e. The lungs have a tremendous reserve capacity; a healthy person can lose 60% of the alveoli and still maintain adequate respiratory function.

Several different classes of medications are used for respiratory disorders.
1. Medications: cough suppressants (antitussives)
   a. Uses
      (1) Centrally suppress nonproductive coughs
      (2) Promote nighttime sleep in adults and children with coughs
   b. Modes of action
      (1) Suppress cough reflex center in the medulla
      (2) General suppression of the central nervous system (CNS)
   c. Key medications
      (1) Codeine sulfate (narcotic) (often in combination with other medications)
      (2) Dextromethorphan (DM) (nonnarcotic) (often in combination with other medications)

   d. Interactions
      (1) Potentiated by other CNS suppressants (alcohol, sedatives, narcotic pain medications)
      (2) Inhibited by narcotic antagonists (naltrexone, naloxone) and CNS stimulants
   e. General side effects
      (1) CNS suppression (drowsiness, depression, decreased respiratory rate, hypotension)
      (2) Constipation
      (3) Potential for abuse with narcotic medications
      (4) Drying and thickening of upper airway sections
   f. Nursing implications
      (1) Instruct client to avoid activities that require alertness or psychomotor coordination.
      (2) Monitor use for signs of dependence or abuse.
      (3) Wait 15 to 20 minutes after taking syrup form of the medication to drink any liquids.
      (4) Monitor bowel elimination for signs of constipation. Encourage diet high in fiber and liquids. Promote exercise.
      (5) Keep room air humidity at 50% to 75% to prevent thick, tenacious secretions.
      (6) Reinforce the need to stop smoking.
2. Medications: bronchodilators
   a. Uses
      (1) Asthma
      (2) Other pulmonary diseases that produce wheezing and dyspnea
      (3) Acute and chronic bronchospasm
      (4) Chronic airway limitations (CAL), COPD
   b. Modes of action
      (1) Stimulate beta$_2$ receptors in the lungs, heart, GI system, CNS, and vascular system
      (2) Inhibit adenosine receptors resulting in an increase in cyclic adenosine monophosphate (cAMP) and bronchodilation
      (3) Positive inotropic effect that increases cardiac output
      (4) Increase urinary output
      (5) Decrease peripheral vascular resistance due to vasodilation
   c. Key medications
      (1) methylxanthine (theophylline) (IV—aminophylline, PO—Theolair) (often in combination with other medications)

  (2) metaproterenol (sympathomimetic) (Alupent)
d. Interactions
  (1) Cimetidine, erythromycin, propranolol, oral contraceptives, verapamil, and furosemide increase levels of methylxanthine medications.
  (2) Nicotine, phenobarbital, phenytoin, and antituberculosis medications decrease levels of methylxanthine medications.
  (3) Caffeine and CNS stimulants increase the side effects.
e. General side effects
  (1) CNS stimulation (tremors, nervousness, insomnia, agitation, convulsions, anxiety)
  (2) GI upset (nausea, vomiting, cramps, diarrhea)
  (3) Cardiovascular stimulation (tachycardia, premature ventricular contractions [PVCs], ventricular tachycardia (VT), angina, hypotension)
f. Nursing implications
  (1) Monitor client for effectiveness and signs of toxicity.
  (2) Monitor theophylline blood levels (therapeutic level = 10–20 μg/mL; toxicity >20 μg/mL).
  (3) Give last dose 6 to 8 hours before bedtime to promote sleep.
  (4) Instruct client to stop smoking because it decreases the effectiveness of the medication.
  (5) Warn client never to crush or chew sustained-release tablets or capsules.
  (6) Instruct client to take medications with milk or food to decrease GI side effects.
  (7) Instruct client in side effects and the need to call the physician if they develop.
  (8) Instruct client on proper use of inhaler-delivered medications.
  (9) Warn client not to exceed the recommended dosage, especially with inhaler-delivered medications.
3. Medications: mucolytics
a. Uses
  (1) Cystic fibrosis
  (2) Emphysema
  (3) Chronic/acute bronchitis
  (4) Acetaminophen overdose (antidote)
  (5) Any respiratory condition producing thick mucus

b. Modes of action
  (1) Directly decrease thickness and tenacity of mucous secretions
  (2) Break the surface tension of the mucus molecules
  (3) Slow the metabolism of acetaminophen to reduce damage to the liver
  (4) Increase the hepatic inactivation of toxic acetaminophen metabolites
c. Key medication: acetylcysteine (Mucomyst)
d. Interactions: few
  (1) Activated charcoal decreases effectiveness in acetaminophen overdose
  (2) Incompatible with certain antibiotics (amphotericin B, erythromycin, tetracycline)
e. General side effects
  (1) "Rotten egg" smell when delivered by nebulization therapy
  (2) Nausea, vomiting
  (3) Irritation and burning in throat; rhinorrhea
  (4) Drowsiness; dizziness
  (5) Bronchoirritation and spasm
  (6) Sticky residue on face after nebulization
f. Nursing implications
  (1) Double-check route of administration; may be given orally, intravenously, by nebulization, or by endotracheal tube.
  (2) Monitor client closely during therapy for bronchospasms.
  (3) Offer client wet washcloth after nebulizer treatments to remove sticky residue.
  (4) Assess lung sounds prior to and after treatments.
  (5) Encourage coughing after treatments; record amount and characteristics of sputum.
  (6) Encourage fluid intake of 2000 to 3000 mL per day.
  (7) Keep suction equipment handy for quick removal of excessive secretions.
  (8) Reinforce the need to stop smoking.
4. Medications: decongestants
a. Uses
  (1) Relief of congestion of upper airways caused by allergies, upper respiratory infections, and sinusitis
b. Modes of action
  (1) Stimulate the CNS, producing vasoconstriction in the nasal passages

(2) Shrink swollen mucous membranes in the nasal airways

(3) Stimulate the whole sympathetic nervous system

c. Key medication: phenylephrine hydrochloride (HCL) (Neo-Synephrine) (often used in combination medications)

d. Interactions

(1) CNS stimulants and caffeine increase side effects

(2) Few other interactions

e. General side effects

(1) CNS stimulation (insomnia, nervousness, tremors)

(2) Nausea, vomiting, abdominal cramping

(3) Cardiovascular (CV) stimulation (tachycardia, transient hypertension, dysrhythmia)

(4) Urinary retention (rare)

(5) Rebound effect if stopped suddenly after prolonged or excessive use

f. Nursing implications

(1) Give medications when client is in the sitting position, because of changes in blood pressure.

(2) Instruct client to use medication as prescribed; there is a tendency to overuse, and it may be habit forming.

(3) Teach client to avoid touching nasal spray bottle to nose or mucous membranes; clean tip of bottle after each use.

(4) Warn client to reduce caffeine intake and avoid diet medications without physician's approval.

(5) Use with caution in clients with hypertension or known cardiovascular disease.

(6) Reinforce the need to stop smoking.

5. Medications: antihistamines

a. Uses

(1) Allergic reactions; itchy, watery eyes; nasal congestion

(2) Anaphylaxis, skin allergies, and allergic reactions in general

(3) Sinusitis

(4) Motion sickness; drug-induced extrapyramidal symptoms

(5) Sedation; nighttime sleep induction

b. Mode of action

(1) General CNS suppressant

(2) Binds with and blocks histamine one (H_1) receptor sites

c. Key medications

(1) Diphenhydramine HCL (Benadryl) (prototype)

(2) Promethazine (Phenergan)

(3) Hydroxyzine (Atarax, Vistaril)

d. Interactions

(1) Potentiate CNS depressants such as alcohol, narcotic analgesics, antianxiety agents

(2) Additive anticholinergic effects with medications that have anticholinergic properties (atropine, antidepressants, phenothiazine, antihistamines)

e. General side effects

(1) CNS suppression (sedation, drowsiness, dizziness)

(2) CV (hypotension, hypertension, palpitations, tachycardia)

(3) Anticholinergic effects (dry mouth, blurred vision, urinary retention, constipation, dilated pupils)

f. Nursing implications

(1) Warn clients to avoid alcohol, over-the-counter cold/allergy medications, and other CNS medications.

(2) Clients should avoid driving or other activities that require concentration or coordination after taking these medications.

(3) Monitor for effectiveness. If client sleeps excessively, nurse may need to reduce or hold dose.

(4) Instruct the client to take at bedtime to avoid sedation during the day.

(5) Caution client to avoid overusage of these medications; client may develop tolerance.

(6) Reinforce the need to stop smoking.

6. Medications: expectorants

a. Uses: lung diseases that produce thick mucus

(1) Cystic fibrosis

(2) Bronchitis

(3) Emphysema

(4) Mucous plugs

(5) Common cold

(6) Pneumonia

b. Modes of action

(1) Decrease surface tension and adhesiveness of thick mucus

(2) Increase the production of liquid in bronchial tracts and in mucus.

c. Key medication: guaifenesin (Robitussin) (often in combination with other medications)
d. Interactions: none significant
e. General side effects
  (1) GI (nausea, vomiting, stomach cramping)
  (2) Abnormal thyroid tests because of iodine
  (3) Rashes, headache, dizziness
f. Nursing implications
  (1) Encourage client to increase fluid intake to 2000 to 3000 mL per day.
  (2) Assess lung sounds, mucous production, and cough while client is taking medication.
  (3) Instruct client in proper method to cough effectively.
  (4) Warn client not to crush or chew sustained-release tablets or capsules.
  (5) Reinforce the need to stop smoking.
  (6) Keep air humidified at 50% to 75%.

8

Endocrine System Medications

SUMMARY OF KEY ASPECTS OF THE ANATOMY AND PHYSIOLOGY OF THE ENDOCRINE SYSTEM

The endocrine system is composed of several different structures.

1. This is a very complex system with many interrelated organs.
   a. The endocrine system is regulated through a negative feedback mechanism of the nervous system.
   b. **The pituitary gland** is called the master gland because of its regulation of the production of other hormones. It has anterior and posterior parts (Fig. 8–1).
   c. The pituitary gland is under the control of the hypothalamus.
   d. The hypothalamus regulates the anterior pituitary gland secretion by release of neurosecretory-releasing and neurosecretory-inhibiting factors.
   e. The pituitary gland is located at the base of the brain in the sella turcica and is attached to the hypothalamus by the hypophyseal stalk.

2. One of the best ways to review and remember this system is by reviewing a chart of the glands and hormones (Table 8–1).
3. Abnormalities of the endocrine system occur when there is either too much hormone being made (hypersecretion) or too little hormone being made (hyposecretion).
   a. Hypersecretion states of glands are most commonly treated by surgical removal, radiation, or other methods to reduce the ability of these glands to secrete hormones.
   b. Only in a very few instances are medications used to treat hypersecretion states.
   c. Hyposecretion states of glands are most commonly treated by supplemental hormones.
   d. In some hyposecretion conditions, transplantation of the affected gland can be performed.

The pancreas is a dual-purpose organ in the body.

1. As an exocrine organ, it produces amylase, lipase, and other powerful enzymes to help in the digestion of protein and fat.
2. As an endocrine organ, it produces
   a. Glucagon in the alpha cells
   b. Insulin in the beta cells

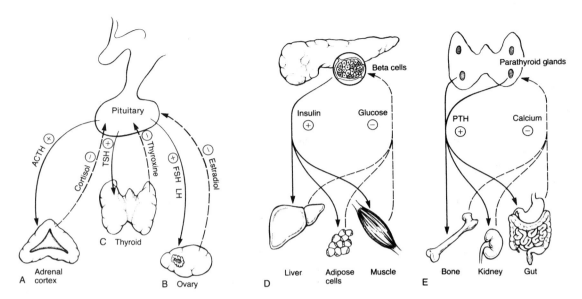

FIGURE 8–1. Diagrammatic representation of several feedback systems. (A), (B), and (C) represent the feedback control in which the hormonal product of the target gland acts on the release of the corresponding pituitary hormone. Solid lines represent direct control, dotted lines represent feedback mechanism. (D) and (E) illustrate feedback control, in which the metabolic substance controlled by the hormone acts directly upon its release.

(A) Corticotropin-releasing factor (CRF) stimulates the pituitary to release corticotropin. Corticotropin stimulates the adrenal cortex to secrete cortisol. Cortisol feeds back to the hypothalamic-pituitary axis and inhibits CRF-ACTH release.

(B) Gonodotropin-releasing hormone (GNRH) stimulates the pituitary to release follicle-stimulating hormone (FSH) and luteinizing hormone (LH). FSH and LH stimulate the ovaries to release estradiol. Estradiol feeds back to the hypothalamic-pituitary axis and inhibits GNRH-FHS/LH release.

(C) Thyroid-releasing hormone (TRH) stimulates the pituitary to release thyroid-stimulating hormone (TSH). TSH stimulates the thyroid to secrete thyroxine. Thyroxine feeds back to the hypothalamic-pituitary axis and inhibits TRH/TSH release.

(D) Insulin release is controlled by glucose in the blood. If glucose increases, insulin is secreted. If glucose decreases, insulin is inhibited.

(E) The parathyroid gland regulates serum calcium. A drop in serum calcium stimulates parathormone (PTH) secretion. Conversely, an increase in calcium shuts off PTH production. (From Mathewson-Kuhn, M: Pharmacotherapeutics: A Nursing Process Approach, ed 3. FA Davis, Philadelphia, 1994, p 902, with permission.)

3. **Insulin** is an anabolic hormone that functions in several different ways.
   a. It facilitates glucose entry into muscle and fat cells.
   b. It helps with the conversion of glucose into glycogen, amino acids into protein, and free fatty acids into triglyceride.
4. When insulin production or use is disrupted in any way, a condition called *diabetes mellitus* develops.
   a. Diabetes mellitus is a disease characterized by the body's inability to use glucose in a normal fashion.
   b. Diabetes mellitus has been a very common topic on NCLEX examinations for many years.
   c. Often questions about diabetes mellitus are integrated with other topics (e.g., a pregnant diabetic client or a child with diabetes).
5. There are two primary categories of diabetes:
   a. Type 1: insulin-dependent diabetes mellitus (IDDM)
      (1) The client is dependent on exogenous insulin for maintenance of life.
      (2) Onset is in youth generally, although it can develop at any age.
      (3) When the client's blood sugar becomes high, the client tends to develop ketoacidosis.
      (4) IDDM seems to be genetic in origin.
      (5) Some diabetic clients make islet cell antibodies, which destroy the insulin.

(6) In some cases IDDM appears to be a type of autoimmune disorder.
b. Type 2: noninsulin-dependent diabetes mellitus (NIDDM)
  (1) Clients are not dependent upon exogenous insulin.
  (2) It is usually controlled with diet, weight loss, exercise, or oral medication.
  (3) 60% to 90% of these clients are obese.
  (4) These clients tend to have a decreased number of receptor cell sites for insulin but produce near normal amounts of insulin.
  (5) Type 2 diabetic clients tend not to develop ketoacidosis when their blood sugars are elevated.
  (6) Onset is normally after 40 years of age but it is possible at any age.
  (7) Clients may require insulin when under stress from surgery, infection, trauma, or when under emotional stress.
  (8) Generally there is a family history of diabetes.
c. Risk factors for diabetes mellitus include:
  (1) Family history of diabetes
  (2) Prolonged exposure to high stress levels
  (3) Long-term corticosteroid use
  (4) Ethnic origin (Native-American)
  (5) Previous episodes of hypoglycemia
d. Classic clinical indications of diabetes mellitus
  (1) Polyuria, polydipsia, polyphagia
  (2) Poor wound healing
  (3) Frequent infections
  (4) Peripheral neuropathy
e. There are several sources for commercially prepared insulins.
  (1) Pork pancreas (very similar to human insulin)
  (2) Beef pancreas
  (3) Genetically modified bacteria (Humalin insulin)
  (4) Semisynthetically manufactured and purified (Humalin insulin)

6. Medications: insulin
a. Uses
  (1) Treatment of type 1 diabetes mellitus
  (2) Treatment of ketoacidosis and coma
  (3) Treatment of type 2 diabetes mellitus when client is in a stress state
  (4) Nondiabetic clients receiving hyperalimentation
  (5) Pregnancy-induced diabetes
  (6) Clients with hyperkalemia

b. Modes of action
  (1) Increases glucose transport into body tissues to be used as energy
  (2) Increases fat and protein metabolism
  (3) Stimulates the formation of fatty tissues (lipogenesis)
  (4) Promotes transport of amino acids into various tissues and converts into protein
  (5) Increases the intracellular migration of potassium and magnesium ions
c. Key medications (Table 8–2)
  (1) Regular insulin (rapid-acting)
  (2) NPH insulin (intermediate-acting)
  (3) Premixed 30/70 insulin (combination)
d. Interactions
  (1) Potentiated by beta-blockers, anabolic steroids, alcohol, monoamine oxidase (MAO) inhibitors, tetracycline, warfarin, and oral hypoglycemic agents
  (2) Inhibited by thiazide diuretics, glucocorticoids, calcium channel blockers, thyroid supplements, estrogen, and smoking
e. General side effects
  (1) Hypoglycemia (insulin reaction) at peak times (weakness, hunger, diaphoresis, nausea, glucose <50, tremors, seizures)
  (2) Allergic reactions at injection site (redness, itching)
  (3) Somogyi effect (rebound phenomenon due to sensitivity to insulin, resulting in hyperglycemia, particularly in the early morning)
  (4) Hypertrophy or atrophy at repeatedly used injection site
  (5) Lipodystrophy
f. Nursing implications
  (1) Always double-check the type and strength of the insulin before administration.
  (2) Double-check the route of administration (only regular insulin can be given IV; insulin cannot be given PO).
  (3) Make sure intermediate-acting and long-acting insulins are mixed well prior to administration (do not shake).
  (4) When mixing regular and intermediate-acting insulins in the same syringe, draw up the regular insulin first.
  (5) Administer mixed insulins within 20 minutes of mixing.
  (6) Monitor clients for hypoglycemic reaction at peak action times of insulins.

TABLE 8–1. SUMMARY OF ENDOCRINE GLANDS, HORMONES, AND THEIR FUNCTIONS

Gland	Hormone	Function	Dysfunction	
			Hyposecretion	Hypersecretion
Pituitary				
Adenohypophysis	Somatotropin or growth hormone (GH)	Regulates growth of body tissues	Dwarfism	Giantism, acromegaly
	Thyrotropin or thyroid-stimulating hormone (TSH)	Regulates growth and secretion of thyroid	Hyperthyroidism	Hypothyroidism
	Corticotropin or adreno-corticotropic hormone (ACTH)	Regulates release of glucocorticoids from adrenal cortex	Addison's disease	Cushing's disease
	Gonadotropins	Regulate development of primary and secondary sex characteristics and secretion of male and female hormones from ovaries and testes		
	Follicle-stimulating hormone (FSH)		Anovulation, aspermatogenesis	Primary gonadal failure
	Luteinizing hormone (LH)			Primary gonadal failure
	Interstitial cell-stimulating hormone (ICSH)			Primary gonadal failure
	Prolactin or luteotropic hormone (LTH)			Amenorrhea, galactorrhea
Neurohypophysis	Antidiuretic hormone (ADH)	Controls water balance of body	Diabetes insipidus	Syndrome of inappropriate ADH
	Oxytocin	Stimulates contraction of uterine musculature		
Thyroid	Thyroxine, tri-iodothyronine	Regulates rate of carbohydrate, fat, and protein catabolism; regulates metabolic rate	Cretinism, myxedema, hypothyroidism	Graves' disease, hyperthyroidism, thyrotoxicosis
	Calcitonin	Decreases blood calcium levels	↑Ca	↓Ca
Parathyroid	Parathormone	Increases blood calcium levels	↓Ca	↑Ca
Pancreas	Glucagon	Increases blood glucose levels	Hypoglycemia	
	Insulin	Decreases blood glucose levels	Diabetes mellitus, ketoacidosis	Hypoglycemia, insulin shock

(7) Schedule snacks for peak action times of insulin.

(8) Instruct client on the necessity of rotating subcutaneous injection sites.

(9) Instruct family members on insulin administration and recognition of hypoglycemia or hyperglycemia.

(10) Stress the need for proper diet, exer-

TABLE 8–1. *(Continued)*

Gland	Hormone	Function	Dysfunction Hyposecretion	Dysfunction Hypersecretion
Adrenals				
Cortex	Mineralocorticoids (aldosterone)	Maintain fluid and electrolyte balance	Addison's disease	Hyperaldosteronism
	Glucocorticoids (cortisol)	Promote positive response to stress by affecting carbohydrate, fat, and protein metabolism	Addison's disease, acute adrenal crisis	Cushing's syndrome
	Sex hormones (androgens, estrogens, progestins)	Influence secondary sex characteristics ONLY in certain disorders; normally, their levels are too low for physiologic activity		Adrenogenital syndrome
Medulla	Epinephrine, norepinephrine	Provide for response to stress	Severe hypotension, cardiovascular collapse	Pheochromocytoma
Gonads				
Ovaries	Estrogen	Regulate development of secondary sex characteristics and sexual maturation and functioning	Sexual dysfunction, infertility	Sexual dysfunction, tion, precocious puberty
	Progesterone	Regulate preparation for and maintenance of pregnancy		
Testes	Testosterone	Regulate development of secondary sex characteristics and sexual maturation and functioning	Delayed male puberty, male hypogonadism	Hirsutism in women, genetic female pseudohermaphroditism

Source: Mathewson-Kuhn, M: Pharmacotherapeutics: A Nursing Approach, ed 3. FA Davis, Philadelphia 1994, pp 901–902, with permission.

cise, weight loss, and care of feet and legs.

(11) Instruct the client that open vials of insulin can be stored at room temperature but that once insulin is refrigerated, it must be kept refrigerated.

(12) Encourage the client to wear a medical-alert bracelet and carry a source of glucose (hard candy) at all times.

7. Medications: oral hypoglycemic agents
   a. Uses: treatment of type 2 diabetes
   b. Modes of action

(1) Increase the effectiveness of insulin

(2) Stimulate pancreatic beta cells to make and release insulin.

(3) Increase insulin receptor sensitivity to the hormone

   c. Key medications
      (1) chlorpropamide (Diabinase) (prototype first-generation oral hypoglycemic)
      (2) glyburide (DiaBeta, Micronase) (prototype second-generation oral hypoglycemic)
   d. Interactions
      (1) Similar to insulin (see above)

TABLE 8–2. INSULINS

Drug Name/Route and Dosage	Pharmacokinetics/ Dynamics	Nursing Implications
All Insulins	**PB:** not bound **B:** mainly in liver, kidney, and muscle tissue (lesser extent) **E:** kidney	**Assesment:** Obtain baseline and periodic assessments of blood glucose levels; blood cell counts; potassium, triglyceride, and cholesterol levels. Assess glycosylated hemoglobin (HbA$_{1C}$) level. If patient has DKA, monitor ECG and assess for cardiac dysrhythmias. Assess the patient's present knowledge of diabetes and basics of care, including meal pattern, hyperglycemia, hypoglycemia, role of exercise, blood glucose monitoring and/or urine testing, and skin and foot care. If patient is on insulin therapy, assess injection technique. Assess injection sites for lipohypertrophy. If patient is on pump therapy, assess abdomen for abscesses at catheter insertion site. Assess insulin injection sites for local or delayed allergy. Continually assess for hyperglycemia and hypoglycemia. **Intervention:** Only regular insulin can be administered by IV route. Dosage is always expressed in USP units. Use only syringes calibrated for particular concentration of insulin. Because no syringes are made for U-500 insulin, it must be administered with U-100 syringe. Dosage adjustments may be required if you interchange different insulin sources. Avoid interchanging. Switching from separate injections to prepared mixture may alter patient response. Monitor blood glucoses closely. Administer insulin as ordered. Double-check type and dosage with another nurse before administration. When administering insulin intravenously, do not mix insulin with any other medication in IV bag. Some insulin adheres to IV bottle as well as IV tubing. Flush 50 mL of solution through tubing to minimize further adherence. IV pumps or controllers should be used to safely monitor intermittent or continuous insulin infusions. Serum potassium levels must be monitored. Give patients their insulin and meals on time. **Patient Teaching**—Educate patient according to needs determined through needs assessment. If mixing insulins, advise patient not to alter order of mixing or to change model or brand of syringe or needle without permission of physician. **Evaluation:** Evaluate patient's blood glucose level and urinary glucose and ketones. Evaluate patient's knowledge of diabetes and basics of treatment. Evaluate all technical skills that will be performed in home setting. Evaluate patient's desire to adhere to prescribed regimen, using verbal and nonverbal cues. Determine if there is need for follow-up care at home.

TABLE 8–2. (*Continued*)

Drug Name/Route and Dosage	Pharmacokinetics/ Dynamics	Nursing Implications

Rapid-Acting Insulins

Regular Insulin (Humalin R) (Novolin R) (Regular Iletin I) (Novolin R PenFill) (Regular Purified Iletin II) (Velosulin BR) (Humulin RU-500)

May be given subcuta- neously (SC), IV, or in insulin pump. Dosage is individuali- zed according to pa- tient's blood glucose values. When given SC, give 15–30 min before meals (ac).	**Onset:** 0.5–1 h **Peak:** 2–5 h **Duration:** 6–8 h ½**L:** NA	Same as for all

Insulin Lispro (Humalog) (Humalog cartridge)

SC route only: give ≤15 min ac.	**Onset:** within 15 min **Peak:** 30–90 min **Duration:** 300 min ½**L:** NA	Same as for all

Semilente Insulin (Semilente Iletin I)

SC route only: give 15–30 min ac break- fast and supper. Dosage is individualized.	**Onset:** 1–1.5 h **Peak:** 5–10 h **Duration:** 12–16 h ½**L:** NA	Same as for all

Intermediate-Acting Insulins

NPH Insulin (Humulin N) (Novolin N) (NPH Iletin I) (NPH Iletin II Purified) (Novolin N PenFill)

SC route only: usually given 15–30 min ac breakfast and supper. Dosage is individualized.	**Onset:** 1–1.5 h **Peak:** 4–12 h **Duration:** 24 h ½**L:** NA	Same as for all

Lente Insulin (Humulin L) (Novolin L) (Lente Iletin I) (Lente Iletin II)

SC route only: usually given 15–30 min ac breakfast and supper. Dosage is individualized.	**Onset:** 1–2.5 h **Peak:** 7–15 h **Duration:** 24 h ½**L:** NA	Same as for all

Insulin Mixtures (Humulin 70/30) (Novolin 70/30) (Humulin 50/50) (Novolin 70/30 PenFill)

SC route only: usually given 15–30 min ac breakfast and supper. Dosage is individualized.	**Onset:** 0.5 h **Peak:** 4–8 h **Duration:** 24 h ½**L:** NA	Same as for all

Long-Acting Insulins

Ultralente insulin (Humulin U)

SC route only: Usually given 15–30 min before breakfast. Dosage is individualized.	**Onset:** 4–8 h **Peak:** 10–30 h **Duration:** >36 h ½**L:** NA	Same as for all

DKA = diabetic ketoacidosis; NA = not available.

Source: Kuhn, M: Pharmacotherapeutics: A Nursing Process Approach, ed 4. FA Davis, Philadelphia, 1998, pp 648–649, with permission.

(2) disulfiram (Antabuse) effect when taken with alcohol
  e. General side effects
    (1) Skin and allergic reactions (pruritic, erythema, urticaria, photosensitivity)
    (2) Gastrointestinal (GI) upset (nausea, anorexia, heartburn, diarrhea, constipation)
    (3) Hypoglycemia
    (4) Headache, weakness, dizziness
  f. Nursing implications (similar for insulin)
    (1) Inform clients that they may require insulin if they become ill or suffer an injury or trauma.
    (2) Encourage clients to follow the prescribed diet and to eat on a regular schedule.
    (3) Clients taking second-generation medications need to eat within 30 minutes of taking the medication.
    (4) Instruct clients to take the medication at the same time each day.
    (5) Stress the need to avoid aspirin and alcohol while taking this medication.
    (6) Caution clients to use sunscreen and protective clothing when outside.

The adrenal glands produce several critical hormones in the body.

1. Normally one adrenal gland is located on top of each kidney.
2. Adrenal medulla (center part) produces two hormones.
  a. Epinephrine
  b. Norepinephrine
3. Adrenal cortex (outer portion) produces three groups of hormones.
  a. Mineralocorticoids (primary = aldosterone)
    (1) Maintain normal blood volume by increasing sodium and water retention in the distal tubules
    (2) Cause potassium excretion and increased excretion of ammonium and magnesium ions
  b. Androgens
    (1) Same functions as testosterone
    (2) Promotes the buildup of muscle mass in the body.
    (3) Few legitimate medical uses but widely used by athletes.
    (4) Many dangerous side effects (cancer, psychosis, depression, rage)
  c. Glucocorticoids (primary is cortisol)
    (1) Regulate the blood glucose level
    (2) Increase gluconeogenesis
    (3) Decrease the rate of glucose utilization by the cells
    (4) Increase protein catabolism
    (5) Promote glucolysis
    (6) Are also important in promoting sodium and water retention
4. Medications: glucocorticoids
  a. Uses
    (1) Treatment of hypercalcemia in clients with bone cancer
    (2) Treatment of autoimmune and collagen diseases (rheumatoid arthritis, lupus, and so forth)
    (3) Suppression of acute allergic/anaphylactic reactions
    (4) Reduction of increased intracranial pressure caused by trauma, disease, or surgery
    (5) Reduction of inflammation of air passages in clients with chronic airway limitations (CAL) (asthma, chronic bronchitis, emphysema)
    (6) Prevention of rejection of transplanted organs
    (7) Stabilization of clients in shock states or post trauma
    (8) Reduction of intraocular pressure in eye disorders
    (9) Topically for localized skin reactions, contact dermatitis, and other skin disorders
    (10) Clients with thrombocytopenia
  b. Modes of action
    (1) Suppress inflammatory response
    (2) Degrade collagen
    (3) Suppress the immune system by decreasing new antibody release and decreasing eosinophile, basophil, and monocyte production
    (4) Reduce scar tissue formation
    (5) Promote red blood cell and platelet formation
    (6) Increase gastric acid and pepsin production
    (7) Help maintain emotional stability
  c. Key medications
    (1) dexamethasone (Decadron)
    (2) hydrocortisone (Cortef)

(3) methylprednisone (Solu-Medrol)

(4) prednisone (Deltasone)

d. Interactions

(1) Increase the need for insulin or oral hypoglycemics

(2) Increase hypokalemia with diuretics, amphotericin B, and some penicillin antibiotics

(3) Inhibited by phenytoin, phenobarbital, and rifampin.

e. General side effects: Cushing's syndrome

(1) Muscle wasting, especially in extremities

(2) Alteration in fat deposition (moon face, buffalo hump, protruding abdomen)

(3) Gluconeogenesis/decreased rate of glucose utilization (hyperglycemia)

(4) Sodium and water retention (edema, hypertension)

(5) Lowered resistance to infection

(6) Emotional instability, psychosis, suicidal behavior, paranoia, euphoria, rage

(7) Changes in secondary sex characteristics

(8) Acne, hirsutism

(9) Menstrual irregularities

(10) Increased appetite

(11) Thin, fragile skin

(12) GI irritation (gastritis, peptic ulcers)

(13) Poor wound healing

f. Nursing implications

(1) Glucocorticoids are unsafe in pregnancy. Avoid giving to children except for short-term therapy.

(2) Assess client frequently for signs of GI bleeding (black, tarry stools; anemia, and so forth).

(3) Warn client about the increased susceptibility to infections and encourage appropriate actions (good hand washing, avoidance of crowds, and of persons with obvious infections).

(4) Oral medications should always be taken with food, antacids, or milk to help reduce GI irritation.

(5) Warn the client to never stop taking the medication suddenly, because of the possibility of rebound effects.

(6) Missed doses should be taken as soon as possible, but client should not double-up on doses.

(7) Inform the client to notify the physician if any of the Cushing's syndrome symptoms develop.

(8) It is best for clients to take corticosteroids at 8:00 A.M. to mimic the body's normal rhythms.

(9) Monitor the client for changes in mood or behavior, particularly euphoria, depression, or paranoia.

(10) Stress the need for frequent checkups to monitor for hypertension, edema, or congestive heart failure (CHF).

(11) Instruct diabetic clients that it may be more difficult to control their blood sugar while they are taking these medications.

The thyroid gland produces several hormones essential for normal metabolism in the body.

1. Hormones synthesized and secreted
   a. Thyroxin (T_3) (highly active)
   b. Triiodothyronine (T_4) (converted into T_3)
   c. Thyroid hormone functions
      (1) Regulate protein and carbohydrate catabolism in all cells
      (2) Regulate metabolic rate of the cells
      (3) Regulate body heat production
      (4) Act as insulin antagonists
      (5) Maintain growth hormone secretion
      (6) Promote skeletal maturation
      (7) Affect central nervous system (CNS) development
      (8) Maintain muscle tone and vigor and secretions of the GI tract
      (9) Increase the respiratory rate, heart rate, utilization of oxygen
      (10) Maintain calcium mobilization in the body
      (11) Increase red blood cell mobilization
      (12) Stimulate lipid turnover, free fatty acid release, and cholesterol synthesis
2. Hypersecretion of the thyroid gland produces hyperthyroidism, or Graves' disease.
   a. Common symptoms associated with Graves' disease
      (1) More common in women 20 to 40 years of age but can occur to anyone at any age
      (2) Exophthalmos
      (3) Increased pulse, blood pressure, respiratory rate, basal metabolism

    (4) Increase in CNS activity (hypertalkativeness, hyperactivity, anxiety, tremors)

    (5) Amenorrhea

3. Medications: antithyroid

  a. Uses

    (1) Hyperthyroidism

    (2) Thyrotoxicosis

  b. Modes of action

    (1) Blocks the conversion of T_4 to T_3

    (2) Interferes with hormone production

  c. Key medication: propylthiouracil (PTU, Propacil)

  d. Interactions

    (1) Potentiated by lithium, potassium iodide, and phenothiazines

    (2) Increased risk for aplastic anemia when taken with antineoplastic agents and radiation therapy

    (3) Increases bleeding effects of warfarin and aspirin

  e. General side effects

    (1) GI upset (nausea, vomiting, anorexia)

    (2) Rash, skin irritation, skin discoloration

    (3) Hypothyroidism

    (4) Agranulocytosis, aplastic anemia

    (5) Excessive thirst

    (6) Depression

  f. Nursing implications

    (1) Monitor clients with cardiac conditions closely for complications.

    (2) Inform clients that it may take 3 to 6 weeks before medication becomes effective.

    (3) Monitor client closely for medication effectiveness.

    (4) Warn clients to avoid taking over-the-counter medications that contain aspirin.

    (5) Stress the need for frequent checkups, thyroid tests, and blood counts.

    (6) Instruct clients to store medications in a tightly closed, dark container in a cool, dry place.

    (7) Warn clients that increases in the amount of iodine in the diet may affect results of medication; avoid shellfish.

    (8) Encourage rest, good nutrition, and avoidance of heat.

4. A lower-than-normal secretion of thyroid hormones produces hypothyroidism that may be indicated by:

  a. Goiter—an enlargement of the thyroid gland indicated by a swelling in the neck area

    (1) May be present with any type of thyroid disorder

    (2) Most often associated with low diet iodine intake

    (3) Rare as a primary disorder in the United States

  b. Myxedema—puffiness and sogginess of the skin, which is dry, nonpitting edema; swollen lips; thickened nose; enlarged tongue; thickened skin

  c. Cretinism—hypothyroidism in children, indicated by:

    (1) Sluggish movements

    (2) Weight gain

    (3) Cold intolerance

    (4) Dry skin

    (5) Brittle hair

    (6) Slow thinking

    (7) Slow, slurred speech

    (8) Decreased heart rate, BP, respiratory rate

5. Medications: thyroid hormone supplements

  a. Uses

    (1) Myxedema

    (2) Cretinism

    (3) Conditions that produce low level of thyroid hormone

  b. Modes of action

    (1) Increase levels of T_3 and T_4

    (2) Suppress thyrotropin-dependent thyroid cancers

  c. Key medication: levothyroxine (Levothroid, Synthroid) (prototype)

  d. Interactions

    (1) Potentiates cardiac effects of sympathetic stimulants, anticholinergic agents

    (2) Inhibits effect of beta blockers

    (3) Increases the need for insulin or oral hypoglycemic agents

  e. General side effects

    (1) CNS stimulation (irritability, insomnia, nervousness, headache)

    (2) Cardiovascular (CV) stimulation (tachycardia, dysrhythmia, hypertension, angina)

    (3) GI stimulation (nausea, abdominal cramps, diarrhea)

    (4) Increased sweating, hair loss

    (5) Weight loss

    (6) Heat intolerance

    (7) Hyperthyroidism

  f. Nursing implications

    (1) Doses are extremely small; always double-check before administration.

(2) Encourage the client to take the medication at the same time in the morning each day to increase compliance.

(3) Teach the client to take pulse before taking medication; hold if pulse is more than 100 beats per minute (BPM).

(4) Warn client not to stop taking the medication without physician's approval.

(5) Inform the client to always check with the physician before taking any other medications.

(6) Monitor for the development of symptoms of hyperthyroidism or thyrotoxicosis.

(7) Stress the need for follow-up examinations and testing of thyroid level and function.

(8) Warn the client that these are slow-acting medications and that several weeks or months may pass before there are any noticeable changes.

(9) Encourage long rest periods, avoidance of the cold, pacing of activity, and a healthy diet.

9

Obstetric Medications

KEY ASPECTS OF SELECTED OBSTETRIC PROBLEMS

Although a potentially wide range of medications is used in the obstetric setting, the NCLEX limits its medication questions to a few selected medications used to treat particular complications.

PREMATURE LABOR

1. Definition
   a. Labor between 20 and 37 weeks
   b. Contractions regular and less than 10 minutes apart
   c. Contractions causing cervical dilation and effacement or changes in the cervix to indicate labor progress
2. Primary modes of treatment
   a. Complete bed rest—usually at home unless having regular contractions
   b. Monitoring of contractions and vital signs
   c. Vaginal examinations only when absolutely necessary
   d. Emotional support—reassurance, explanations, and support
   e. Pelvic rest—avoidance of pelvic movement and compressions; lying on side
   f. Administration of narcotic or sedative medications
   g. Use of uterine relaxants
3. Medications: uterine relaxant; tocolytic
   a. Uses
      (1) Prevention of premature labor
      (2) Abatement of premature labor
   b. Modes of action
      (1) Stimulation of primary beta$_2$-adrenergic receptors
      (2) Reduction in the force and frequency of uterine contractions
   c. Key medications
      (1) ritodrine (Yutopar)
      (2) magnesium sulfate (see below)
   d. Interactions
      (1) Glucocorticoids increase risk of maternal pulmonary edema.
      (2) Inhibited by beta-blockers.

(3) Potentiated by magnesium sulfate, narcotic analgesics, diazoxide, and general anesthetics.
  e. General side effects
    (1) Central nervous system (CNS) stimulation (headache, tremors, anxiety, insomnia)
    (2) Cardiovascular (CV) stimulation (tachycardia, premature ventricular contractions [PVCs], ventricular tachycardia [VT], chest pain)
    (3) Gastrointestinal (GI) stimulation (nausea, vomiting, abdominal cramping)
  f. Nursing implications
    (1) Follow package insert for dilution and intravenous administration; avoid mixing with normal saline.
    (2) Monitor maternal blood pressure (BP), pulse, and cardiac rhythm every 15 minutes during administration.
    (3) Monitor fetal heart rate every 15 minutes during administration.
    (4) Position mother on left side to reduce hypotension.
    (5) Provide a calm, subdued atmosphere to reduce feelings of anxiety.

PREGNANCY-INDUCED HYPERTENSION, OR PREECLAMPSIA

1. Definition
  a. Hypertensive disorder occurring after 20 weeks gestation
  b. Identification
    (1) Blood pressure increases to 30/15 above baseline
    (2) Proteinuria
    (3) Rapid weight gain
    (4) Edema of face and fingers
    (5) Hyperreflexia
    (6) Headache, epigastric pain
  c. Left untreated, may lead to eclampsia (convulsions, coma, and death)
2. Primary modes of treatment
  a. Monitor fetal heart rate closely.
  b. Monitor maternal BP, input and output (I&O), mental status, reflexes every 1 to 4 hours.
  c. Strict bed rest (home or hospital) on left side.
  d. Reduce environmental stimulation.
  e. Decrease sodium intake, increase fluids.

f. Good nutrition, especially calcium; protein (1g/kg/day).
g. Stop smoking.
h. Reduce stress.
i. Monitor for worsening condition (headache, visual disturbances, epigastric pain).
j. Sedative and/or antihypertensive medications (Valium, Serax, sedation, hydralazine—Apresoline).
k. Use of neuromuscular blocking agents.
3. Medications: neuromuscular blocking agent; antidysrhythmic; antiseizure
  a. Uses
    (1) Prevent seizures in preeclampsia or eclampsia.
    (2) Reduction of BP in pregnancy-induced hypertension (side effect of medication).
    (3) Treat magnesium-deficiency states.
    (4) Antidote for barium poisoning.
    (5) Treatment of multifocal ventricular tachycardia.
    (6) Treatment for premature labor (see above).
  b. Modes of action
    (1) General depression of the CNS
    (2) Produces peripheral neuromuscular blockade
    (3) Relaxes smooth muscles; dilates blood vessels
    (4) Decreases or stops uterine contractions
  c. Key medication: magnesium sulfate
  d. Interactions
    (1) Potentiated by narcotics, barbiturates, and other CNS depressants
    (2) Inhibited CNS stimulants
  e. General side effects
    (1) General CNS depression (loss of deep tendon reflexes, flaccid paralysis, hypothermia, drowsiness)
    (2) CV depression (bradycardia, heart blocks, severe hypotension, circulatory collapse, and shock)
    (3) Respiratory depression/arrest
    (4) Urinary retention
  f. Nursing implications
    (1) Keep the antidote (calcium gluconate IV) at the bedside during administration.
    (2) Assess fetal well-being continuously with fetal monitor during administration.
    (3) Monitor maternal knee jerk reflex and output hourly; BP and respirations (>12) every 15 minutes.

(4) Follow directions exactly for administration; use pump or controller.

(5) Discontinue at least 2 hours prior to the time of expected delivery.

(6) Evaluate for effectiveness by decreased blood pressure, reduction in strength of uterine contractions, and reduction in hyperflexia.

Uterine stimulants are used in two primary situations.

1. Dystocia of labor
   a. Refers to a difficult or an abnormal labor due to:
      (1) Ineffective uterine activity
      (2) Abnormal presentation
      (3) Excessive size of the baby
      (4) Inadequate pelvis
      (5) Combination of above factors
   b. Dystocia of the powers is the most common type.
      (1) Hypotonic uterine contractions produce no or inadequate cervical effacement and dilatation.
      (2) Contractions are of low intensity.
      (3) Intervals between contractions become longer.
      (4) Duration of contractions is short.
2. Induction of labor
   a. Used to start labor or augment a slow labor due to inadequate uterine contractions.
   b. Indications for induction
      (1) Elective induction (social considerations, convenience)
      (2) Medical induction (fetal distress, postmaturity, uteroplacental insufficiency, toxemia, diabetes, inadequate contractions).
3. Medications: uterine stimulants, posterior pituitary hormone
   a. Uses
      (1) Induction of labor
      (2) Dystocia
      (3) Promotion of milk letdown reflex postpartum
      (4) Control of postpartum uterine bleeding
      (5) Promotion of uterine involution postpartum
   b. Modes of action
      (1) Promote contraction of smooth muscles in the uterus and blood vessels
      (2) Produce peripheral vasoconstriction

(3) Block alpha receptors
(4) Increase sodium and water retention
(5) Simulate mammary gland smooth muscles
   c. Key medications
      (1) oxytocin (Pitocin)
      (2) methylergonovine maleate (Ergometrine)
   d. Interactions
      (1) Potentiated by vasopressors (severe hypertension)
      (2) Inhibited by CNS depressants
   e. General side effects
      (1) Hypertension
      (2) Hypertonic uterine contractions, uterine rupture
      (3) Nausea, vomiting
      (4) Fluid retention, water intoxication
      (5) Allergic reactions
      (6) Maternal seizures
      (7) Fetal hypoxia, intracranial hemorrhage
   f. Nursing implications
      (1) Administer oxytocin by intravenous pump or controller.
      (2) Increase rate slowly until effective uterine contractions are evident.
      (3) Monitor client and fetus continuously during infusion of medication.
      (4) Prior to administration, the client must be assessed for adequate pelvis; cervical dilation of 2 to 3 cm, effacement of 50% before starting.
      (5) The baby's head must be engaged prior to administration to prevent injury.
      (6) If a significant change in fetal heart rate (FHR) occurs, stop infusion and turn mother on left side.
      (7) Keep magnesium sulfate at bedside as antidote.

ABNORMALITIES OF THE MENSTRUAL CYCLE

1. Premenstrual syndrome (PMS) is a diffuse, loosely defined set of physical and behavioral symptoms.
   a. Physical symptoms
      (1) Begins 7 to 10 days before menses; ends at the onset of menses
      (2) Edema of legs and feet
      (3) Abdominal bloating

    (4) Feeling of pelvic fullness
    (5) Breast tenderness
    (6) Weight gain (fluid)
    (7) Insomia, fatigue, headache, backache
  b. Psychological symptoms
    (1) Heightened creativity
    (2) Increased ability to concentrate
    (3) Increased mental or physical activity
    (4) Emotional instability (irritability, depression, crying spells)
    (5) Feelings of unreality and panic

2. Dysmenorrhea is painful menstruation; it is one of the most common gynecologic problems in women of all ages.
  a. Primary dysmenorrhea occurs when there is no organic disease.
    (1) Initially it occurs when ovulation begins about 6 to 12 months after menarche.
    (2) Excessive secretion and subsequent excessive release of prostaglandin during menstrual shedding of the endometrium increase the amplitude and frequency of uterine contractions.
    (3) Pain is described as low abdominal aching or cramping pain in back and upper thighs.
  b. Secondary dysmenorrhea is associated with organic pelvic disease (endometriosis/uterine fibroids).
    (1) Endometriosis is a disease characterized by the presence and growth of glands and stroma identical to the lining of the uterus, found outside the uterus attached to other organs or tissue.
    (2) Most common sites are the ovaries, cul-de-sac, uterosacral ligaments, rectovaginal septum, sigmoid colon, round ligaments, pelvic peritoneum, and urinary bladder.
    (3) The cause is unknown.
3. Amenorrhea is the absence of menstrual periods.
4. Oligomenorrhea is light or irregular menses.
5. Menorrhagia is excessive uterine bleeding occurring at the regular intervals of menstruation.
  a. The period of flow is of greater amount and longer than usual duration.
  b. It is usually a symptom associated with secondary dysmenorrhea (endometriosis).
6. Metrorrhagia is uterine bleeding, usually of normal amount, occurring at completely irregular intervals.
  a. The period of flow is sometimes prolonged.
  b. It is many times associated with secondary dysmenorrhea or hormonal problems.

6. Medications: female sex hormone
  a. Uses
    (1) Abnormalities of the menstrual cycle
    (2) Controls symptoms of menopause
    (3) Reduces osteoporosis in postmenopausal women
    (4) Cancer of breast and prostate
    (5) Contraception (oral)
    (6) Lactation suppression
    (7) Acne in females
  b. Modes of action
    (1) Promotes growth and development of the female reproductive organs
    (2) Prepares the uterus to receive the fertilized ova
    (3) Stimulates development of female secondary sexual characteristics
    (4) Maintains regularity of menstrual cycle
  c. Key medications: estrogen (Premarin)
  d. Interactions
    (1) Cardiovascular effects potentiated by nicotine
    (2) Inhibited by barbiturates or rifampin
  e. General side effects
    (1) Sodium and water retention (edema, bloating, hypertension)
    (2) Blood clots (especially with smoking)
    (3) Breast swelling and tenderness
    (4) Nausea, vomiting, anorexia
    (5) Headache, dizziness, depression
  f. Nursing implications
    (1) Stress the need to stop smoking while taking estrogen preparations.
    (2) Stress the need for frequent follow-up visits to monitor BP and weight.
    (3) Instruct the client to report any breakthrough bleeding.
    (4) Instruct the client in the proper use of the medication according to the route prescribed (oral, vaginal suppository, transdermal).
    (5) If nausea is problematic, instruct the client to take the medication with solid food.
    (6) Caution client to use sunscreen to prevent hyperpigmentation of skin.

CHAPTER

10

Gastrointestinal System Medications

KEY ASPECTS OF THE ANATOMY AND PHYSIOLOGY OF THE GASTROINTESTINAL (GI) SYSTEM

1. The GI system is composed of a number of organs.
   a. Stomach
      (1) The second step in the digestive process
      (2) Secretes gastrin, pepsin, hydrochloric acid
      (3) Stores food, fluids for gradual release into small intestine
   b. Small intestine
      (1) Location of most digestion and absorption
      (2) Composed of the duodenum, jejunum, and ileum
      (3) Mixes food with pancreatic enzymes, bile, bacteria
   c. Liver
      (1) Converts ammonia into urea
      (2) Forms plasma proteins (maintains colloid osmotic pressure)
      (3) Synthesizes blood clotting factors, vitamin K

   (4) Metabolizes/detoxifies drugs and toxins
   (5) Synthesizes bile
   (6) Synthesizes and stores glycogen
   (7) Metabolizes fats, carbohydrates, and proteins
   d. Gall bladder
      (1) Stores and concentrates bile
      (2) Releases bile into small intestine when fat is present
   e. Pancreas
      (1) Both an exocrine and an endocrine gland
      (2) As an endocrine gland it produces insulin/glucagon
      (3) As an exocrine gland it produces amylase and lipase to help digest fat and protein
   f. Large intestine
      (1) Reabsorbs electrolytes and H_2O
      (2) Holds digested food matter for bowel movement
2. Selected GI disorders
   a. **Pancreatitis** is an acute inflammation of the pancreas brought on by digestion of the

organ by its own enzymes secondary to blockage of the common bile duct by tumors or stones. Symptoms include:
- (1) Acute left upper quadrant/midepigastric pain and back pain
- (2) Nausea and vomiting
- (3) Elevated serum amylase (normal 0–130), elevated lipase (normal 0–1)
- (4) Internal bleeding, shock, hypotension, tachycardia

b. **Gastritis** is the inflammation of the mucosal lining of the stomach caused by alcohol, salicylate, infection, oral steroid medications, or stress. Symptoms include:
- (1) Bloated feeling in abdomen after eating
- (2) Headache, lassitude
- (3) Nausea, vomiting, hiccupping, diarrhea, colic
- (4) GI bleeding (black stools/vomiting blood)

c. Peptic ulcer disease (gastric, duodenal, and stress ulcers) exists when there are ulcerations of the gastrointestinal mucosa and underlying tissue caused by gastric acid secretions resulting from either an increase in secretion of hydrochloric acid or from tissues that have decreased resistance to the acid itself. Symptoms include:
- (1) Gnawing or burning epigastric pain 2 to 3 hours after eating
- (2) Pain decreases or subsides with food or antacids
- (3) GI bleeding (tarry stools, melena [maroon, digested blood in stools], vomiting bright red blood)
- (4) Loss of appetite, weight loss

3. Medications: antacids
a. Uses
- (1) Gastritis; indigestion
- (2) Peptic ulcer disease
- (3) Reflux esophagitis
- (4) Prevention of peptic ulcers
- (5) Phosphate binders in chronic renal failure

b. Modes of action
- (1) Increase the pH of gastric stomach secretions
- (2) Neutralize gastric hydrochloric acid
- (3) If taken with meals, bind with phosphate in food to lower serum phosphate levels

c. Key medications
- (1) aluminum hydroxide (Amphogel)
- (2) calcium carbonate (Tums)
- (3) magnesium hydroxide (Maalox)

d. Interactions: numerous
- (1) Slow the absorption of most medications
- (2) Inactivate tetracycline medications
- (3) Increase blood levels of quinidine, flecainide, and amphetamine

e. General side effects
- (1) Constipation (aluminum and calcium preparations)
- (2) Diarrhea (magnesium preparations)
- (3) Electrolyte imbalances (hypermagnesemia, hyperaluminumenia, hypophosphatemia)
- (4) Sodium and water retention
- (5) Rebound hyperacidity of stomach secretions
- (6) Metabolic alkalosis

f. Nursing implications
- (1) Instruct client to take 1 hour after meals.
- (2) Instruct the client to avoid taking antacids for 2 hours when taking other medications.
- (3) Inform clients that they may experience better relief with liquid preparations than with tablets.
- (4) Monitor for side effects; if excessive diarrhea/constipation develops, medication may need to be changed.
- (5) Inform client to shake liquids well before using.
- (6) Instruct clients on sodium-restricted diets to use low-sodium preparations.
- (7) Reinforce need to alter lifestyle (stop smoking; reduce stress; increase exercise; avoid spicy or greasy foods; avoid alcohol; limit intake of aspirin, oral steroids, and ibuprofen).

4. Medications: cytoprotective, antiulcer agent
a. Uses
- (1) Gastritis; indigestion
- (2) Peptic ulcer disease
- (3) Reflux esophagitis
- (4) Prevention of peptic ulcers

b. Mode of action
- (1) Reacts with hydrochloride (HCL) to form a viscous, pastelike substance that adheres to the GI mucosa.

(2) Coats the lining of the lower esophagus and stomach to form a protective barrier to the effects of gastric secretions.

(3) Promotes healing of ulcerated areas of mucosa.

c. Key medication: sucralfate (Carafate)

d. Interactions

(1) Delays the absorption of most medications

(2) Inhibited by concurrent use of antacids

e. General side effects

(1) Extreme constipation

(2) Metallic taste in mouth; dry mouth

(3) Nausea

(4) Dizziness; drowsiness (rare)

f. Nursing implications

(1) Instruct client that medication works best on empty stomach (1 hour before or 2 hours after meals).

(2) Stress the need to continue the full course of therapy (4–8 weeks) even if symptoms are gone to ensure healing of ulcers.

(3) Advise clients to increase their intake of high-fiber foods, fluids, and to increase exercise to prevent constipation.

5. Medications: histamine$_2$ (H$_2$) receptor antagonists

a. Uses

(1) Gastritis; indigestion

(2) Peptic ulcer disease

(3) Reflux esophagitis

(4) Prevention of peptic/stress ulcers

(5) Control/prevention of GI bleeding

(6) Pancreatitis

b. Modes of action

(1) Competitively blocks the stimulation of receptor sites by histamine H$_2$

(2) Decreases production of gastrin-induced and histamine-induced acid secretions

(3) Reduces overall gastric acidity in the stomach

(4) Reduces production of pancreatic secretions

c. Key medications

(1) cimetidine (Tagamet) (prototype)

(2) ranitidine (Zantac)

d. Interactions: numerous

(1) Increases blood levels of benzodiazepines, beta-blockers, calcium channel blockers, and most central nervous system (CNS) medications

(2) Inhibited by smoking, antacids, and sucralfate

e. General side effects

(1) CNS (headache, drowsiness, dizziness, disorientation)

(2) GI (diarrhea, constipation)

(3) Hematologic (anemia, blood dyscrasias)

(4) Genitourinary (GU) (gynecomastia, impotence)

(5) Severe bradycardia after intravenous administration

f. Nursing implications

(1) Instruct client that the best time to take these medications is just before meals and at bedtime, although food has little effect on absorption.

(2) Warn clients never to stop taking this medication suddenly because of rebound effect.

(3) Stress the need to avoid alcohol and other CNS medications while on these medications.

(4) Monitor the client for disorientation and dizziness, particularly the elderly.

(5) Instruct client to avoid taking medications at the same time as antacids.

(6) Reinforce need to alter lifestyle (reduce stress; increase exercise; avoid spicy or greasy foods; avoid alcohol; limit intake of aspirin, oral steroids, and ibuprofen).

6. Constipation is a condition that exists when a client has decreased frequency and/or passage of hard, dry stools.

a. Common causes of constipation include:

(1) Weakness of abdominal muscles

(2) Pregnancy; postpartum status

(3) Diet low in fiber, insufficient fluid intake, and lack of exercise

(4) Side effect of medications

(5) Decreased motility of GI tract (elderly, diabetics)

(6) Intestinal obstruction

(7) Abuse of laxatives

(8) Fear, anxiety, psychiatric disorders

7. Hepatic encephalopathy—hepatic coma

a. One function of the liver is to form urea from ammonia.

b. When cirrhosis is present, the liver is unable to make urea, and the serum ammonia levels increase.

c. Ammonia is toxic to the CNS. Symptoms include:
- (1) Disorientation
- (2) Tremors
- (3) Wandering at night
- (4) Motor disturbances
- (5) Coma

d. Goals of treatment are to reduce the digestion of protein in the GI tract and to lower ammonia levels. It can be accomplished by:
- (1) Using antibiotics such as Neomycin to destroy bacteria in intestines
- (2) Placing the client on a low-protein diet
- (3) Using lactulose to rid the intestines of the bacteria and undigested protein

8. Medications: laxatives, cathartics, purgatives, stool softeners
   a. Uses
   - (1) Relief of constipation
   - (2) Prevention of constipation in immobile clients
   - (3) Treatment of hepatic encephalopathy
   - (4) Cleaning of bowel prior to GI tests

   b. Modes of action
   - (1) Bulk-forming laxatives increase the amount of stool in the intestines by absorbing water into the GI tract.
   - (2) Surfactant laxatives (stool softeners) decrease the surface tension of the stool, allowing water to enter and soften the stool.
   - (3) Stimulant cathartics cause irritation of the intestinal mucosa, resulting in an increase in intestinal mucus and increased peristalsis in the colon.
   - (4) Disaccharide cathartics (used only in liver failure and hepatic coma) pull water into the intestine to soften stool, absorb and inactivate ammonia in the GI tract, and convert to lactic acid by bacteria to reduce bacterial flora.

   c. Key medications
   - (1) psyllium (Metamucil) (bulk laxative)
   - (2) bisacodyl (Dulcolax) (stimulant cathartic)
   - (3) docusate calcium (Surfak) (surfactant laxative)
   - (4) lactulose (Cephulac, Chronulac) (disaccharide cathartic)

   d. Interactions
   - (1) Decrease the absorption of most medications

- (2) Inhibited by antidiarrheals and narcotic medications

   e. General side effects
   - (1) GI (abdominal cramping, flatus, diarrhea, nausea, esophageal obstruction with bulk laxatives)
   - (2) Electrolyte imbalances
   - (3) Burning sensation with suppositories

   f. Nursing implications
   - (1) Monitor bowel elimination pattern for effectiveness.
   - (2) Inform client to use only as directed and avoid abuse of medications.
   - (3) Instruct the client to discontinue use if there is persistent diarrhea. Electrolyte imbalances and dehydration may occur or may be a sign of intestinal obstruction.
   - (4) Stress the need to increase exercise, drink plenty of fluids, and eat a high-fiber diet.
   - (5) Warn the client to avoid taking surfactant stool softeners with mineral oil; promotes systemic absorption of mineral oil.
   - (6) Warn the client that some laxatives may turn the urine pink/red color.
   - (7) Instruct the client to avoid chewing enteric-coated pills or taking laxatives with antacids.
   - (8) Warn the client not to take laxatives with H_2 inhibitors.
   - (9) Stress the need to take bulk laxatives with 1 to 2 full glasses of water; avoid mixing ahead of administration time.

9. Vomiting occurs when the chemoreceptor trigger zone (CTZ) in the medulla of the brain is stimulated, in turn stimulating the vomiting center (VC), also located in the medulla (Fig. 10–1). Causes include:
   a. Bacterial or viral infections; food poisoning
   b. Medication reactions
   c. Effects of radiation or chemotherapy
   d. Intolerance to foods
   e. Early pregnancy
   f. Motion sickness
   g. GI disorders (ulcers, obstructions)
   h. Fear, anxiety, tension, vertigo
   i. Postoperative status

10. Medications: antiemetics
    a. Uses
    - (1) Vomiting

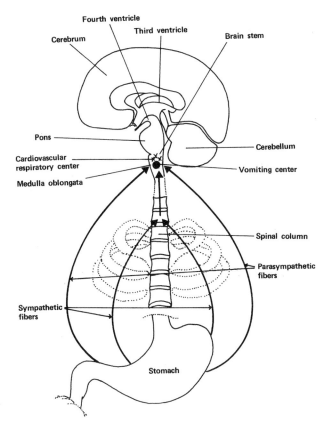

FIGURE 10–1. *Vomiting sequence. Stimuli leave the stomach or other sensory centers, follow the afferent parasympathetic fibers or the sympathetic fibers, and travel via the spinal column to the vomiting center in the medulla oblongata. (From Kuhn, M: Pharmacotherapeutics: A Nursing Process Approach, ed 4. FA Davis, Philadelphia, 1998, p 755, with permission.)*

    (2) Severe nausea
    (3) Prophylactically for chemotherapy
    (4) Prophylactically for motion sickness
  b. Mode of action: depends on category of medication
    (1) Antihistamine—blocks H_1 receptors, inhibiting vestibular stimulation
    (2) Phenothiazine—inhibits dopamine receptors in the CTZ and suppresses the cardiovascular (CV) response
    (3) GI stimulants—block dopamine receptors in the CTZ and accelerate gastric emptying time
  c. Key medications
    (1) dimenhydrinate (Dramamine) (antihistamine) (prototype)

    (2) trimethobenzamide (Tigan) (antihistaminelike)
    (3) prochlorperazine (Compazine) (phenothiazine)
    (4) metoclopramide (Reglan) (GI stimulant)
  d. Interactions
    (1) Potentiated by most CNS depressants, including alcohol, antidepressants, sedatives, and hypnotics.
    (2) Inhibited by CNS stimulants and antacids.
  e. General side effects
    (1) Drowsiness, dizziness, headache, blurred vision, tinnitus
    (2) Dry mouth, anorexia, constipation
    (3) Tachycardia, hypertension, hypotension
    (4) Respiratory depression
  f. Nursing implications
    (1) Warn client to avoid alcohol and other CNS medications while taking antiemetics.
    (2) To prevent motion sickness or vomiting due to chemotherapy, medication should be taken 30 to 60 minutes prior to activity.
    (3) Assess for effectiveness by noting number of vomiting episodes.
    (4) Advise the client to avoid driving or other activities requiring alertness while taking medication.
    (5) Encourage good oral hygiene to control dry mouth side effect.
    (6) Warn client to change position slowly to limit effects of postural hypotension.
11. Diarrhea is a sudden increase in the number of stools, which are often liquid and may be greenish in color.
  a. Causes include
    (1) Bacteria (*Shigella, Salmonella, Escherichia coli*) or viral infections
    (2) Anatomic or mechanic abnormalities (Hirschsprung's disease, malabsorption syndromes, food allergy)
    (3) Inflammatory bowel disorders
  b. Symptoms include
    (1) Frequent, liquid stools
    (2) Listlessness
    (3) Abdominal cramping, pain
12. Medications
  a. Uses
    (1) Short-term for diarrhea due to infections

(2) Long-term for diarrhea due to disease processes

b. Mode of action
  (1) Suppresses GI motility
  (2) Decreases production of gastric and pancreatic secretions

c. Key medication: diphenoxylate HCL plus atropine (Lomotil)

d. Interactions
  (1) Potentiated by most CNS depressants, including alcohol, antidepressants, sedatives, and hypnotics
  (2) Hypertensive crisis when used with monoamine oxidase (MAO) inhibitors

e. General side effects
  (1) Dizziness, drowsiness, headache, insomnia, anticholinergic effects
  (2) Constipation, dry mouth, nausea, vomiting
  (3) Urinary retention

f. Nursing implications
  (1) Assess the client for number of stools, consistency, and hydration status
  (2) Instruct the client to take the medication as directed and avoid exceeding recommended dosages.
  (3) Warn client to avoid alcohol and other CNS medications while taking antiemetics.
  (4) Advise the client to avoid driving or other activities requiring alertness while taking medication.
  (5) Instruct the client that if the diarrhea persists, or if a fever or signs of dehydration/electrolyte imbalance develop, notify the physician immediately.

11

Sensory System Medications

KEY ASPECTS OF THE ANATOMY AND PHYSIOLOGY OF SELECTED SENSORY SYSTEMS

EYE DISORDERS

1. Glaucoma is an eye disease characterized by increased intraocular pressure associated with progressive loss of the peripheral visual fields.
   a. Normal intraocular pressure: 13 to 22 mm Hg
   b. Glaucoma diagnosed if greater than 30
   c. Types of glaucoma
      (1) Wide or open angle (chronic simple glaucoma) is indicated by few symptoms, slow onset, gradual narrowing of visual fields (tunnel vision), poor night vision, loss of color discrimination, misty appearance of cornea, blurred vision, and fixed and dilated pupils.
      (2) Narrow angle/acute glaucoma is an emergency situation indicated by sudden onset, severe eye pain, nausea/vomiting, blurred vision, colored halos around lights, dilated pupils, reddened sclera, and blindness if not treated in 72 hours.

   d. Several different groups of medications are used to treat glaucoma.
2. Medications: miotics
   a. Uses
      (1) Long-term management of chronic glaucoma
      (2) Short-term control of symptoms of acute glaucoma
      (3) Esotropia (crossed eyes)
   b. Modes of action
      (1) Parasympathetic stimulant causes constriction of the pupil, drawing the fused muscle away from the canal of Schlemm
      (2) Allows aqueous humor to drain
      (3) Produces contraction of the accommodative muscles
   c. Key medication: pilocarpine hydrochloride (HCL) (Isopto Carpine, Pilocar) (prototype)
   d. Interactions
      (1) Potentiated by concurrent use of beta-blockers (cardiovascular effect)
      (2) Inhibited by anticholinergic medications
   e. General side effects
      (1) Eye irritation, blurred vision, reduced night vision (eyedrops)

(2) Nausea, vomiting, sweating, flushing (oral)

f. Nursing implications

(1) Instruct client in proper administration of eyedrop preparations (Fig. 11–1).

(2) If eyedrops are to be used daily, instruct client to administer at bedtime to decrease blurring of vision.

(3) Advise client of the need for regular eye examinations to evaluate effectiveness of medications.

(4) Instruct the client that if vision becomes severely limited or if eye pain should develop, to contact the physician immediately.

3. Medications: carbonic anhydrase inhibitor (acetazolamide NA [Diamox]) (See Chapter 6.)

4. Medications: beta-adrenergic blocking agent (timolol maleate [Timoptic]) (See Chapter 3.)

Inflammation is a nonspecific immune response that occurs in reaction to any type of tissue/organ injury no matter what the cause.

1. Prostaglandins are chemical substances that are released whenever there is trauma or injury to tissues that produce:

a. Pain—a subjective sensation of discomfort

b. Fever—an elevation in body temperature due to stimulation of the hypothalamus

c. Tissue inflammation—redness, warmth, swelling, and pain at the site of the injury due to vasodilation and increased tissue permeability.

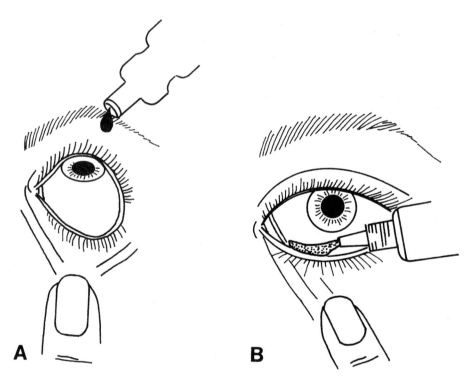

FIGURE 11–1. Administration of eye medications. (A) Eyedrops are administered onto the lower lid, which has been pulled down with the forefinger. The eye is then closed for 30 seconds to allow the medication to flow over the entire eye. The medication applicator approaches the eye from below and outside the patient's field of vision. Do not let the dropper tip touch any surface, including eye lashes. (B) Eye ointment is administered onto the lower lid, which is pulled down with the forefinger. Only a small amount (one-fourth of an inch) of ointment need be used. The eye is then closed to allow the medication to flow over the entire eye. (From Kuhn, M: Pharmacotherapeutics: A Nursing Process Approach, ed 4. FA Davis, Philadelphia, 1998, p 975, with permission.)

2. Common causes of inflammation
   a. Physical trauma
   b. Radiation
   c. Electrical energy
   d. Extreme temperature
   e. Autoimmune diseases (lupus rheumatoid arthritis)
   f. Viral or bacterial infections
   g. Allergic reactions
   h. Inflammatory disease processes (gout, emphysema, dysmenorrhea)
3. Medications: nonsteroidal anti-inflammatory drugs (NSAIDs)
   a. Uses
      (1) Mild to moderate pain
      (2) Rheumatoid arthritis, osteoarthritis, gout
      (3) Reduction of fever
      (4) Reduction of inflammation caused by a variety of disease processes
   b. Modes of action
      (1) Inhibit the formation of prostaglandins
      (2) Suppress the hypothalamus, reducing body temperature
      (3) Block the transmission of pain impulses across the synapses of the pain receptors
      (4) Reduce platelet aggregation and tissue permeability, reducing swelling
      (5) Suppress white blood cell functions in initiating the immune response
   c. Key medications
      (1) acetylsalicylic acid (aspirin, ASA)
      (2) orphenadrine citrate (Norflex)
      (3) ibuprofen (Motrin)
      (4) indomethacin (Indocin)
      (5) colchicine (Novocolchine)
   d. Interactions
      (1) Potentiate anticoagulants
      (2) Inhibit absorption of some vitamins, especially vitamin B_{12}.
   e. General side effects
      (1) Thrombocytopenia, bleeding tendencies
      (2) Gastrointestinal (GI) irritation (gastritis, ulcers, bleeding)
      (3) Tinnitus, ototoxicity
      (4) Reye's syndrome when ASA is used to treat viral infections in children under 18
   f. Nursing implications
      (1) Instruct client to take these medications with milk or food and a full glass of water.
      (2) Warn parents to avoid the use of ASA in children with viral infections or fevers.

      (3) Monitor client for bleeding or GI complications.
      (4) Stress the need to avoid alcohol when taking these medications.
      (5) Instruct the client about the need for frequent follow-up assessment by the physician.
4. Medications: nonsteroidal antipyretic analgesic
   a. Uses
      (1) Mild to moderate pain in noninflammatory diseases
      (2) Reduction of fever
   b. Modes of action
      (1) Lower prostaglandin production by inhibiting the enzyme needed for its synthesis
      (2) Suppresses the activity of the hypothalamus to decrease body temperature
      (3) Blocks the transmission of pain at receptor sites
      (4) Has NO anti-inflammatory effects.
   c. Key medications: acetaminophen (Tylenol)
   d. Interactions
      (1) Potentiated hepatic effects by diflunisal and alcohol
      (2) Inhibited by acetylcysteine (Mucomyst) (antidote for overdose)
   e. General side effects
      (1) Liver damage with high-dose, long-term use
      (2) Rash, urticaria
   f. Nursing implications
      (1) Instruct the client that this medication is not effective for inflammatory disorders such as rheumatoid arthritis.
      (2) Evaluate the temperature and degree of pain relief after administration.
      (3) Warn client to avoid alcohol while taking this medication.
      (4) Advise the client that exceeding the recommended maximum dosage (1000 mg) does not increase the effectiveness of the medication.
      (5) Inform diabetic clients that use of this medication may affect blood glucose testing results.

Gout is a hereditary form of arthritis in which serum uric acid levels increase to a point where uric acid crystals are deposited in the joints (normal uric acid = 2.3–7 mg/dL).

1. Affects primarily men over 30

2. Usually a family history of the disease
3. Characterized by hyperuricemia
4. Abnormal purine metabolism or excessive intake of purines results in the formation of uric acid crystals.
   a. Purines are nitrogenous substances found in many foods.
   b. The uric acid crystals precipitate from the body fluid and are deposited in the joints and connective tissue, producing the symptoms of the disease.
   c. It can affect any joint in the body but is most commonly seen in the great toe (90%).
   d. Symptoms
      (1) Tight, reddened skin over affected joint.
      (2) Joint swelling/severe pain
      (3) Elevated temperature
      (4) Permanent joint malformation
      (5) Renal failure
      (6) Tophi (nodular formations of uric acid crystals on the ear lobes, fingers, and hands)
      (7) Uric acid is greater than 8
   e. Acute gout attacks commonly begin at night and may last from 3 to 7 days. Attacks may be precipitated by:
      (1) Trauma
      (2) Increased alcohol consumption
      (3) High-purine diet
      (4) Diuretics (cause systemic fluid depletion which results in increased reabsorption of uric acid crystals)
5. Medications: uricostic agents
   a. Uses
      (1) Long-term management of chronic gout
      (2) Control the production of uric acid resulting from the use of antineoplastic medications and thiazide diuretics
      (3) Increase the half-life of penicillin and other anti-infectives
   b. Modes of action
      (1) Inhibit the renal tubular reabsorption of uric acid
      (2) Promote excretion of uric acids and lower uric acid levels
      (3) Prevent formation of new urate deposits and produce a gradual reduction of old deposits
   c. Key medications: probenecid (Benemid)
   d. Interactions

      (1) Potentiates barbiturates, penicillamine, benzodiazepines, and heparin
      (2) Inhibited by large doses of aspirin
   e. General side effects
      (1) Headache, dizziness
      (2) GI upset (nausea, vomiting, diarrhea)
      (3) Uric acid calculi (kidney stones)
      (4) Aplastic anemia, anemia
   f. Nursing implications
      (1) Instruct the client to take the medication with food or milk to reduce the GI side effects.
      (2) Instruct the client to increase the fluid intake (water) to 2–3 L/d to reduce the chance of developing renal calculi.
      (3) Instruct the client to avoid vitamin C or cranberry juice.
      (4) Warn diabetic clients that blood glucose monitoring may be inaccurate while taking this medication.
      (5) Inform the client to avoid taking aspirin while on this medication.
      (6) Stress the need to follow a low-purine diet (avoid red meats, fowl, fish/shell fish, sardines, anchovies, organ meats [kidney, liver]), meat extracts, and legumes.
      (7) Instruct the client that alcohol will increase uric acid levels and the symptoms of gout.
      (8) Teach the client the necessity of weight loss.
6. Medications: uric acid production inhibitors (xanthine oxidase inhibitors)
   a. Uses
      (1) Chronic gout or severe tophaceous gout
      (2) Renal calculi associated with high uric acid levels
      (3) Hyperuricemia resulting from cancer chemotherapy or other medications
   b. Modes of action
      (1) Inhibit the action of the enzyme xanthine oxidase in the conversion of xanthine to uric acid
      (2) Lower the uric acid level in both the blood and the urine
   c. Key medications: allopurinol (Zyloprim)
   d. Interactions
      (1) Potentiates oral hypoglycemics and warfarin
      (2) Bone marrow depression increased with

concurrent use of mercaptopurine and azathioprine

e. General side effects

(1) Rashes (pruritic maculopapular, exfoliate, urticarial)

(2) GI upset (nausea, vomiting, diarrhea)

(3) Aplastic anemia, bone marrow depression

(4) Renal failure

f. Nursing implications

(1) Instruct the client to report the development of rashes (a toxic reaction).

(2) Stress the need for frequent follow-up evaluations for liver, blood, and renal function testing.

(3) Instruct the client to take the medication with food or milk to reduce the GI side effects.

(4) Instruct the client to increase the fluid intake (water) to 2 to 3 liters per day to reduce the chance for developing renal calculi.

(5) Warn diabetic clients that blood glucose monitoring may be inaccurate while taking this medication.

(6) Inform the client to avoid taking aspirin while on this medication.

(7) Stress the need to follow a low-purine diet (avoid red meats, fowl, fish/shellfish, sardines, anchovies, organ meats [kidney, liver]), meat extracts, and legumes.

(8) Instruct the client that alcohol will increase uric acid levels and the symptoms of gout.

(9) Teach the client the necessity of weight loss.

7. Medications: NSAID during acute attacks, especially indomethacin (Indocin) and colchicine (Novocolchicine) (See NSAID above.)

CHAPTER

12

Immune System Medications

KEY CONCEPTS IN CANCER MEDICATIONS

Cancer is a general term that describes a group of diseases marked by uncontrolled growth and spread of abnormal cells.

1. Key definitions
   a. **Neoplasm** (new growth) is the property of cancer cells to grow and reproduce without the normal restraints found in noncancerous cells.
   b. **Differentiation** is the property normal cells have that allows them to reproduce cells identical to the parent cells.
   c. **Anaplasia** is the loss of cell differentiation found in cancer cells, which allows them to reproduce cells different from the parent cells, often more primitive in structure.
   d. **Pleomorphism** is the changes that occur in the size and shape of cancer cells, as well as in the size and shape of the nucleus.
   e. **Mitosis** is the splitting of one cell into two identical cells when the genetic material in the nucleus is sufficient to support two cells.

(1) **Transfer ribonucleic acid (RNA)** transfers the genetic material from an enzyme into an amino acid.
(2) **Messenger RNA** transfers the genetic information from the deoxyribonucleic acid (DNA) to the protein-forming substances in the cell for reproduction.
(3) *DNA* is the primary genetic material found in the nucleus.

   f. A **carcinogen** is anything that can alter the RNA or DNA in cells.
   (1) Altered DNA or RNA will produce mutant cells.
   (2) Mutant cells are usually identified by the immune system and destroyed before they can reproduce.
   (3) All mutant cells have the potential to become cancer cells if they are allowed to reproduce.
   g. Common carcinogens
   (1) Ultraviolet light, x-ray radiation
   (2) Radioactive materials
   (3) Polycyclic hydrocarbons (soot, tars, oil, cigarette smoke, dioxin)

(4) Industrial products (asbestos, benzine, cleaners, insecticides, chromium compounds, nickel)

(5) Food products (saccharin, smoked foods, nitrosamine in meat, other preservatives)

(6) Medications (oral contraceptives, estrogen, aminoglycoside antibiotics, all anticancer medications)

(7) Hereditary genetic predispositions (breast, colon, eye, skin cancers)

(8) Viruses (hepatitis B)

h. **First-order kinetics (kill rate)** refers to the percentage of cancer cells that are killed each time the medication is given.

(1) A first-order kinetic of 95% means that 95% of the cancer cells are killed the first time the medication is given.

(2) The second time the medication is given, 95% of the remaining 5% of cancer cells are killed.

(3) Cancer is considered cured only when all (100%) of the malignant cells are killed.

(4) Sometimes malignant cells may be reduced to a number where they are no longer detectable, but if any are still alive, the cancer is not cured.

2. Chemotherapy is the primary mode of treatment for many types of cancer.

a. Principles of combination therapy

(1) Most of the antineoplastic medications work on parts of the cell-reproduction cycle.

(2) Antineoplastic medications destroy or interfere with either the RNA or the DNA during the reproduction process.

(3) Two medications given together should work on different parts of the growth cycle.

(4) This combination therapy reduces the chance for resistance and increases the first-order kinetics.

(5) It also lessens the side effects to some degree from high doses of one medication.

b. Combination therapy is based on the following principles:

(1) Only medications that are known to be partially effective when used alone are selected.

(2) Medications with differing toxic effects are selected to decrease a potentially lethal side effect.

(3) Optimal doses and scheduling usually involve cyclical administration in which high doses are given for a time, then stopped, then repeated.

(4) The medication combinations are given as consistently and as frequently as possible while allowing normal tissue to recover between cycles.

(5) Long-term, indwelling central lines (e.g., Hickman catheter) are usually inserted for medication administration and frequent blood sampling.

c. Anticancer medications also destroy the DNA/RNA in normal cells.

(1) They affect the fastest reproducing cells first.

(2) One of the characteristics of cancer cells is rapid, uncontrolled reproduction (neoplastic growth).

d. Because of the chemical nature of antineoplastic agents, they may produce various levels of tissue irritation.

(1) Medications classified as *vesicant* are capable of producing blisters on the skin and, if they become infiltrated, tissue necrosis.

(2) Medications classified as *irritant* are capable of producing cell excitation, causing damage to cells, cellulitis, thrombophlebitis, and sensitivity similar to an allergic reaction.

(3) Medications classified as *nonvesicant* do not cause blisters on the skin nor tissue necrosis when infiltrated, but they may be a mild irritant capable of producing thromboembolism.

3. Medications: antineoplastic, alkylating agents

a. Uses

(1) Nonresectable tumors

(2) Clients who are poor surgical risks

(3) Adjunct therapy with surgery

(4) Primary treatment with hematologic cancers, cancers of the breast, lungs, and ovaries

b. Modes of action

(1) Interfere with cell division

(2) Block the formation of new DNA

c. Key medications

(1) chlorambucil (Leukeran) (nonvesicant)

(2) cyclophosphamide (Cytoxin) (nonvesicant)

d. Interactions

(1) Potentiated by bone marrow depressants

(2) Inhibit effect of vaccines

e. General side effects: see below.

f. Nursing implications: see below.

4. Medications: antineoplastic, antimetabolites

  a. Uses

    (1) Treatment of many types of cancers (colon, breast, rectal, gastric, and pancreatic)

    (2) Topical treatment of multiple actinic keratoses and superficial basal cell carcinoma

    (3) Nonresectable tumors

    (4) Clients who are poor surgical risks

    (5) Adjunct therapy with surgery

  b. Modes of action

    (1) Simulate the nutrients the cancer cells need to grow and reproduce

    (2) Enter the cells and inhibit absorption of the normal cell nutrients

    (3) Inhibit RNA and DNA synthesis by preventing thymidine production

  c. Key medication: fluorouracil (Adrucil, 5-FU) (prototype) (nonvesicant)

  d. Interactions: same as above

  e. General side effects: see below.

  f. Nursing implications: see below.

5. Medications: antineoplastic, anthracycline, antibiotic

  a. Uses

    (1) Used to treat leukemia; breast, bladder, ovarian and lung cancer; Wilm's tumor; and Kaposi sarcoma.

    (2) Nonresectable tumors

    (3) Clients who are poor surgical risks

    (4) Adjunct therapy with surgery

  b. Modes of action

    (1) Bind to DNA, forming an insoluble complex that prevents further DNA and RNA synthesis

    (2) Suppress both immune system and bone marrow

    (3) Actions similar to aminoglycoside antibiotics but too toxic for simple infections

  c. Key medication: doxorubicin (Adriamycin) (prototype) (vesicant)

  d. Interactions

    (1) Potentiate bone marrow suppression of other antineoplastic agents and radiation therapy

    (2) Inhibit effects of vaccines

  e. General side effects: see below.

  f. Nursing implications: see below.

6. Medications: antineoplastic, vinca alkaloids

  a. Uses

    (1) Treat many types of cancers (Hodgkin's disease, leukemia, neuroblastoma, Wilm's tumor)

    (2) Nonresectable tumors

    (3) Clients who are poor surgical risks

    (4) Adjunct therapy with surgery

  b. Modes of action

    (1) Bind to the proteins of mitotic spindle

    (2) Inhibit the separation of the chromosomes during reproduction

    (3) Prevent cell division

    (4) Immunosuppression, but little effect on bone marrow

  c. Key medication: vincristine (Oncovin) (prototype) (vesicant)

  d. Interactions: same as above

  e. General side effects of all antineoplastic agents

    (1) Bone marrow suppression (leukopenia, thrombocytopenia, anemia, aplastic anemia)

    (2) Gastrointestinal (GI complications—nausea, vomiting, diarrhea (constipation with vincristine), stomatitis

    (3) Skin alterations (photosensitivity, tissue necrosis and sloughing if infiltrated)

    (4) Toxicity to organs and failure (liver, lungs, kidneys)

    (5) Alopecia (loss of hair)

    (6) Secondary infections

    (7) Sterility

    (8) Abnormal cell growth, cancer

  f. Nursing implications

    (1) Monitor cell counts and protect the client from injury and bleeding.

    (2) Platelet and packed red blood transfusions may be required because of the bone marrow suppression.

    (3) Monitor the client for signs of infection at the indwelling central line and for candidial and other bacterial infections.

    (4) Encourage nystatin oral care to prevent the development of stomatitis.

    (5) Use measures to prevent infection (good hand washing, reverse isolation, limit exposure to organisms).

    (6) Give phenothiazines and other antiemetics 30 minutes *before* treatment is started.

    (7) Instruct the client in relaxation techniques, imagery, and alterations in diet

to reduce frequency or severity of GI symptoms.

    (8) Use antacids (Mylanta) around the clock to minimize ulcerations of the stomach.

    (9) Monitor infants for severe diaper rashes caused by excretion of chemotherapeutic agents in the urine.

    (10) Warn the client to protect the skin from direct sunlight because of photosensitivity.

    (11) Encourage the client to increase fluid intake to 2–3 L/d to prevent kidney damage.

    (12) Advise the client for frequent follow-up assessments to monitor liver enzymes, blood urea nitrogen (BUN), creatinine, complete blood count (CBC), and oxygen saturation.

    (13) Monitor the client for cardiac dysrhythmias and congestive heart failure (CHF).

    (14) During chemotherapy wrap the scalp in a tourniquet to decrease circulation so the agents will not readily circulate to the scalp; this can reduce hair loss.

    (15) Use care in handling of antineoplastic agents (wear gloves, gown, mask, use laminar flow hood during preparation, dispose of materials properly, avoid contact if pregnant or breast feeding).

    (16) Monitor intravenous sites of vesicant medications closely during infusion to prevent infiltration and tissue necrosis.

GENERAL INFORMATION CONCERNING ANTI-INFECTIVES

1. **Infection** is a general term that describes the presence and growth in the body of a foreign organism that usually produces some degree of tissue damage.
2. Infection normally triggers an immune response with symptoms similar to inflammation, including:
   a. Pain
   b. Fever, or localized warmth
   c. Redness
   d. Swelling
   e. Purulent drainage

3. Types of infective organisms
   a. **Bacteria** are single-cell organisms without a true nucleus or functionally specific components of metabolism and require a host to supply food and a supportive environment for reproduction.
    (1) **Aerobic** bacteria need a fresh and continuous supply of oxygen in order to reproduce.
    (2) **Anaerobic** bacteria can reproduce in an environment that is oxygen free.
    (3) **Gram-positive** bacteria absorb gram stain and are often aerobic.
    (4) **Gram-negative** bacteria do not absorb gram stain and tend to be anaerobic.
   b. **Protozoa** are modified bacteria that retain some of the properties of animals and some properties of plants.
   c. **Viruses** are obligate intracellular parasites that cannot live outside of cells because of their inability to obtain food or replicate DNA without a host.
    (1) They are composed of a central core of DNA or RNA.
    (2) When they enter a cell, they use the DNA and RNA of the cell to reproduce.
    (3) They block the ability of the cell to synthesize protein, damaging or killing the cell.
   d. **Fungi** are plant-type organisms that take the form of yeast, mold, or mushroom.
    (1) In the body, the growth of fungi is controlled by the normal bacteria present (normal flora).
    (2) Destroying bacteria in the body often allows fungi to grow unchecked, resulting in fungal infections.
    (3) Yeast infections are the most common form of fungal infections, usually found on the mucous membranes or skin, but can become systemic.
   e. **Parasitic helminths** are worms that invade the body, usually through the fecal-oral route, and damage tissues as they grow and reproduce.
    (1) Most commonly helminths infect the GI system, but they may infect the blood, nervous system, or vital organs.
    (2) Common types of helminths include roundworms, tapeworms, flatworms, and flukes.
   f. **Parasitic arthropods** include a number of

creatures that infest humans and other mammals and often are vectors for a number of infectious diseases, including typhus, trench fever, and bubonic plague.

(1) **Pediculosis** (lice) affect the hairy parts of the body and are a common problem in the United States.

(2) **Sarcoptes scabiei** (scabies) is a microscopic itch mite that infects the warm, moist skin-fold areas of the body (between the fingers and toes, under the breasts).

4. Key definitions used with anti-infectives

a. **Indigenous flora** refers to bacteria that normally live on or in certain parts of the body (skin, respiratory tract, GI tract) and normally do not cause infection.

b. **Opportunistic organisms** are bacteria or fungi that are normally found in the indigenous flora and may produce infection when the host defense mechanisms are damaged or impaired.

c. **Mode of transmission** is the way the infectious organisms are spread from one person to another.

(1) **Airborne route** generally refers to infections spread by the respiratory system through the air.

(2) **Direct-contact route** refers to infections spread through touching the organism, someone who has the organism, or an object that has been contaminated with the organism.

(3) **Sexual-contact route** is the spread of infectious organisms that have infected the genital areas of the body through direct sexual contact or intercourse.

(4) **Vector route** is the spread of infections through some mediary, which may be an insect, animal, or object.

d. **Prodromal symptom** is the first symptom that indicates the onset of a particular disease. It is not always the most typical symptom.

e. **Incubation period** refers to the time interval between exposure to the organism and the development of the disease.

(1) Many common viral infections (colds, flu, varicella) have an incubation period of 5 to 10 days.

(2) Most bacteria have incubation periods of 24 to 38 hours.

(3) The length of the incubation period can be affected both by the nature of the organism and by the status of the host's immune system.

f. **Resistant organisms** are bacteria, viruses, or parasites that are no longer able to be destroyed by the usual amounts and types of anti-infective medications.

(1) Resistance occurs when the genetic makeup of the organism is altered.

(2) It is often the result of prolonged subclinical exposure to anti-infectives.

g. **Nosocomial infections** are infections acquired after the person has entered the health-care system.

(1) They are often the result of poor hygiene practices on the part of health-care providers (improper or no hand washing, breaks in sterile technique).

(2) Nosocomial infections tend to be serious because of the often resistant nature of organisms found in health-care facilities and the debilitated state of many clients.

h. **Antibiotic** generally refers to a medication used to control or eliminate bacterial infections.

(1) **Broad-spectrum (extended-spectrum)** antibiotic is a medication that can be used to treat a large number of bacteria or a whole class of bacteria and is used when the infective organism is unknown.

(2) **Narrow-spectrum** antibiotic refers to a medication that is useful against only a specific or few particular bacteria and is used when the organism has been identified by a culture.

(3) **Bactericidal** antibiotics actually kill the bacteria outright.

(4) **Bacteriostatic** antibiotics prevent the bacteria from reproducing and eventually will lead to the death of the organism.

i. **Superinfection** is the unrestrained growth of an organism (usually fungi) that occurs when the normal flora is altered because of treatment with antibiotics.

j. **Peak and trough** is a laboratory test that establishes the maximum blood level of a medication (peak) and the lowest blood level of a medication (trough) to determine whether the blood levels of the medication are within the therapeutic range.

(1) Although this test can be performed with any medication, it is usually done for antibiotics.

(2) The peak medication level is drawn 30 minutes after the medication is administered intravenously.

(3) The trough level is drawn 30 minutes before the next dose of medication is to be given intravenously.

5. Medications: anti-infective; antibiotic (penicillins)

a. Uses: broad-spectrum

(1) Most infections with gram-positive cocci, rods, aerobic bacteria, and some anaerobic

(2) Respiratory/airway infections (pharyngitis, pneumonia, otitis media, sinusitis)

(3) Genitourinary (GU) infections (urinary tract infection [UTI], syphilis, gonorrhea)

(4) Cardiovascular (CV) infections (endocarditis, rheumatic heart disease)

(5) GI infections (salmonella, shigella, dysentery)

(6) Do not penetrate the blood-brain barrier (limited use with infections of the brain, spinal cord, eye)

b. Modes of action

(1) Bacteriocidal

(2) Interfere with the synthesis of an enzyme necessary to maintain the integrity of the cell walls

(3) Inhibits cell wall synthesis

c. Key medications

(1) ampicillin (Omnipen)

(2) amoxicillin (Amoxil)

d. Interactions: see below.

e. General side effects: see below.

f. Nursing implications: see below.

6. Medications: anti-infective; antibiotic (cephalosporin)

a. Uses: broad-spectrum

(1) Same organisms as the penicillins

(2) Classified by generations—the spectrum of the medication widens as the generation increases (e.g., third-generation medications have a broader spectrum than first-generation medications)

(3) Do not penetrate the blood-brain barrier

(4) Second- and third-generation medications work better on gram-negative bacteria than first-generation and penicillins

b. Modes of action

(1) Both bacteriostatic and bacteriocidal

(2) Inhibit cell-wall synthesis

c. Key medications

(1) cephalexin (Keflex) (first generation)

(2) cephadrine (Anspor, Velosef) (first generation)

(3) cefaclor (Ceclor) (second generation)

(4) cefoxitin (Mefoxin) (second generation)

(5) ceftazidime (Fortaz) (third generation)

d. Interactions: see below.

e. General side effects: see below.

f. Nursing implications: see below.

7. Medications: anti-infectives; antibiotic (aminoglycosides)

a. Uses: broad-spectrum

(1) Most effective against gram-negative bacilli and anaerobic organisms

(2) Tuberculosis

(3) GI organisms (klebsiella, proteus, *Escherichia coli*, pseudomonas)

(4) Also effective against many gram-positive organisms

(5) Poorly distributed to the central nervous system

b. Modes of action

(1) Bacteriocidal (high doses); bacteriostatic (low doses)

(2) Interfere with the replication of the RNA in the cell

(3) Prevent the bacteria from synthesizing proteins it requires to maintain its integrity and reproduce

c. Key medications

(1) gentamicin (Garamycin)

(2) streptomycin

d. Interactions: see below.

e. General side effects: see below.

f. Nursing implications: see below.

8. Medications: anti-infective: antibiotic (tetracycline)

a. Uses: broad-spectrum

(1) Rocky Mountain spotted fever and Lyme disease

(2) Sexually transmitted diseases (chlamydia, syphilis, gonorrhea, pelvic inflammatory disease [PID])

      (3) Respiratory infections (chronic bronchitis, Legionnaires' disease)

      (4) Most infections treated by penicillin when the client is allergic to penicillin

      (5) Not a first-line antibiotic in most infections except Rocky Mountain spotted fever and Lyme disease

      (6) Does not cross the blood-brain barrier

  b. Modes of action

      (1) Bacteriostatic

      (2) Interferes with the functioning of transfer and messenger RNA

      (3) Inhibits protein synthesis in the cell, preventing reproduction

  c. Key medications

      (1) tetracycline (Sumycin, Achromycin) (prototype)

      (2) doxycycline (Vibramycin)

  d. Interactions: see below.

  e. General side effects: see below.

  f. Nursing implications: see below.

9. Medications: anti-infective; antibiotic (sulfonamide)

  a. Uses: broad-spectrum

      (1) UTI, bacterial vaginal infections, prostatitis

      (2) Ulcerative colitis, toxoplasmosis

      (3) Burn trauma (topically)

      (4) Effective against wide range of gram-negative and gram-positive organisms

      (5) Penetrates the blood-brain barrier (meningitis)

  b. Modes of action

      (1) Bacteriostatic

      (2) Blocks the action of para-aminobenzoic acid (PABA) to prevent the synthesis of folic acid

      (3) Interferes with the formation of DNA in newly divided cells

  c. Key medications

      (1) sulfadiazine (Microsulfon)

      (2) sulfamethoxazole plus trimethoprim (Bactrim, Septra)

      (3) silver sulfadiazine (Silvadene)

  d. Interactions: see below.

  e. General side effects: see below.

  f. Nursing implications: see below.

10. Medications: anti-infective; antibiotic (macrolides)

  a. Uses: broad-spectrum

      (1) Effective against most gram-positive and some gram-negative organisms

      (2) Staph aureus infections

      (3) Respiratory infections (pneumonia)

      (4) Back-up medication for clients who are allergic to penicillin

      (5) Does not penetrate the blood-brain barrier

  b. Modes of action

      (1) Bacteriostatic

      (2) Binds to ribosomes to inhibit protein synthesis

  c. Key medication: erythromycin (EES)

  d. Interactions: see below.

  e. General side effects: see below.

  f. Nursing implications: see below.

11. Medications: anti-infective; antibiotic (miscellaneous)

  a. Uses: broad-spectrum

      (1) Both gram-positive and gram-negative organisms

      (2) Used when organisms are resistant to other antibiotics

  b. Modes of action

      (1) Bacteriocidal

      (2) Combines two medications: imipenem is the antibiotic, and cilastatin is added to slow the metabolism of the antibiotic

      (3) Inhibits cell-wall synthesis

  c. Key medication: imipenem/cilastatin (Primaxin)

  d. Interactions: see below.

  e. General side effects: see below.

  f. Nursing implications: see below.

12. Medications: anti-infective; antibiotic (miscellaneous)

  a. Uses: broad-spectrum

      (1) Serious infections; infections resistant to other antibiotics

      (2) First-line medication in typhoid fever only

      (3) Most gram-negative and gram-positive organisms

      (4) Crosses the blood-brain barrier (meningitis, brain abscesses, eye infections)

  b. Modes of action

      (1) Bacteriostatic

      (2) Inhibits protein synthesis in bacteria and rapidly growing cells (especially bone marrow)

      (3) Prevents replication of DNA during mitosis

  c. Key medication: chloramphenicol (Chloromycetin)

d. Interactions: see below.
e. General side effects: see below.
f. Nursing implications: see below.

13. General interactions for antibiotics
    a. Potentiated by medications that decrease urine output and other classes of antibiotics
    b. Decreased effectiveness when used with diuretics
    c. Decrease the effectiveness of birth control pills

14. General side effects for antibiotics
    a. Allergic reactions, rashes
    b. Superinfection (black, hairy tongue; thrush; vaginal yeast infections)
    c. GI upset (nausea, vomiting, diarrhea, abdominal bloating)
    d. Nephrotoxicity, renal failure (particularly with cephalosporins, aminoglycosides, sulfonamides, chloramphenicol)
    e. Hepatotoxicity (most antibiotics)
    f. Staining of the teeth in children when taken in a liquid form (tetracycline)
    g. Photosensitivity (tetracycline, sulfonamides)
    h. Ototoxicity (hearing loss, tinnitus) (aminoglycosides)
    i. Bone marrow suppression, aplastic anemia (cephalosporins, chloramphenicol)
    j. Neuromuscular damage, respiratory arrest (aminoglycosides)

15. Nursing implications for antibiotics
    a. Encourage the client to increase fluid intake to 2 to 3 liters of fluid per day while on antibiotic.
    b. Obtain culture and sensitivity before administration of antibiotics.
    c. Instruct clients to take all of the prescribed medication even if they are symptom free.
    d. Evaluate the client for effectiveness; if symptoms do not improve in 3 to 5 days, client may require a different antibiotic.
    e. Warn the client that GI symptoms (nausea, abdominal cramping and diarrhea) are common because of the alteration in the intestinal flora. Instruct the client to continue taking the medication but to also drink buttermilk or eat yogurt to replace the flora.
    f. Monitor the blood levels of the antibiotics, particularly when the client is using the aminoglycosides.
    g. Monitor CBC closely, especially when on chloramphenicol.

h. Always monitor the client closely for the first 15 minutes when receiving an intravenous antibiotic for the first time.
i. Encourage the client to wear sunscreen or stay covered when outdoors while taking sulfonamides or tetracycline.
j. Have children drink tetracycline liquid preparations through a straw to prevent staining of teeth.
k. Instruct clients to take all oral antibiotics with 1 to 2 full glasses of liquid.
l. Most oral antibiotics are more effective if taken on an empty stomach, but they can be taken with food to decrease GI upset.

Tuberculosis (TB) is an infection of the lungs caused by the mycobacterium tuberculosis.

1. The TB bacterium is a gram-positive acid-fast bacteria.
   a. It produces fibrosis and calcification within the lung tissue.
   b. It is transmitted by direct contact or airborne routes.
   c. Clients who are debilitated, have poor nutritional status, or are immune suppressed (human immunodeficiency virus [HIV]) are most susceptible.
   d. Symptoms include:
      (1) Weakness, chronic fatigue
      (2) Localized chest pain
      (3) Fever, night sweats
      (4) Cough, hemoptysis
      (5) Weight loss, malnutrition
   e. Diagnosis made by:
      (1) Positive purified protein derivative (PPD)
      (2) Sputum positive for acid-fast bacillus (AFB)
      (3) Chest x-ray
      (4) C & S of sputum (take 6–8 weeks to grow organism)
   f. Outbreaks of resistant TB organisms are becoming more common.

2. The TB organism is difficult to treat.
   a. It becomes resistant to one antibiotic very quickly.
   b. Treatment for active TB requires the use of two or more medications at the same time.
   c. Treatment lasts 6 to 12 months.
   d. Clients who have converted from a negative PPD test to positive but who do not have the active disease will be prescribed one medication isonicotine hydrazine (INH) usually for 12 months.

e. The organism may lie dormant for long periods of time (months to years).
3. Medications: anti-infective; antibiotics (antitubercular)
   a. Uses
      (1) Treatment of active tuberculosis
      (2) Treatment of leprosy
      (3) Prophylactic treatment of persons with positive TB skin tests or known exposure but no active disease
   b. Modes of action
      (1) Bacteriocidal
      (2) Inhibit the production of mycolic acid, disrupting the metabolism of the organism
      (3) Inhibits cell-wall synthesis
   c. Key medications
      (1) isoniazid (INH) (narrow-spectrum)
      (2) rifampin (Rifadin) (broad-spectrum)
      (3) aminoglycoside antibiotics (see above)
   d. Interactions
      (1) Potentiate hepatotoxic effects with alcohol and other hepatotoxic medications
      (2) Inhibit metabolism of phenytoin
      (3) Decreased absorption when taken with antacids
   e. General side effects
      (1) GI irritation (nausea, vomiting, diarrhea, pancreatitis)
      (2) Liver toxicity and failure
      (3) Central nervous system (CNS) toxicity (ototoxicity, peripheral neuropathy, seizures, psychosis, blurred vision)
      (4) Renal failure
      (5) Reddish-orange urine, sweat, and tears
      (6) Rashes and irritation of skin
   f. Nursing implications
      (1) Stress the need for frequent (monthly) follow-up assessments to monitor liver function studies; x-ray should be repeated in 6 months.
      (2) Warn clients about the common side effects of medications.
      (3) Stress the need to avoid alcohol altogether as well as other hepatotoxic medications.
      (4) Inform clients taking isoniazid that the peripheral neuropathy side effects (numbness, tingling in the extremities) can be reduced by taking pyridoxine (vitamin B$_6$).
      (5) Stress the importance of taking the medications as prescribed and not skipping

doses. Even a few days of missed doses may cause the organism to become resistant to the current medications.
      (6) Instruct the client in monitoring temperature and weight daily and recording the results.
      (7) Reinforce the need to dispose of secretion-contaminated items (tissues, clothes, sheets) properly. May remain contagious for several weeks to a month after treatment is started.
      (8) Stress the need for a diet high in protein, vitamins, and carbohydrates, as well as the need for extended rest periods.

FUNGAL INFECTIONS (SEE ABOVE)

1. There are two types of fungal infections.
   a. Topical (superficial) infections affect the skin and mucous membranes of the mouth, rectum, and vagina.
      (1) **Candida albicans** is the most common organism.
      (2) Yeasts occur commonly.
      (3) Ringworm is another common fungal infection.
   b. Systemic infections may affect the lungs, blood, and CNS.
      (1) They are very serious, difficult to treat, and often fatal.
      (2) They are rarely seen in healthy individuals, but common in clients with compromised immune systems (HIV, immunosuppressives).
2. Clients taking antibiotics are at high risk for topical fungal infections.
3. Medications: anti-infective; antifungal
   a. Uses
      (1) Systemic and topical fungal infections
      (2) Histoplasmosis
      (3) Thrush (oral candidiasis)
      (4) Intravenous preparations effective against gram-negative bacteria
   b. Modes of action
      (1) Destroy the cell wall of the fungus by increasing its permeability.
      (2) Allow the protoplasm to leak out and kill the organism.
   c. Key medications
      (1) nystatin (Mycostatin) (topical)
      (2) metronidazole (Flagyl) (systemic)

(3) triacetin (Fungoid, Ony-Clear Nail) (topical)

d. Interactions: few

(1) Corticosteroids may inhibit effectiveness.

e. General side effects

(1) Nephrotoxicity

(2) Thrombophlebitis at intravenous site

(3) GI upset (nausea, vomiting, diarrhea)

(4) Electrolyte imbalance (hypokalemia, hypomagnesemia)

(5) Fever, chills

f. Nursing implications

(1) Teach client proper method of administration (topical, suppository, oral liquid).

(2) Instruct the client to swish the oral mycostatin liquid in the mouth before swallowing.

(3) Monitor for effectiveness and relief of symptoms.

(4) Attempt to determine the source/cause of the infection and eliminate it.

(5) Stress the need for good personal hygiene.

PARASITIC WORMS

1. The Centers for Disease Control (CDC) has determined that 15% of the U.S. population is afflicted at any given time.

a. Approximately one half of all school children will have pinworms (enterobiasis/helminths) at some time during their childhood.

b. Parasitic worms are contracted through the fecal/oral route by ingesting food or substances contaminated with worm eggs.

c. Symptoms of enterobiasis (pinworms)

(1) Intense anal itching, worsens at night

(2) Vaginitis, enuresis

(3) Irritability/restlessness

(4) "Sleep walking" at night/insomnia

(5) Abdominal pain, diarrhea, anorexia

(6) Stools positive for ova and parasites (O & P)

(7) Cellophane-tape test positive for eggs

d. Symptoms of ascariasis (roundworms)

(1) Anorexia, irritability, nervousness

(2) Enlarged, bloated abdomen

(3) Fever, weight loss

(4) Intestinal colic

(5) Appendicitis, bowel obstruction

(6) Jaundice, pneumonitis

(7) Worms visible in stools

(8) Stool positive for O&P

2. Medications: anthelmintic

a. Uses

(1) Treatment of roundworms, tapeworms, flatworms, and flukes

(2) Treatment of parasites, eggs, and hydatid cysts

b. Modes of action

(1) Interferes with the absorption of glucose in the worm

(2) Disrupts functioning of worm's nervous system

c. Key medication: mebendazole (Vermox) (prototype)

d. Interactions

(1) Potentiated by carbamazepine and phenytoin

(2) Inhibited by antacids and cathartics

e. General side effects

(1) GI irritation (nausea, vomiting, diarrhea, abdominal cramping as worms die) (common)

(2) CNS (headache, dizziness, numbness) (rare)

f. Nursing implications

(1) Instruct the client that the tablet may be chewed (especially with children), crushed, swallowed whole, or mixed with food.

(2) Instruct client that for best results, it should be taken with a high-fat meal (increases absorption).

(3) Stress the need for follow-up examinations for evidence of reinfestation.

(4) Identify close contacts for possible infestation and treatment (family members, school, day care).

(5) Stress the need for good hand washing and general hygiene and proper disposal of feces.

(6) Instruct mothers of infants to make sure infants wear tight-fitting diapers/panties and to change linen/underwear daily.

(7) Fingernails should be cut short, or the child should wear mittens-socks on hands to prevent scratching and contamination.

(8) Instruct parents not to allow dogs to play in the sandbox.

(9) Find and eliminate source of worms.

PARASITIC ARTHROPOD INFESTATIONS: SEE ABOVE

1. Medications: pediculicide, scabicide
   a. Uses
      (1) Treatment of parasitic arthropod infestations
      (2) Elimination of scabies, head lice, body lice, crab lice, and their eggs
   b. Modes of action
      (1) Neurotoxic to the nervous system of parasitic arthropods
      (2) Produces seizures, paralysis, and death of the infecting creature
   c. Key medications
      (1) lindane (Kwell)
      (2) permethrin (Nix)
   d. Interactions
      (1) Potentiated by simultaneous use of shampoo or skin preparations (increased systemic absorption).
      (2) CNS medications may increase neurotoxic side effects.
   e. General side effects
      (1) CNS (seizures, paralysis, death)
      (2) Skin (local irritation, contact dermatitis)
   f. Nursing implications
      (1) Stress the need to follow the directions on the bottle exactly. Exceeding the recommended dosage or frequency can cause neurotoxicity in children.
      (2) Prior to application of creams or lotions, wash area and allow to cool and dry. Apply enough lotion or cream to cover the entire body surface with a thin film. Leave on for 6 to 8 hours.
      (3) Instruct clients to cut long hair, comb hair with a fine-tooth comb dipped in vinegar to remove nit, discard contaminated combs/brushes after use.
      (4) Teach clients not to exchange personal items (hats, gloves, shirts).
      (5) Instruct clients to launder bed linens, towels, clothes, and anything with which the client has come in contact.

(6) Identify close contacts for examination and possible treatment.

(7) Nurses and other hospital personnel applying the shampoo or lotion should wear gloves.

HUMAN IMMUNODEFICIENCY VIRUS (HIV)

1. Acquired immune deficiency syndrome (AIDS) is the disease syndrome caused by HIV.
   a. HIV produces changes in the genetic structure of the cells of the immune system.
   b. Different white blood cells play different roles in protecting against disease.
      (1) Lymphocytes are divided into B cells and T cells. There are two types of T cells.
      (2) Type 1 helps B cells destroy disease-causing organisms (helper T cells).
      (3) Type 2 helps T cells stop or suppress the B cells and helper T cells once the infection has been stopped (suppressor T cells).
      (4) Normal ratio is 2 helper T cells for each 1 suppressor T cell.
      (5) HIV attacks and either destroys or inhibits the production of the helper T cells, leaving an overabundance of suppressor T cells.
      (6) This leaves the immune system weak and unable to identify and fight off infection from bacteria or other viruses.
   c. Modes of transmission
      (1) Direct sexual contact is the primary mode.
      (2) Contact with contaminated needles and blood products is much less common.
      (3) Mother to unborn child either through the placenta or during the birth process.
   d. Incubation period may be from 2 months to over 5 years or more before any signs of infection appear.
   e. Early symptoms include severe and prolonged:
      (1) Recurrent fever
      (2) Rapid weight loss
      (3) Swollen lymph glands
      (4) Constant fatigue
      (5) Diarrhea and diminished appetite
      (6) White spots and sores in the mouth

f. Later symptoms include:
 (1) Kaposi's sarcoma
 (2) *Pneumocystic carinii pneumonia* (PCP)
 (3) Central nervous system damage (infections of CNS, memory loss, inability to make decisions, loss of coordination and body functions, blindness)
2. Medications: antiviral, anti-HIV
 a. Uses
  (1) Delay and suppression of symptoms associated with AIDS
  (2) Reduction of discomfort associated with symptoms of AIDS
  (3) Prevention of HIV in infants born to HIV-infected mothers
  (4) Other viral infections (herpes simplex, influenza)
 b. Modes of action
  (1) Inhibit enzymes responsible for DNA replication in the viral cell
  (2) May inhibit viral penetration of the host cell
 c. Key medications
  (1) zidovudine (AZT)
  (2) didanosine (ddI)
 d. Interactions
  (1) Potentiate bone marrow depression with antineoplastic agents

 (2) Increased side effects/toxicity with probenecid
 e. General side effects
  (1) GI upset (nausea, abdominal cramping, vomiting, diarrhea)
  (2) CNS (seizures, headache, weakness, anxiety, disorientation, tremors)
  (3) Anemia, granulocytopenia
 f. Nursing implications
  (1) Monitor for effectiveness of medication by decrease in symptomology and reduction in opportunistic infections.
  (2) Encourage client to continue follow-up visits for monitoring of blood work and viral load.
  (3) Instruct client to take medication exactly as prescribed and not to skip doses or double up on doses.
  (4) Caution clients to avoid driving or other activities that require mental alertness until effects of medication are known.
  (5) Warn clients that this medication does not cure the disease and that they are still contagious even though asymptomatic.
  (6) Instruct clients to contact the physician immediately if they should develop a fever, sore throat, or other symptoms of infection.

13

Nutritional Supplements

1. Nutrients are substances necessary for the promotion and maintenance of health and growth of the person.
2. Medications are pharmacological agents that are capable of interacting with a living organism to produce a biologic effect.
   a. Nutrients
      (1) Water
      (2) Carbohydrates
      (3) Proteins
      (4) Fats
      (5) Vitamins
      (6) Minerals
      (7) Combinations of the above
   b. Some substances classified as nutrients may also be classified as medications. For example:
      (1) Lithium is a mineral that is used as a medication.
      (2) Potassium is a mineral that is used as a medication.
   c. Medications are regulated by the Food and Drug Administration (FDA), whereas substances classified as nutrients generally are not.

NUTRITIONAL SUPPLEMENTS

1. Supplemental feedings may be given:
   a. Orally
   b. Nasogastric tube feeding
   c. Gastric percutaneous endoscopic gastrostomy (PEG) tube feeding (Figs. 13–1, 13–2)
2. Uses
   a. Debilitated clients who have additional nutrition requirements that cannot be met by their prescribed diet
   b. Clients who are unable to eat normally because of disease or injury
   c. Promotion of healing and recovery in postoperative or severely ill clients
3. Modes of action
   a. Delivered in a concentrated form, supplemental vitamins, carbohydrate, protein, fat, and minerals
   b. Promote healing and recovery by supplying nutrients necessary for tissue rebuilding
4. Key supplements
   a. Ensure, Isocal, Sustical
      (1) Milky, thick fluids

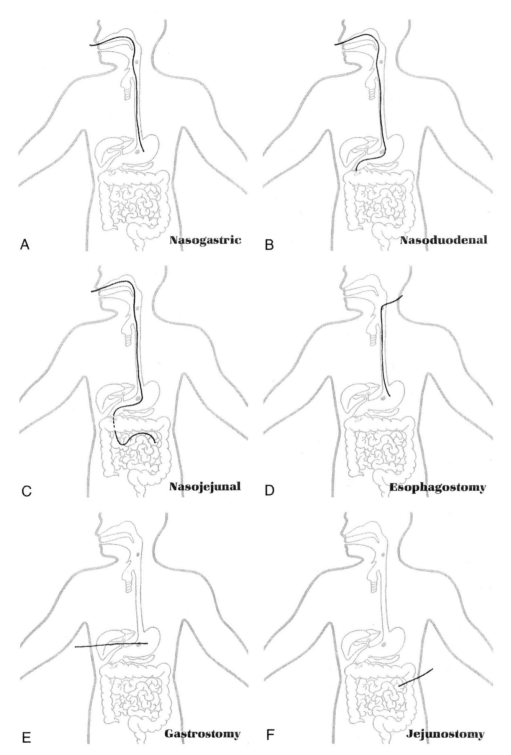

A Nasogastric   B Nasoduodenal

C Nasojejunal   D Esophagostomy

E Gastrostomy   F Jejunostomy

FIGURE 13–1. Enteral feedings can be administered via various routes. For short-term therapy a nasogastric (*A*), nasoduodenal (*B*), or nasojejunal (*C*) tube may be used. For long-term therapy an esophagostomy (*D*), gastrostomy (*E*), or jejunostomy (*F*) tube may be used. A percutaneous endoscopic gastrostomy (*E*) tube does not require general surgery or laparotomy. It is inserted under endoscopic visualization. (Courtesy of Ross Laboratories, Columbus, OH, with permission.)

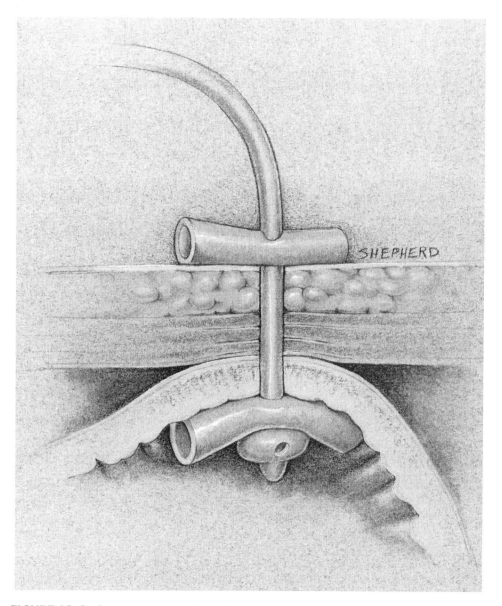

FIGURE 13–2. Percutaneous endoscopic gastrostomy (PEG tube). (Courtesy of Ross Laboratories, Columbus, OH, with permission.)

(2) Provide 1 cal/mL
(3) High in carbohydrates
(4) Require functioning gastrointestinal (GI) tract for digestion
b. Vivonex
(1) Kool-Aid–like fluid
(2) High in protein
(3) Requires no digestion
(4) Leaves no GI residue

5. General side effects/complications
a. Diarrhea, abdominal bloating, vomiting, gastric retention
b. Electrolyte imbalances
c. Aspiration
d. Drying of oral cavity
e. Irritation of nares
f. Dumping syndrome
6. Nursing implications

a. Nasogastric (NG) tube supplemental feedings
  (1) Select smallest diameter of tube that will allow for feeding to flow.
  (2) Formulas that supply 1 kcal/mL will meet most client requirements.
  (3) The supplement should be kept refrigerated but then allowed to warm to room temperature prior to administration.
  (4) May be administered by intermittent gravity flow or continuous feeding with a pump.
  (5) Keep the head of the bed elevated 35 to 45 degrees during feedings to prevent aspiration.
  (6) Weigh the client daily, maintain accurate input and output (I&O), and assess hydration status.
  (7) Maintain good nasal and oral care.
  (8) Assess tube placement before intermittent gastric feedings and every 4 hours for continuous feedings.
b. Gastric tube (G-tube; PEG tube) supplemental feedings
  (1) Intermittent feedings should not exceed 500 mL at a time, given over 30 minutes.
  (2) Solution should be warmed to near body temperature prior to administration (cold feedings cause cramping and diarrhea).
  (3) Stimulate the digestive tract by having the client suck on a hard candy just before and during the feeding.
  (4) Good skin care around tube insertion site is important—hydrochloric acid may seep around the tube and cause breakdown of the skin.
  (5) G-tube may be permanent for some clients; evaluate client for problems with alteration in body image.

HYPERALIMENTATION/TOTAL PARENTERAL NUTRITION (TPN)

1. TPN solution makeup
  a. D50W is usually the base solution.
  b. Aminosyn is added to the D50W.
    (1) Contains essential amino acids
    (2) Requires no digestion, and the body can use it immediately to rebuild tissues
  c. Vitamins.
  d. Minerals.
  e. Electrolytes.
  f. Essential trace elements.
2. The solution is highly hypertonic.
  a. Administration is required by central indwelling venous catheter (central venous pressure [CVP] catheter; jugular vein catheter).
  b. Use of peripheral veins is possible for short term but quickly leads to thrombophlebitis.
3. Uses
  a. Restore/maintain normal body composition and nutrition in individuals who are unable to meet their needs via the GI tract
  b. Promote healing and recovery of clients postoperatively by supplementing nutrients taken orally
4. General side effects/complications
  a. Hyperglycemia
  b. Fluid volume overload; hypertension; congestive heart failure (CHF)
  c. Air embolism
  d. Infections (catheter site; systemic)
  e. Renal failure
5. Nursing implications
  a. Assess clients' nutritional and hydration status daily.
    (1) Daily weights
    (2) Accurate I&O
  b. Monitor blood glucose every 4 hours with finger-stick blood sugars because of high glucose content in the solution.
    (1) Start TPN solutions slowly and increase gradually.
    (2) Supplemental insulin may be required initially, even in nondiabetics.
    (3) Monitor for signs and symptoms of hyperglycemia and diabetic ketoacidosis (DKA).
    (4) Never increase the rate of infusions of TPN if they get behind for some reason.
    (5) When discontinuing solution, do so slowly. *Never* stop suddenly—this may lead to insulin shock.
  c. Monitor for and prevent infection.
    (1) Often clients receiving TPN are malnourished and at risk for infection because of their condition.
    (2) High-glucose-content solution is excellent culture medium for bacteria and yeast.

(3) Use strict aseptic technique when handling catheter, tubing, and solution bottle.

(4) Check client's temperature every 4 hours (earliest sign of infection is an elevated temperature).

(5) Culture purulent catheter drainage.

(6) Refrigerate TPN until 1 hour before administration.

(7) Inspect solution for turbidity, precipitates, or cracks in bottle.

(8) Administer solution via intravenous tubing with 0.22 micron in-line filter, and change tube with each bottle.

(9) Do not allow solution to hang more than 12 hours (check hospital policy).

(10) If connections should come apart, the entire system must be replaced as a unit.

(11) Never "break the system" to add medications to the line.

(12) The TPN should have its own line with nothing else running through it.

d. Monitor for and avoid fluid volume overload.

(1) Always use an infusion pump/controller.

(2) Assess the client, particularly the elderly client, every 4 hours for signs of fluid overload (elevated blood pressure [BP], rales, increasing CVP, shortness of breath, edema, urine output).

e. Monitor for, prevent, or treat air embolus.

(1) Put the head of the bed down flat when changing TPN tubing.

(2) Instruct client to bear down and/or hold breath when changing intravenous tubing to increase the pressure in the subclavian vein.

(3) Clamp the subclavian or central catheter during tubing changes.

(4) Purge the line of ALL air before connecting.

(5) Monitor client for signs and symptoms of air embolism (short of breath, chest pain, coughing, cyanosis, tachycardia, or a churning noise in the chest upon auscultation).

(6) If an air embolism is suspected, clamp catheter and position on left side with the head lower than the body to keep air from going into pulmonary circulation, left heart, and into arterial circulation.

(7) Report suspected air embolism immediately, treat shock, relieve hypoxia with oxygen.

f. Provide catheter site care.

(1) Check hospital policy for site care; usually change dressing on site every 24 hours. Use an antibiotic ointment at site, and use sterile gloves.

(2) Have client turn face away from insertion site during dressing change to prevent contamination from airway organisms.

(3) If in policy, flush catheter with heparin solution between infusions if treatment is intermittent.

(4) Monitor for catheter-site infections (redness, drainage at site).

6. Infusion of lipids

a. Lipids are fat emulsion fluids that can be administered directly into the circulatory system through a central intravenous line.

(1) They require no digestion and are in a ready-to-use form by the body.

(2) Usually 500 mL are administered every other day.

(3) Solution appears as a milky-white liquid in a glass bottle.

b. Uses

(1) Clients receiving TPN who are unable to take nutrients through the GI tract

(2) Markedly malnourished clients

c. General side effects/complications of lipid infusions

(1) Allergic reactions

(2) Chills, fever, flushing

(3) Diaphoresis

(4) Nausea, vomiting

(5) Headache, vertigo

(6) Pressure over eyes

(7) Other complications similar to TPN

d. Nursing implications for lipid solutions

(1) Use an electronic infusion pump and monitor rate of infusion closely.

(2) If at all possible, use a separate subclavian line for administration (sometimes given while TPN is turned off).

(3) Use the special vented tubing that comes with solution.

(4) Do not use intravenous line filters with lipids, inasmuch as particles are too large to pass through and will clog the tubing.

(5) Take baseline vitals. Repeat every 10 minutes during first 30 minutes of infusion.

(6) Discontinue and notify physician if side effects occur.

(7) Other complications similar to TPN.

VITAMINS

1. Vitamins include several types of substances that are required in small amounts for normal development and functioning of the body.
   a. These are generally considered food supplements and not regulated by the FDA.
   b. Some vitamins are used like medications to treat and cure certain disease processes.
   c. Fat-soluble vitamins include vitamins A, D, E, K.
      (1) These can become toxic in the body if taken in excessive amounts.
      (2) Clients with liver or renal disorders are at risk for toxicity.
   d. Water-soluble vitamins are B-complex and C.
      (1) Excreted by the kidneys
      (2) Necessary for the healing process and rebuilding of damaged tissues
2. Pyridoxine (vitamin B_6)
   a. Uses
      (1) Treatment of vitamin B_6 deficiency states (seborrheic dermatitis on face, stomatitis, glossitis)
      (2) Adjunct therapy for nausea and vomiting associated with morning sickness and radiation therapy
      (3) Treatment of central nervous system (CNS) complications of isoniazid (INH) therapy (depression, peripheral neuropathy, convulsions)
   b. Modes of action
      (1) Enhances certain metabolic steps involving amino acid metabolism
      (2) Suppresses lactation in breast-feeding mothers
      (3) Increases the peripheral decarboxylation of levodopa, decreasing its availability
   c. Interactions
      (1) Inhibits the effect of levodopa therapy in clients with Parkinson's disease
      (2) Inactivated by high-temperature food preparation

d. General side effects: few
   (1) Excess vitamin B_6 is metabolized by the liver and excreted in the urine.
e. Nursing implications
   (1) Give supplemental medication as ordered for treatment of deficiency states caused by INH therapy.
   (2) Avoid high-temperature preparation of foods containing vitamin B_6 (soybeans, wheat germ, fish, liver, kidney, nuts).
   (3) Instruct breast-feeding mothers to avoid vitamin supplements with B_6 and foods containing large amounts of the vitamin.

MINERALS/ELECTROLYTES

1. Minerals are substances found in the earth that generally combine with other minerals to form compounds.
2. Ions are electrically charged elements.
   a. Cations are ions with a positive charge.
   b. Anions are ions with a negative charge.
3. Electrolytes are formed when ions mix with water.
   a. Sodium (Na) is the most common electrolyte found in the body.
      (1) It is present in most foods.
      (2) It is necessary for maintenance of normal hydration status and function of muscles and neurons.
   b. Potassium (K) is the second most common electrolyte found in the body.
      (1) It is vital for the functioning of muscles and the nervous system.
      (2) The heart is especially sensitive to abnormal levels of potassium.
      (3) Normal serum potassium is 3.5 to 5.5 mEq/L.
      (4) It is excreted freely by the kidneys.
4. Medications: electrolyte supplements (potassium)
   a. Uses
      (1) Clients taking diuretics
      (2) Clients with chronic diarrhea, ileostomies, or colostomies
      (3) Clients with adrenal gland abnormalities
      (4) Clients with diabetes insipidus (DI)
   b. Modes of action
      (1) Interact with sodium in the cells to produce depolarization

(2) Maintain acid/base balance, isotonicity, and electrophysiologic balance of the cell

c. Key medications: potassium chloride (KCL) (K-tabs)

d. General side effects

(1) GI irritation (nausea, vomiting, abdominal cramping, gastritis, ulcers)

(2) Dysrhythmia, electrocardiogram (ECG) changes

(3) Disorientation, weakness

(4) Irritation at the intravenous site

e. Nursing implications

(1) Monitor client for signs of toxicity (ECG changes, bradycardia/tachycardia).

(2) Monitor serum potassium levels closely for effectiveness.

(3) Instruct client to take medication with food to reduce GI irritation.

(4) Warn clients not to chew or crush extended-release tablets or capsules; take with a full glass of liquid.

(5) Monitor intravenous sites closely when administered for redness, pain, or irritation.

(6) Always administer potassium-containing intravenous medications on a controller or pump.

(7) Intravenous infusion rates should not exceed 1 mEq per minute in adults; rate should be no more than 40 mEq in 1000 mL of intravenous solution.

(8) Instruct clients to avoid using salt-substitute products while taking potassium supplements.

(9) Teach clients about food sources of potassium.

three

Practice Tests

TEST 1

1. A client asks the nurse about taking two medications together. The nurse recognizes that there will be an antagonistic medication interaction and explains that when the two medications are taken together:
   A. Medication absorption will be increased.
   B. There will be a decrease in stomach acid and decreased absorption.
   C. One medication will decrease or eliminate the effect of the other medication.
   D. One medication produces the same effects as the other.

2. A physician orders an IV nitroglycerin drip to be titrated. Which of the following would be the most likely parameters for this medication?
   A. Chest pain and level of consciousness (LOC)
   B. Respirations and urine output
   C. Blood pressure and pulse
   D. Headache pain and blood pressure

3. In teaching a client about the side effects of a beta-blocker medication to be taken at home, the nurse explains that the atrioventricular (A-V) node is often affected because the function of the A-V node in the heart is to:
   A. Initiate depolarizing impulses
   B. Increase the force of myocardial contraction and increase myocardial oxygen demand
   C. Delay and block out extra impulses
   D. Allow for bypass of the normal conduction system

4. Two medications taken at the same time produce an effect that is the sum of the effects of both medications. This interaction is called:
   A. Additive
   B. Antagonistic
   C. Indifference
   D. Synergistic

5. A 78-year-old client is hospitalized and receives digoxin (Lanoxin) IV. The nurse should withhold the drug and notify the physician if the patient's:
   A. Respiratory rate falls below 14.
   B. History reveals liver failure.
   C. Pulse is 54 beats per minute.
   D. Blood pressure is 72/40 mm Hg.

6. For which of the following reasons would a client be receiving furosemide (Lasix)?
   A. Hypotension
   B. Myxedema
   C. Anasarca
   D. Cerebral aneurysm

7. The physician orders an IV heparin drip to run at 1200 U/h. The heparin is mixed 20,000 U in 500 mL of D5W. The tubing has a drip factor of 10. The nurse would set the IV pump at:
   A. 3 mL/h
   B. 30 mL/h
   C. 300 mL/h
   D. 30 gtt/min

8. A hospitalized client with terminal cancer has been receiving morphine sulfate 5 mg IV q 4 h for the past 3 weeks for pain relief. She now states that the pain is still present, even after the medication is given. The nurse recognizes that this client:
   A. Has developed a physical dependency to the medication
   B. Is seeking attention for herself because of poor self-image
   C. Resents the fact that the nurse is healthy
   D. Has developed tolerance to the narcotic

9. A client asks a nurse what a medication is called that increases the force of the cardiac muscle. The best response by the nurse is, "This medication is known as a:
   A. Positive chronotropic medication"
   B. Positive inotropic medication"
   C. Negative inotropic medication"
   D. Negative dromotropic medication"

10. Which of the following would be the most desirable diet for a patient taking cardiac glycosides?
    A. High-sodium, low-potassium, high-fat
    B. Low-sodium, low-potassium, low-fat
    C. High-iron, high-calcium, high-potassium
    D. Low-sodium, high-potassium, low-fat

11. A nurse assess a client to be developing the late signs of lanoxin (Digoxin) toxicity, which include:
    A. Junctional dysrhythmia, A-V block
    B. Anorexia, headache
    C. Renal failure, aplastic anemia
    D. Disorientation, vomiting

12. In assessing a client prior to administration of a calcium channel blocker, which of the following elements from the client's history would be a contraindication for the use of these medications? A history of:
    A. Liver failure
    B. Severe hypertension
    C. Increased intracranial pressure
    D. Asthma

13. An important nursing consideration when administering nitroglycerin (NTG) IV is:
  A. Place the medication in a glass bottle.
  B. Moisten the patient's mucous membranes first.
  C. Follow the medication with a full glass of water.
  D. Piggyback other medications directly into the NTG line.

14. What is a major advantage of dobutamine (Dobutrex) over dopamine (Intropine) for clients in cardiogenic shock?
  A. It produces less hypotension as a side effect.
  B. Acute renal failure is rarely seen with this medication.
  C. It does not produce vasoconstriction.
  D. The dosage of the medication is much smaller.

15. A medication is to be given by injection within the subdural space and into the cerebrospinal fluid for the treatment of meningitis. This route is called:
  A. Intraspinal
  B. Intracutaneous
  C. Intra-articular
  D. Intrathecal

16. A client is receiving IV heparin 4500 U q 4 h. A partial thromboplastin time (PTT) is drawn a half hour before his 8:00 A.M. dose. The results come back at 7:55 A.M. with the PTT at 92 seconds. The most appropriate action for the nurse would be to:
  A. Give the next two doses at the same time
  B. Give the next dose and call the results to the physician
  C. Immediately check the patient's vital signs and LOC
  D. Hold the dose, and call the results to the physician

17. A client is to receive a loading dose of digoxin (Lanoxin). The nurse would recognize that the physician ordered the correct dose if it was:
  A. 10 mg PO q 4 h
  B. 0.25 mg PO q 8 h × 3
  C. 0.125–0.25 mg PO qd
  D. 100–150 mg IM q 12 h

18. A client is to receive 1 L of 1/4 NS in 10 hours. No IV pumps are available at this time. The drop factor for the tubing is 10 gtt/mL. At what rate should the fluid run?
  A. 100 mL/h
  B. 100 gtt/min
  C. 17 gtt/min
  D. 17 mL/h

19. A client is to receive furosemide (Lasix) 60 mg IV push. The medication comes in a vial labeled "Lasix—100 mg in 10 mL." How much of the medication should the nurse give?
  A. 16.6 mL
  B. 0.6 mL
  C. 6 mL
  D. 6.6 mL

20. A 54-year-old female client is receiving captopril (Capoten) for which of the following problems?
   A. Chronic hypertension
   B. Venous thrombosis
   C. Hypertensive crisis
   D. Unstable angina pectoris

21. A client admitted to the hospital in hypertensive crisis is ordered to receive hydralazine (Apresoline) 20 mg IV for a blood pressure greater than 190/100. The best response of the nurse to this order is to:
   A. Call the physician because the dose is too small
   B. Give the medication as ordered
   C. Give half the dose first to see how it affects the blood pressure
   D. Hold the medication, and call the physician because the dose is too large

22. In teaching a client about methyldopa (Aldomet), the nurse would be correct in stating that it is classified as a(n):
   A. Direct vasodilator
   B. Antiadrenergic, alpha$_2$-blocker
   C. Diuretic, antihypertensive
   D. Anticholinergic, beta$_1$-blocker

23. The most common process by which drugs cross the membranes of the cells of the body is called:
   A. Passive diffusion
   B. Active filtration
   C. Active transport
   D. Passive pinocytosis

24. A 23-year-old female college student who takes birth control pills and is a heavy smoker develops a thrombus in her leg. She is admitted to the hospital and is started on heparin. Which of the following nursing actions would be the most important for this client?
   A. Allow her to go to the designated smoking area to prevent nicotine withdrawal.
   B. Give her aspirin for headaches and joint pain.
   C. Maintain her on strict bed rest.
   D. Have her walk every 4 hours to prevent pneumonia and joint stiffness.

25. A client is to take furosemide (Lasix) at home. The nurse would know that the client requires more teaching if she states:
   A. "This medication should be taken just before bedtime."
   B. "I need to eat lots of fresh fruits and vegetables."
   C. "I need to continue taking the medication even when I start feeling really good."
   D. "If I feel really dizzy or weak, I need to call the physician."

26. Which of the following would be an indication that the nurse is giving IV push furosemide (Lasix) too rapidly?
   A. The client has a sudden urge to void.
   B. The IV pump begins to alarm "occlusion."
   C. The client states that his or her ears are "plugged up."
   D. The nurse administers 40 mg over 4 minutes.

27. A client is to receive tissue plasminogen activator (t-PA). The nurse under-stands that this client probably is:
    A. In congestive heart failure
    B. Experiencing an acute myocardial infarction
    C. Developing a blood clot in his leg
    D. Bleeding from a gastric ulcer

28. A nursing student who just gave her client 50,000 U heparin IV could ex-pect to administer which of the following?
    A. protamine sulfate
    B. diltiazem (Cardizem)
    C. aquamephytin (vitamin K)
    D. atropine sulfate

29. The nurse recognizes that a client who is receiving the medication hy-drochlorothiazide (HCTZ) most likely has:
    A. Hypertension
    B. Pulmonary embolism
    C. Increased intracranial pressure
    D. Chronic bronchitis

30. A client is started on prazosin (Minipress). The most important action to be included in the nursing care plan related to this medication is:
    A. Monitoring the client's intake and output (I & O) and daily weight
    B. Making sure the client takes the medication with milk or food
    C. Watching for signs of cardiogenic shock
    D. Monitoring the client's blood pressure and heart rate

31. Which of the following routes of administration would have the fastest rate of absorption?
    A. PO
    B. SC
    C. IM
    D. Inhalation

32. A student working in the emergency room (ER) is asked by the registered nurse (RN) to draw up an IV injection of aminocaproic acid (Amicar) for a client. Which condition is the patient most likely experiencing?
    A. Hypertensive crisis
    B. Cardiogenic shock
    C. Acute respiratory distress
    D. Hemorrhage

33. Common side effects that may occur when a client is taking furosemide (Lasix) for hypertension include:
    A. Tachycardia, respiratory stimulation
    B. Restlessness, insomnia
    C. Abdominal and leg cramps
    D. Weakness, edema

34. When giving medications, the nurse recognizes that responses other than the expected clinical responses that occur at higher than normal doses are called:
    A. Idiosyncratic reactions
    B. Toxic effects
    C. Side effects
    D. Therapeutic effects

35. In assessing a client with hyperthyroidism, the nurse would most likely note which of the following symptoms?
    A. Tachycardia, exophthalmos, and labial moods
    B. Anorexia, bradycardia, and depression
    C. Weight gain, buffalo hump, and immunosuppression
    D. Mental slowness, slurred speech, and obesity

36. In a toddler, the nurse should consider which of the following factors most important in the administration of a medication?
    A. Sex of the child
    B. Age of the child
    C. Weight of the child
    D. Developmental level of the child

37. While teaching a client with hypothyroidism about her home medications, the nurse includes the fact that levothyroxine (Synthroid) is a synthetic form of:
    A. Thyrocalcitonin
    B. Triiodothyronine
    C. Thyroxine
    D. Thyrocortropine

38. When assessing a client who is taking levothyroxine (Synthroid), the nurse would expect to see which of the following side effects?
    A. Nervousness, tachycardia, and tremors
    B. Somnolence, bradycardia, and paraesthesia
    C. Hyperglycemia, hypertension, and edema
    D. Buffalo hump, constipation, and sodium loss

39. A client with hyperthyroidism is receiving propylthiouracil (Propacil) for the condition. The nurse recognizes that the primary mode of action for this medication is to:
    A. Destroy part of the thyroid gland so that it will not produce as much thyroid hormone
    B. Inhibit the conversion of T_4 to T_3
    C. Suppress the anterior pituitary gland to slow down its hormonal secretions
    D. Sedate the CNS and suppress the cardiac function

40. Plant sources of medications that are composed of carbon, hydrogen, nitrogen, and oxygen are called:
    A. Glycosides
    B. Gums
    C. Alkaloids
    D. Resins

41. Which of the following statements about the effects of insulin on the body made by a client who has recently been diagnosed with type 1 diabetes would indicate that additional teaching was needed?
    A. Insulin allows the cells to absorb and use glucose.
    B. Insulin increases the stores of fat and glycogen.
    C. Insulin is made in the alpha cells of the pancreas.
    D. Insulin increases fat and protein metabolism.

42. A distinguishing characteristic of a type 1 diabetic client is:
    A. The blood sugar can be controlled with diet.
    B. Exogenous insulin is required for life.
    C. Insulin to maintain normal blood sugar can be taken orally.
    D. Type 1 diabetes always starts in childhood.

43. The physician orders an IV of D51/2NS started at 200 mL/h on a client in diabetic ketoacidosis (DKA) with a blood sugar of 550. An initial dose of 75 U insulin is given IV. What type of insulin is used?
    A. NPH insulin
    B. Lente insulin
    C. Ultralente insulin
    D. Regular insulin

44. A 52-year-old client was diagnosed as having type 2 diabetes 5 years ago. His blood sugar has been controlled by diet and chlorpropamide (Diabinese). After a recent illness, his physician changed him to glyburide (DiaBeta). An important teaching measure the nurse should emphasize for this client in relation to this new medication is:
    A. It is less potent, so he needs to take a larger dose.
    B. It stimulates insulin production, so he needs to eat shortly after taking the medication.
    C. It is more potent and can be taken every other day.
    D. The two medications are really the same.

45. A set of written guidelines for treating certain diseases or sets of symptoms, often found in hospital special-care units, is called:
    A. Single orders
    B. Physician orders
    C. Stat orders
    D. Standing orders

46. The nurse tells a postoperative client that she is administering a medication that will reduce the pain of surgery. With this statement, the nurse recognizes the importance of the client's:
    A. Attitude about narcotic medications
    B. Ability to control his environment
    C. Expectations about the medication's effects
    D. Culture and value system

47. In teaching a newly diagnosed type 1 diabetic client who is also an alcoholic, the nurse includes the fact that alcohol in moderate mounts will:
    A. Increase the blood sugar
    B. Be absorbed more rapidly because of the diabetes
    C. Increase the risk of vascular complications
    D. Decrease the blood sugar

48. Which of the following is the most appropriate nursing measure when administering transdermal nitroglycerin to a client? Place the patch:
    A. In the same spot each time to increase absorption
    B. Only at the fifth intercostal space, left midclavicular line over the heart for maximum effectiveness
    C. On the left arm only
    D. At a different location with each application

49. A client's serum digoxin level is 3.1 ng/mL. The most appropriate action for the nurse would be to:
    A. Administer the next dose of digoxin as scheduled.
    B. Assess the client's pulse and blood pressure before administering the next dose.
    C. Hold the next digoxin dose and call the physician.
    D. Call a code, and begin CPR.

50. A client who is seen in the outpatient clinic for hypertension is started on methyldopa (Aldomet). The nurse instructs the client that the most common early side effect of methyldopa therapy is:
    A. Sedation
    B. Persistent cough
    C. Tachycardia
    D. Hypotension

ANSWERS/RATIONALES

1. **Correct Answer: C.** This defines antagonistic interaction.

Rationales for Other Answer Choices: A. Generally decreases absorption. **B.** No effect on stomach acid. **D.** Not an antagonistic reaction.
Nursing Process Phase: implementation; client need: safe and effective care environment; concern area: medical/surgical

2. **Correct Answer: C.** These two are affected by NTG; usual parameters are systolic BP <90, pulse >110.

Rationales for Other Answer Choices: A. Pain relief is a secondary consideration, LOC not affected. **B.** Not directly affected by NTG. **D.** Not commonly used as parameters.
Nursing Process Phase: assessment; client need: safe and effective care environment; concern area: medical/surgical

3. **Correct Answer: C.** These functions are enhanced by beta-blockers sometimes to the point of causing bradycardia and A-V blocks.

Rationales for Other Answer Choices: A. Function of the S-A node. **B.** MOA of lanoxin. **D.** Function of the bundles of Kent.
Nursing Process Phase: implementation; client need: safe and effective care environment; concern area: medical/surgical

4. **Correct Answer: A.** Defines the term; for example, tylenol with codeine.

Rationales for Other Answer Choices: B. Two medications cancel each other out. **C.** Two medications have no influence on each other. **D.** The end result is greater than an additive effect (e.g., alcohol and valium).
Nursing Process Phase: planning; client need: health promotion and maintenance; concern area: medical/surgical

5. **Correct Answer: C.** Usual parameter is <60 BPM.

Rationales for Other Answer Choices: A. Has no effect on respirations. **B.** Liver failure is not a contraindication. **D.** BP not directly affected by this medication; this may be the client's normal pressure.
Nursing Process Phase: assessment; client need: safe and effective care environment; concern area: medical/surgical

6. **Correct Answer: C.** This is generalized body edema, often treated with diuretics.

Rationales for Other Answer Choices: A. Hypertension is treated with diuretics. **B.** This is a nonpitting sogginess of the skin found in hypothyroidism. **D.** Not treated with diuretics.
Nursing Process Phase: analysis; client need: health promotion and maintenance; concern area: medical/surgical

7. **Correct Answer: B.** $\text{Concentration} = \dfrac{20,000}{500} = 40 \text{ U/mL}$

$$\text{rate} = 1200 : x :: 40 : 1$$

$$x = 1200/40 = 30 \text{ mL/h}$$

Rationales for Other Answer Choices: A, C, D are incorrect; tubing drip factor not necessary when a pump is used. All pumps are in mL/h.
Nursing Process Phase: implementation; client need: safe and effective care environment; concern area: medical/surgical

8. **Correct Answer: D.** Long-term use of central nervous system (CNS) medications can lead to tolerance, when more and more of the medication is required to achieve the same effect.

Rationales for Other Answer Choices: A. Lack of relief does not indicate dependency. **B.** Not indicated by the symptoms. **C.** Cannot conclude this from the information in the question.
Nursing Process Phase: planning; client need: safe and effective care environment; concern area: medical/surgical

9. **Correct Answer: B.** These medications are used in CHF.

Rationales for Other Answer Choices: A. Increases the rate of the heart. **C.** Decreases the force of contraction. **D.** Decreases the rate at which the impulses travel through the conduction system of the heart.
Nursing Process Phase: implementation; client need: health promotion and maintenance; concern area: medical/surgical

10. **Correct Answer: D.** These medications often increase urinary output, promoting the loss of potassium. Low-sodium and low-fat diets are recommended for clients with cardiac diseases.

Rationales for Other Answer Choices: A. Just the opposite of the best diet. **B.** Need more potassium. **C.** Iron and calcium not affected by these medications.
Nursing Process Phase: implementation; client need: health promotion and maintenance; concern area: medical/surgical

11. **Correct Answer: A.** Cardiac blocks and dysrhythmias are late signs of lanoxin toxicity.

Rationales for Other Answer Choices: B. Early signs of lanoxin toxicity. **C.** Not associated with lanoxin toxicity. **D.** Early signs of lanoxin toxicity.
Nursing Process Phase: assessment; client need: safe and effective care environment; concern area: medical/surgical

12. **Correct Answer: A.** These medications are converted by the liver into an active form. Liver failure may render the medications ineffective, or the medications may cause more damage to the liver.

Rationales for Other Answer Choices: B. Are often used to lower blood pressure. **C.** Not a contraindication. **D.** Not a contraindication.
Nursing Process Phase: assessment; client need: safe and effective care environment; concern area: medical/surgical

13. **Correct Answer: A.** The PVC in plastic IV bottles leaches the NTG out of the solution.

Rationales for Other Answer Choices: B. No effect on IV NTG. **C.** IV medications do not need to be followed by water. **D.** NTG is incompatible with most IV medications; never piggyback anything into it.
Nursing Process Phase: planning; client need: safe and effective care environment; concern area: medical/surgical

14. **Correct Answer: C.** Both increase cardiac output, but dobutamine is less likely to cause tissue or organ damage caused by vasoconstriction.

Rationales for Other Answer Choices: A. Hypertension is a side effect of both. **B.** Renal failure not a complication of either medication. **D.** Dosage is based on client response (cardiac output, BP, urine).
Nursing Process Phase: planning; client need: safe and effective care environment; concern area: medical/surgical

15. **Correct Answer: D.** Defines the term; used with meningitis.

Rationales for Other Answer Choices: A. Injected into the spinal cord (e.g., anesthesia). **B.** Made-up term, has no meaning. **C.** Injected into a joint.
Nursing Process Phase: planning; client need: safe and effective care environment; concern area: medical/surgical

16. **Correct Answer: D.** Therapeutic PTT is 50 to 70 seconds. PTTs over 90 place the client at high risk for bleeding. It is likely the physician will decrease the dose or even hold the next dose.

Rationales for Other Answer Choices: A. Totally inappropriate action. **B.** The next dose should be held. **C.** No need for this action at this time.
Nursing Process Phase: implementation; client need: safe and effective care environment; concern area: medical/surgical

17. **Correct Answer: B.** Normal loading dose for lanoxin is three times the maintenance dose, divided, in 24 hours.

Rationales for Other Answer Choices: A. This is an excessive dosage. **C.** Usually not given in a range. **D.** Dosage is excessive.
Nursing Process Phase: planning; client need: safe and effective care environment; concern area: medical/surgical

18. **Correct Answer: C.** $\dfrac{\text{amount to infuse} \times \text{drop factor}}{\text{time (min)}}$

$$\frac{1000 \times 10}{600} = 16.6 \ (17) \ \text{gtt/min}$$

Rationales for Other Answer Choices: A, B, D are incorrect.
Nursing Process Phase: planning; client need: safe and effective care environment; concern area: medical/surgical

19. **Correct Answer: C.** $100 : 10 :: 60 : x$

$$100x = 600$$

$$x = 600/100 = 6 \ \text{mL}$$

Rationales for Other Answer Choices: A, B, D are incorrect.
Nursing Process Phase: implementation; client need: safe and effective care environment; concern area: medical/surgical

20.   **Correct Answer: A.**   This is an ACE inhibitor commonly used for chronic hypertension.

Rationales for Other Answer Choices: B. Use heparin.   **C.** Only in oral form, not effective for crisis.   **D.** Not used for this condition.
Nursing Process Phase: analysis; client need: health promotion and maintenance; concern area: medical/surgical

21.   **Correct Answer: B.**   Normal dosage range for crisis is 10 to 20 mg.

Rationales for Other Answer Choices: A. Dose is correct.   **C.** This is not an acceptable nursing practice.   **D.** Dose is correct.
Nursing Process Phase: implementation; client need: safe and effective care environment; concern area: medical/surgical

22.   **Correct Answer: B.**   This medication reduces the sympathetic stimulation of the heart and produces vasodilation.

Rationales for Other Answer Choices: A. Incorrect classification.   **C.** No diuretic effect.   **D.** Anticholinergics tend to increase blood pressure.
Nursing Process Phase: planning; client need: safe and effective care environment; concern area: medical/surgical

23.   **Correct Answer: A.**   Medications move from an area of higher concentration to an area of lower concentration.

Rationales for Other Answer Choices: B. Process does not occur in the body.   **C.** Very few medications move across membranes this way.   **D.** This way bacteria are destroyed.
Nursing Process Phase: planning; client need: health promotion and maintenance; concern area: medical/surgical

24.   **Correct Answer: C.**   Bed rest is important to prevent dislodgement of the clot, which could become a pulmonary emboli.

Rationales for Other Answer Choices: A. Need to maintain bed rest; smoking constricts blood vessels and may contribute to clot formation.   **B.** Aspirin potentiates anticoagulants and should be avoided.   **D.** Need to maintain bed rest.
Nursing Process Phase: implementation; client need: safe and effective care environment; concern area: medical/surgical

25.   **Correct Answer: A.**   This medication should be taken early in the day. If taken before bed, client would be up during the night voiding.

Rationales for Other Answer Choices: B. Tends to wash out potassium.   **C.** For long-term use for hypertension (HTN) or congestive heart failure (CHF).   **D.** Side effects of the medication that may require reduction of its dose.
Nursing Process Phase: evaluation; client need: safe and effective care environment; concern area: medical/surgical

26. **Correct Answer: C.** Too rapid administration of this medication can cause a transient deafness.

Rationales for Other Answer Choices: A. A desired effect of the medication. **B.** Need to put the pump in reset. **D.** Appropriate rate of administration (10 mg/min).
Nursing Process Phase: assessment; client need: health promotion and maintenance; concern area: medical/surgical

27. **Correct Answer: B.** The most common use of this potent thrombolytic medication is to dissolve clots in the coronary arteries, which can cause a myocardial infarction (MI).

Rationales for Other Answer Choices: A. Not used for this condition. **C.** Not used for clots in peripheral blood vessels. **D.** Would make the bleeding worse.
Nursing Process Phase: analysis; client need: health promotion and maintenance; concern area: medical/surgical

28. **Correct Answer: A.** This is antidote for heparin toxicity; 50,000 U is 10 times the normal dose.

Rationales for Other Answer Choices: B. Not used for this problem. **C.** This is the antidote for coumadin overdose. **D.** Not used for this condition.
Nursing Process Phase: implementation; client need: safe and effective care environment; concern area: medical/surgical

29. **Correct Answer: A.** The common use for this diuretic is the control of blood pressure.

Rationales for Other Answer Choices: B. Not an appropriate use. **C.** Does not affect increased intracranial pressure (ICP). **D.** No respiratory effects.
Nursing Process Phase: analysis; client need: safe and effective care environment; concern area: medical/surgical

30. **Correct Answer: D.** This is a potent antihypertensive and can cause marked hypotension and tachycardia.

Rationales for Other Answer Choices: A. Not a diuretic; these measures are used with diuretics. **B.** Does not need to be taken with food. **C.** It is unlikely it would cause cardiogenic shock.
Nursing Process Phase: planning; client need: safe and effective care environment; concern area: medical/surgical

31. **Correct Answer: D.** The large surface area of capillaries in the lungs provides for rapid absorption of medications.

Rationales for Other Answer Choices: A. Generally provides slow absorption. **B.** Absorption is slow from SC—poor circulation in fat. **C.** Faster than **A** or **B**, but slower than **D.**
Nursing Process Phase: implementation; client need: health promotion and maintenance; concern area: medical/surgical

32. **Correct Answer: D.** This medication is used as an antidote to streptokinase and heparin or can be used with general bleeding disorders.

Rationales for Other Answer Choices: A. Does not affect blood pressure. **B.** Does not affect cardiac output.   **C.** No effect on the respiratory system.
Nursing Process Phase: analysis; client need: safe and effective care environment; concern area: medical/surgical

33.   **Correct Answer: C.**   These result when large amounts of calcium are lost with the increased urination.

Rationales for Other Answer Choices: A. Not common side effects of this medication. **B.** Not common side effects of this medication. **D.** Not common side effects of this medication.
Nursing Process Phase: assessment; client need: safe and effective care environment; concern area: medical/surgical

34.   **Correct Answer: B.**   These tend to be more severe than side effects and occur when the blood levels are excessive.

Rationales for Other Answer Choices: A. These are reactions that are the opposite of what is expected. **C.** These occur at normal, therapeutic blood levels. **D.** These are the desired effects of the medication.
Nursing Process Phase: planning; client need: safe and effective care environment; concern area: medical/surgical

35.   **Correct Answer: A.**   Increased thyroid levels increase metabolism and stimulate the CNS.

Rationales for Other Answer Choices: B. May indicate anorexia nervosa or severe depression. **C.** Symptoms of Cushing's syndrome. **D.** Symptoms of hypothyroidism.
Nursing Process Phase: assessment; client need: safe and effective care environment; concern area: medical/surgical

36.   **Correct Answer: C.**   Weight (body mass) is the single most important factor in determining the dosages of child medications.

Rationales for Other Answer Choices: A. Has little effect on absorption in children. **B.** Only in so far as it helps determine size. **D.** Has little effect on the absorption of medications.
Nursing Process Phase: planning; client need: safe and effective care environment; concern area: pediatrics

37.   **Correct Answer: C.**   Same as T_4, the less active form of the thyroid hormone that is converted to T_3.

Rationales for Other Answer Choices: A. This hormone affects calcium use in the body. **B.** This is T_3. **D.** Not a hormone.
Nursing Process Phase: implementation; client need: safe and effective care environment; concern area: medical/surgical

38.   **Correct Answer: A.**   These symptoms are similar to what is seen in hyperthyroidism.

Rationales for Other Answer Choices: B. Not associated with this medication. **C.** Not associated with this medication. **D.** Not associated with this medication.
Nursing Process Phase: assessment; client need: health promotion and maintenance; concern area: medical/surgical

39. Correct Answer: B.   This medication does not directly affect the thyroid gland but lowers the levels of the more active T$_3$.

Rationales for Other Answer Choices: A. Mechanism of action (MOA) of radioactive iodine.   **C.** No effect on the pituitary.   **D.** No effect on the CNS.
Nursing Process Phase: planning; client need: safe and effective care environment; concern area: medical/surgical

40. Correct Answer: C.   Defines the term.

Rationales for Other Answer Choices: A. Medications composed of glucose and steroid molecules.   **B.** Sticky resins produced by plants.   **D.** Amorphous organic substances that are insoluble in water but soluble in alcohol.
Nursing Process Phase: planning; client need: health promotion and maintenance; concern area: medical/surgical

41. Correct Answer: C.   Insulin is made in the beta cells of the pancreas.

Rationales for Other Answer Choices: A. Correct statement.   **B.** Correct statement.
D. Correct statement.
Nursing Process Phase: evaluation; client need: safe and effective care environment; concern area: medical/surgical

42. Correct Answer: B.   Without insulin blood sugars become elevated, and client develops DKA.

Rationales for Other Answer Choices: A. Diet restrictions are necessary but insufficient by themselves.   **C.** There is no such thing as oral insulin.   **D.** Diabetes may start at any time in a person's life but often does start in childhood.
Nursing Process Phase: planning; client need: safe and effective care environment; concern area: medical/surgical

43. Correct Answer: D.   Regular insulin is the only type that can be given IV.

Rationales for Other Answer Choices: A. Cannot be given IV.   **B.** Cannot be given IV.   **C.** Cannot be given IV.
Nursing Process Phase: planning; client need: safe and effective care environment; concern area: medical/surgical

44. Correct Answer: B.   This is a second-generation oral hypoglycemic and needs similar nursing considerations as insulin.

Rationales for Other Answer Choices: A. It is more potent; requires a smaller dose.
C. It needs to be taken every day.   **D.** The medications are different; chlorpropamide is a first-generation oral hypoglycemic.
Nursing Process Phase: planning; client need: safe and effective care environment; concern area: medical/surgical

45. Correct Answer: D.   Defines the term.

Rationales for Other Answer Choices: A. One-time orders that are no longer valid after the medication is given once.   **B.** General term that covers all orders written by a physician.   **C.** Order should be carried out immediately.
Nursing Process Phase: planning; client need: safe and effective care environment; concern area: medical/surgical

46. **Correct Answer: C.** Positive expectations by the client tend to enhance the effectiveness of the medication.

Rationales for Other Answer Choices: A. Does not address this issue. **B.** Does not directly address this issue. **D.** Does not directly address these factors.
Nursing Process Phase: evaluation; client need: safe and effective care environment; concern area: medical/surgical

47. **Correct Answer: D.** Moderate amounts of alcohol decrease blood sugar levels. In diabetic clients, it may lead to hypoglycemia or insulin shock.

Rationales for Other Answer Choices: A. Large amounts of alcohol will increase the blood sugar. **B.** Absorption is the same in diabetic clients. **C.** May actually decrease vascular complications in the short term.
Nursing Process Phase: implementation; client need: safe and effective care environment; concern area: medical/surgical

48. **Correct Answer: D.** Sites should be rotated to prevent skin irritation from the medication.

Rationales for Other Answer Choices: A. Same location does not increase absorption. **B.** Placing the patch over the heart does not increase its effectiveness. **C.** Sites should be rotated.
Nursing Process Phase: implementation; client need: safe and effective care environment; concern area: medical/surgical

49. **Correct Answer: C.** Therapeutic range is 0.5 to 1.5 ng/mL. This level is toxic.

Rationales for Other Answer Choices: A. This would make the client even more toxic. **B.** Assessment of vital signs is appropriate, but the medication should not be given. **D.** Unnecessary unless the client is in cardiac arrest.
Nursing Process Phase: implementation; client need: safe and effective care environment; concern area: medical/surgical

50. **Correct Answer: A.** Drowsiness is common in early therapy but usually lessens later.

Rationales for Other Answer Choices: B. Side effect of angiotensin-converting enzyme (ACE) inhibitors. **C.** Not a common side effect. **D.** Occurs only with excessive doses.
Nursing Process Phase: planning; client need: safe and effective care environment; concern area: medical/surgical

1. A client is to receive doxorubicin (Adriamycin) 120 mg in 250 mL D5W intravenous piggyback (IVPB) to run over 2½ hours. At what rate should the nurse run this medication on a volumetric pump?
   A. 125 gtt/min
   B. 150 mL/h
   C. 100 mL/h
   D. 75 mL/min

2. The lack of control in cancer cells' growth rate is called:
   A. Anaplasia
   B. Pleomorphism
   C. Neoplasm
   D. Proliferation

3. Which of the following is classified as an alkylating anticancer drug?
   A. fluorouracil (5-FU)
   B. doxorubicin (Adriamycin)
   C. chlorambucil (Leukeran)
   D. vincristine (Oncovan)

4. Anticancer medications that work by entering the cancer cell and inhibiting the absorption of the needed nutrients are classified as:
   A. Alkylating drugs
   B. Antimetabolites
   C. Antibiotics
   D. Antiembolitics

5. An anticancer medication is classified as a vesicant. The nurse knows that this medication:
   A. Is capable of causing irritation to the skin
   B. Is capable of causing blisters on the skin
   C. Can only be given PO
   D. Must be given by deep IM injection

6. An oncology nurse is preparing several medications for administration. She recognizes that the one that is classified as a vesicant medication is:
   A. vincristine (Oncovan)
   B. fluorouracil (5-FU)
   C. cyclophosphamide (Cytoxin)
   D. chlorambucil (Leukeran)

7. A medication is to be given AU. The nurse would:
    A. Give the medication every day
    B. Place the medication in both eyes
    C. Give the medication IV slowly
    D. Place the medication in both ears

8. Antineoplastic medications are commonly combined in the treatment of cancer. Combinations of these medications are used to:
    A. Decrease the development of cell resistance
    B. Increase the length of treatment
    C. Increase the quantity of each medication used
    D. Decrease the amount of side effects of each medication

9. The normal pattern for the administration of antineoplastic medications is usually:
    A. Low doses given continuously over a long period of time
    B. Massive doses given only once
    C. Relatively high doses on a cyclic schedule
    D. IV medications alternating with PO medications

10. Medications that are used medically and have the highest abuse potential are usually classified as:
    A. Schedule I
    B. Schedule II
    C. Schedule IV
    D. Schedule V

11. After taking a medication, a client begins to vomit and breaks out in a sweat. Which type of reaction is he most likely having?
    A. Idiosyncratic
    B. Unpredictable
    C. Hypersensitive
    D. Adverse

12. A physician orders a client to receive dextromethrophan for which of the following conditions?
    A. Excessively thick mucous secretions
    B. Cough that interferes with sleep
    C. Nasal congestion due to allergy
    D. Cough related to a suppurative lung disease

13. When a client is suddenly taken off a drug, he or she has a craving for the drug and physical symptoms. The client most likely has a:
    A. Physical dependence
    B. Tolerance to the drug
    C. Psychological dependence
    D. No dependence on the substance

14. A 14-year-old client receives acetylcysteine (Mucomyst) for which of the following conditions?
    A. Severe cough
    B. Congestive heart failure
    C. Cystic fibrosis
    D. Peptic ulcer

15. A postpartum client is to receive meperidine (Demerol) 35 mg IV for pain. The medication comes in a vial labeled "50 mg/mL." How much of this medication will the nurse give?
    A. 0.7 mL
    B. 0.14 mL
    C. 1.4 mL
    D. 7 mg

16. Diphenhydramine (Benadryl) is used primarily for:
    A. Relief of allergic reactions
    B. Relief of chronic angina pain
    C. Dilation of the bronchiolus in asthma
    D. Stimulation of the cardiac muscles

17. A client asks the nurse, "Why am I taking an enteric-coated medication?" The best answer by the nurse is:
    A. They dissolve in the acid environment of the stomach and prevent ulcers.
    B. They can be crushed without any effect on their absorption.
    C. You can chew them so that they are easier to swallow.
    D. They prevent gastric irritation because they dissolve in the alkaline environment of the small intestine.

18. Neurotransmitters are released from a neuron's:
    A. Dendrites
    B. Axons
    C. Cell body
    D. Precursor

19. A contraindication for the use of antitussives is when the cough:
    A. Interferes with the activities of daily living
    B. Causes complications such as rib fractures or bradycardia
    C. Begins to act as an irritant
    D. Is related to a suppurative lung disease

20. A female client has bronchitis, so the physician orders guaifenesin (Robitussin). Which of the following client-teaching points should the nurse cover with her?
    A. Avoid becoming pregnant during guaifenesin therapy.
    B. Tell other physicians about the guaifenesin therapy; it could alter thyroid function test results.
    C. Restrict fluids to 300 mL per day.
    D. Take the medication on an empty stomach.

21. In teaching a 64-year-old client about acetylcysteine (Mucomyst), the nurse should include the fact that the effectiveness of this drug results from its ability to:
    A. Alter the molecular composition of mucus and decrease its viscosity
    B. Enter the bronchial glands and stimulate their cells to secrete watery mucus
    C. Stimulate ciliary activity and the salivary glands
    D. Increase the viscosity of bronchial secretions

22. While taking care of a client who is receiving IV antibiotics, the nurse suspects that he is having a delayed hypersensitive reaction. The nurse understands that delayed hypersensitive reactions:
    A. Are usually fatal and must be treated immediately
    B. Occur within 3 to 6 hours after administration of the medication
    C. Are produced by T lymphocytes
    D. Always produce anaphylactic shock

23. The nurse assesses a client who is receiving a theophylline medication. Which of the following assessments would indicate that the client was responding positively to the medication?
    A. Respiratory rate of 18 breaths per minute
    B. Urine output of 450 mL per shift
    C. Heart rate of 92 beats per minute (BPM)
    D. Blood pressure of 138/82

24. Which of the following statements made by a client who is to take an antitussive with codeine at home would indicate to the nurse that her teaching about the medication had been effective?
    A. "I should take this anytime I start to cough."
    B. "This medication may make me anxious and nervous."
    C. "I should call the physician if I develop diarrhea while taking this medication."
    D. "Driving my car after taking this medication could be dangerous."

25. Which of the following complaints would the nurse expect from a client who is receiving acetylcysteine (Mucomyst) by nebulizer treatment?
    A. "This medication makes my heart beat really fast."
    B. "I lose my ability to cough after taking the treatment."
    C. "The mist I breathe in smells like rotten eggs."
    D. "I get a really bad headache every time I do the treatment."

26. A client asks the nurse why the physician prescribed an antihistamine for his upper respiratory viral infections. The best answer by the nurse is that these medications:
    A. Suppress the central nervous system (CNS) and help the client sleep at night
    B. Decrease the permeability to capillary fluid, thus reducing nasal congestion
    C. Reduce pain sensation and promote client comfort
    D. Decrease the production of stomach acid, thereby preventing an ulcer from forming

27. Which of the following orders by a physician for promethazine (Phenergan) for a 35-year-old hospitalized client should the nurse question?
    A. 25 mg q 4 h prn IM
    B. 50 mg q 6 h prn IM nausea
    C. 100 mg q 4 h prn PO
    D. 25 mg q 6 h prn PO

28. What implications does the blood-brain barrier have for the administration of medications?

    A. Only IV medications can penetrate into the brain tissues.

    B. The barrier is highly resistant to water, oxygen, and carbon dioxide.

    C. Many medications are unable to penetrate the brain for their therapeutic effect.

    D. There is no significant implication because the molecules of all medications are so small they can penetrate the barrier.

29. A hospitalized client with chronic obstructive lung disease asks the nurse why the physician will not order diphenhydramine hydrochloride (HCL) (Benadryl) for her nasal congestion. Which of the following responses by the nurse is most appropriate?

    A. "Benadryl can cause bronchoconstriction that may make your breathing more difficult."

    B. "Benadryl and theophylline interact in such a way as to produce excessive agitation and sleep loss."

    C. "Because Benadryl tends to dry up secretions, it may make it more difficult for you to cough out your mucus."

    D. "The physician does not think your congestion is severe enough for this medication."

30. A client has just received morphine sulfate 5 mg IV for chest pain. Which of the following would be the most important side effect of the medication to monitor her for?

    A. Diaphoresis and flushing

    B. Constipation

    C. Hypotension

    D. Suppressed cough reflex

31. A client has both morphine sulfate (MS) and meperidine (Demerol) ordered for pain. Which of the following client assessments would lead the nurse to decide to give the morphine instead of the meperidine?

    A. Pain is much more severe than the last time the medication was given.

    B. BP 110/58, pulse 60.

    C. Temp 97.9, respirations 12/min.

    D. Peripheral pulses weak, skin color flushed.

32. Medications that suppress the limbic system would tend to:

    A. Decrease the body temperature

    B. Suppress sleep and rest

    C. Lessen feelings of anger and anxiety

    D. Increase heart and respiratory rates

33. A physician orders temazepam (Restoril) 15 mg PO prn for a client. Which of the following would be the best response by the nurse to this order?

    A. Question the order because the dose is too large.

    B. Give it as ordered when the patient is restless.

    C. Schedule the medication for HS.

    D. Question the order because the dose is too small.

34. The nurse would know that the teaching plan for a client who was to be discharged with a prescription for chloral hydrate (Noctec) was successful if the client states:
    A. "I shouldn't take any cold medications while I'm taking these pills."
    B. "If one pill doesn't work, I can take up to three more pills over a 1-hour period."
    C. "A few sips of alcohol after I take a pill will help it work better."
    D. "I need to take these pills before I leave for work in the morning so that I won't become so upset by all the traffic."

35. In instructing a client about the home use of the medication acetaloamide (Diamox), which would be the most important element for the nurse to include in the teaching plan?
    A. The medication is safe to use and has few side effects.
    B. Two drops should be put in each eye twice a day.
    C. If the client develops weakness, heart palpitations, or paresthesia, he or she should notify the physician.
    D. The medication may cause dim vision in low light, so night driving could be dangerous.

36. For which of the following conditions would a client most likely be receiving timolol maleate (Timoptic)?
    A. Gastric ulcer
    B. Glaucoma
    C. Lung cancer
    D. Urinary tract infection

37. Medications that cause the pupil of the eye to constrict are called:
    A. Mydriatics
    B. Vasoconstrictors
    C. Miotics
    D. Diuretics

38. A 28-year-old female client is to receive her first dose of chlordiazepoxide (Librium) after her admission. She says to the nurse: "Is that Librium? I can't take Librium!" The nurse's best response would be:
    A. "It's the hospital policy not to tell the patients what medications they are receiving."
    B. "Go ahead and take the pill now. It'll make you feel better."
    C. "You have to take this pill—the doctor ordered it."
    D. "What happens when you take Librium?"

39. All of the following are important considerations when providing tube feedings to clients, except:
    A. Increase the rate of the feeding to "catch up" if it should get behind.
    B. Keep the head of the bed elevated 30 to 45 degrees.
    C. Monitor the client for weight and hydration status.
    D. Change the tubing every 24 hours.

40. The base solution for TPN is usually:
    A. D5W
    B. NS
    C. LR
    D. D50W

41. Because of its osmotic nature, one important consideration of TPN solutions is:
    A. It needs to be run through a central vein.
    B. It is a good growth medium for bacteria.
    C. It provides all the nutrients a client needs.
    D. The tubing should be changed every 24 hours.

42. Which of the following clients would most likely be put on an increased potassium diet?
    A. One who is in renal failure
    B. One who has developed diabetes insipidus
    C. One who is taking aspirin for rheumatoid arthritis
    D. One who has chronic constipation

43. The physician orders potassium chloride (KCL) 40 mEq to be added to the IV for a client. The client's serum potassium is 2.2 mEq/L. The nurse should:
    A. Give the medication as ordered because of the client's low potassium level
    B. Hold the medication, and notify the physician that the client's potassium level is too high
    C. Hold the medication, and contact the physician about the route of administration
    D. Give half the dose now and the other half in 2 hours to prevent irritation of the veins

44. A client who needs 2200 calories per day via tube feeding should receive how much regular, full-strength Isocal in a 24-hour period?
    A. 1100 mL
    B. 2200 mL
    C. 4400 mL
    D. It is impossible to get this many calories from this substance.

45. If all of the following IV solutions are available to an emergency room nurse, which would be best for her to select for use with a client who is severely dehydrated?
    A. D5W
    B. D5W with a 0.9% normal saline
    C. LR
    D. 0.45% normal saline

46. A client asks the nurse, "When are these chemotherapy drugs I'm taking going to cure me?" The best answer by the nurse is that an antineoplastic medication regimen is considered successful when:
    A. 90% of the cancer cells are killed
    B. 95% of the cancer cells are killed
    C. 99% of the cancer cells are killed
    D. 100% of the cancer cells are killed

47. Which of the following statements by a client would indicate to the nurse that more teaching is required concerning cancer?
    A. Anything that can alter the RNA or DNA in a cell can produce mutant cells.
    B. Everyone has some mutant cells in the body at any given time.
    C. Cancer cells follow an orderly progression in reproduction.
    D. Anything that will suppress the immune system will make an individual more susceptible to cancer.

48. A client has heard his physician talking about "first-order kinetics" and asks the nurse to explain the term. The nurse explains that the term "first-order kinetics" refers to the effectiveness of antineoplastic drugs and means that:
    A. The potency of the medication is related to how rapidly it is given.
    B. A specific medication dose kills a specific percentage of cells with each administration.
    C. The medication works on only one specific part of the cell.
    D. The first time the medication is given, it is least effective.

49. The nurse would recognize that her client was having a paradoxical reaction to antihistamine therapy if he displayed which symptoms?
    A. Drowsiness, dryness of mouth and throat
    B. blurred vision, urinary retention
    C. Restlessness, insomnia
    D. Skin rashes, photosensitivity

50. A client with a tumor of the esophagus has difficulty swallowing and is receiving continuous feeding by nasogastric feeding tube. The nurse recognizes that the advantage of a continuous feeding over intermittent feedings is:
    A. Reduced incident of aspiration
    B. Less diarrhea and stomach cramping
    C. Similarity to normal patterns of food intake
    D. Increased absorption of nutrients

ANSWERS/RATIONALES

1. **Correct Answer: C.** $\dfrac{\text{volume to infuse}}{\text{time (in hours)}} = \dfrac{250}{2.5} = 100$

Rationales for Other Answer Choices: A, B, D are incorrect.
Nursing Process Phase: implementation; client need: safe and effective care environment; concern area: medical/surgical

2. **Correct Answer: C.** Defines the term and is a characteristic of cancer cells that make them susceptible to certain medications.

Rationales for Other Answer Choices: A. Loss of cell differentiation. **B.** Changes in cancer cells' size, shape, and nuclei. **D.** Internal mechanism that allows cells to reproduce at the same rate as their death.
Nursing Process Phase: planning; client need: safe and effective care environment; concern area: medical/surgical

3. **Correct Answer: C.** These medications work by interfering with cell division and formation of DNA.

Rationales for Other Answer Choices: A. An antimetabolite. **B.** An antibiotic. **D.** A vinca alkaloid.
Nursing Process Phase: planning; client need: safe and effective care environment; concern area: medical/surgical

4. **Correct Answer: B.** Defines the term.

Rationales for Other Answer Choices: A. Interfere with cell division and formation of DNA. **C.** Interfere with the formation of RNA or DNA. **D.** Prevent the formation of clots.
Nursing Process Phase: planning; client need: safe and effective care environment; concern area: medical/surgical

5. **Correct Answer: B.** Defines the term; these medications can cause extensive tissue damage if they infiltrate.

Rationales for Other Answer Choices: A. Definition of an irritant. **C.** Can be given only IV. **D.** Can never be given IM.
Nursing Process Phase: planning; client need: safe and effective care environment; concern area: medical/surgical

6. **Correct Answer: A.** This is a vesicant medication.

Rationales for Other Answer Choices: B. Nonvesicant. **C.** Nonvesicant. **D.** Nonvesicant.
Nursing Process Phase: planning; client need: safe and effective care environment; concern area: medical/surgical

7. **Correct Answer: D.** AU means both ears.

Rationales for Other Answer Choices: A. QOD. **B.** AO. **C.** Slow push.
Nursing Process Phase: planning; client need: safe and effective care environment; concern area: medical/surgical

   8. **Correct Answer: A.** Cancer cells develop resistance quickly when only one medication is used. Use of medications with different MOA decreases resistance.

Rationales for Other Answer Choices: B. May help shorten length of treatment. **C.** Quantity usually stays the same or is lessened. **D.** Side effects of each individual medication stay the same.
Nursing Process Phase: planning; client need: safe and effective care environment; concern area: medical/surgical

   9. **Correct Answer: C.** These medications are given in high doses until bone marrow suppression occurs, then stopped, then repeated.

Rationales for Other Answer Choices: A. Low doses are generally not effective. **B.** Massive doses produce too many side effects and may leave some cancer cells viable. **D.** Not usually a treatment course.
Nursing Process Phase: implementation; client need: safe and effective care environment; concern area: medical/surgical

  10. **Correct Answer: B.** Defines this class of medications.

Rationales for Other Answer Choices: A. Highly addictive—no medical use. **C.** Relatively low addiction potential. **D.** Slight potential for abuse; usually combination medications.
Nursing Process Phase: planning; client need: safe and effective care environment; concern area: medical/surgical

  11. **Correct Answer: D.** These are side effects (adverse reactions) to many medications.

Rationales for Other Answer Choices: A. Opposite from what is expected (e.g., a sleeping pill causes a client to be excited and confused). **B.** An unusual side effect not seen before. **C.** An allergic reaction manifested by itching, hives, bronchospasms.
Nursing Process Phase: assessment; client need: health promotion and maintenance; concern area: medical/surgical

  12. **Correct Answer: B.** This is a cough suppressant that will reduce coughing so the client can sleep.

Rationales for Other Answer Choices: A. Does not affect viscosity of mucus. **C.** Has no effect on nasal congestion. **D.** Should not be used with these clients—they need to cough out their large quantities of thick secretions.
Nursing Process Phase: analysis; client need: health promotion and maintenance; concern area: medical/surgical

  13. **Correct Answer: A.** Defines the term.

Rationales for Other Answer Choices: B. This is the need for increased quantities of the medication to produce the same effects. **C.** A craving without physical symptoms. **D.** No craving or symptoms.

Nursing Process Phase: assessment; client need: safe and effective care environment; concern area: medical/surgical

14. Correct Answer: C. This is a mucolytic that breaks down thick mucus so it can be coughed out. Thick mucus is common in cystic fibrosis (CF).

Rationales for Other Answer Choices: A. Has no cough suppressant effects. **B.** Has no effect on congestive heart failure (CHF). **D.** May make peptic ulcers worse.
Nursing Process Phase: analysis; client need: safe and effective care environment; concern area: pediatrics

15. Correct Answer: A. $50 : 1 :: 35 : x$

$$50x = 35$$
$$x = \frac{35}{50} = 0.7$$

Rationales for Other Answer Choices: B, C, D are incorrect.
Nursing Process Phase: planning; client need: safe and effective care environment; concern area: maternity

16. Correct Answer: A. This is a histamine blocker used for allergic reactions.

Rationales for Other Answer Choices: B. Has no effect on chest pain. **C.** Has no bronchodilating effects. **D.** Does not directly stimulate cardiac muscle tissue.
Nursing Process Phase: analysis; client need: health promotion and maintenance; concern area: medical/surgical

17. Correct Answer: D. The coating is not affected by the acid in the stomach.

Rationales for Other Answer Choices: A. Statement is not true. **B.** Enteric-coated (EC) medications should never be crushed. **C.** Enteric-coated (EC) medications should never be chewed.
Nursing Process Phase: planning; client need: psychosocial integrity; concern area: medical/surgical

18. Correct Answer: B. The ends of the long axons release neurotransmitters into the synapses.

Rationales for Other Answer Choices: A. The receptor sites are located on the dendrites. **C.** Cell body keeps the neuron alive. **D.** Precursor is converted into a neurotransmitter.
Nursing Process Phase: planning; client need: safe and effective care environment; concern area: medical/surgical

19. Correct Answer: D. Suppurative lung disease indicates a great deal of mucous secretions that need to be coughed out. Antitussives will prevent the client from coughing them out.

Rationales for Other Answer Choices: A. An appropriate use for antitussives. **B.** An appropriate use for antitussives. **C.** An appropriate use for antitussives.
Nursing Process Phase: assessment; client need: safe and effective care environment; concern area: medical/surgical

20. Correct Answer: B. This medication affects iodine usage by the thyroid and may lead to false test results.

Rationales for Other Answer Choices: A. No contraindication for pregnancy. **C.** Should increase fluids to 2 to 3 L/d. **D.** This medication should be taken with food.
Nursing Process Phase: planning; client need: safe and effective care environment; concern area: medical/surgical

21. Correct Answer: A. It decreases the surface tension of the mucus, making it easier to cough up.

Rationales for Other Answer Choices: B. Not the mechanism of action (MOA) of this medication. **C.** Not the MOA of this medication. **D.** Has the opposite effect on bronchial secretions.
Nursing Process Phase: planning; client need: safe and effective care environment; concern area: medical/surgical

22. Correct Answer: C. These are called cell-mediated reactions, with the T lymphocytes as the mediator.

Rationales for Other Answer Choices: A. Usually are not fatal but may be severe. **B.** Can occur from a few minutes to 24 hours after. **D.** Anaphylactic shock can occur, but not usually.
Nursing Process Phase: planning; client need: safe and effective care environment; concern area: medical/surgical

23. Correct Answer: A. The goal is to achieve a normal respiratory rate.

Rationales for Other Answer Choices: B. Has no effect on urine output. **C.** May increase heart rate but is not a goal of treatment. **D.** May increase BP but is not a goal of treatment.
Nursing Process Phase: assessment; client need: safe and effective care environment; concern area: medical/surgical

24. Correct Answer: D. Codeine is a narcotic that can cause drowsiness, slowing of reflexes, and poor judgment. Activities involving complex psychomotor skills should be avoided.

Rationales for Other Answer Choices: A. May lead to abuse of the medication. **B.** Side effects cause drowsiness and sedation. **C.** Narcotics tend to produce constipation.
Nursing Process Phase: evaluation; client need: health promotion and maintenance; concern area: medical/surgical

25. Correct Answer: C. It has a rotten egg smell due to the sulphur content of the medication. There are no other major side effects.

Rationales for Other Answer Choices: A. No direct cardiac effects with this medication. **B.** Has no effect on the cough reflex; may increase coughing as mucous secretions become thinner. **D.** Headache not a common side effect.
Nursing Process Phase: assessment; client need: safe and effective care environment; concern area: medical/surgical

26. Correct Answer: B. This is one of the effects of antihistamines.

Rationales for Other Answer Choices: A. This is a side effect, not the desired effect. **C.** Has no effect on pain. **D.** Antihistamines are H₁ inhibitors; they have no effect on acid.
Nursing Process Phase: implementation; client need: safe and effective care environment; concern area: medical/surgical

27. Correct Answer: C. Normal dosage range 25–50 mg IM, IV, PO.

Rationales for Other Answer Choices: A. Dose is appropriate. **B.** Dose is appropriate. **D.** Dose is appropriate.
Nursing Process Phase: implementation; client need: safe and effective care environment; concern area: medical/surgical

28. Correct Answer: C. This inability to penetrate the brain and CSF makes treating infections and cancers more difficult.

Rationales for Other Answer Choices: A. Many IV medications will not penetrate, some oral medications will. **B.** These substances cross easily. **D.** Untrue statement.
Nursing Process Phase: planning; client need: health promotion and maintenance; concern area: medical/surgical

29. Correct Answer: C. Clients with COPD need to remove the secretions from their lungs.

Rationales for Other Answer Choices: A. Is not a broncho-active medication. **B.** Tend to counteract each other with CNS effects. **D.** Cannot draw this conclusion from the information given.
Nursing Process Phase: implementation; client need: safe and effective care environment; concern area: medical/surgical

30. Correct Answer: C. Hypotension may make the client weak or unsteady when getting up, causing him to fall.

Rationales for Other Answer Choices: A. Common but less serious side effects. **B.** Common but less serious side effect. **D.** Common but less serious side effect.
Nursing Process Phase: assessment; client need: safe and effective care environment; concern area: medical/surgical

31. Correct Answer: A. MS is much more potent than meperidine and used for more severe pain.

Rationales for Other Answer Choices: B. These are normal; no significance. **C.** These are normal; no significance. **D.** Side effects of MS.
Nursing Process Phase: assessment; client need: health promotion and maintenance; concern area: medical/surgical

32. Correct Answer: C. The limbic system is responsible for strong feelings of rage, anger, anxiety, and fear.

Rationales for Other Answer Choices: A. Does not affect the hypothalamus. **B.** Tend to induce sleep. **D.** Tend to decrease heart rate and respiratory rate.
Nursing Process Phase: implementation; client need: psychosocial integrity; concern area: psychiatric nursing

33. **Correct Answer: C.** This is a hypnotic used for inducing sleep, and hour of sleep (HS) would be an appropriate time to give it.

Rationales for Other Answer Choices: A. Normal dose: 15–30 mg. **B.** Incorrect use of the medication. **D.** Dose is correct.
Nursing Process Phase: implementation; client need: safe and effective care environment; concern area: medical/surgical

34. **Correct Answer: A.** This is a CNS depressant used for sleep, and taking other CNS depressants like antihistamines in cold preparations will potentiate it.

Rationales for Other Answer Choices: B. Three or four pills is an excessive dose. **C.** Alcohol should be avoided. **D.** This drug may cause the client to fall asleep while driving.
Nursing Process Phase: evaluation; client need: health promotion and maintenance; concern area: medical/surgical

35. **Correct Answer: C.** It can cause significant electrolyte imbalances that are indicated by these symptoms. Dosage may need to be adjusted.

Rationales for Other Answer Choices: A. It is safe to use but has many side effects. **B.** Is given PO, IV, or IM only—no eyedrops. **D.** Has no miotic effects.
Nursing Process Phase: planning; client need: health promotion and maintenance; concern area: medical/surgical

36. **Correct Answer: B.** This is a beta-adrenergic blocker used in glaucoma to reduce intraocular pressure.

Rationales for Other Answer Choices: A. Not effective for this condition. **C.** Not used to treat this disease. **D.** Has no antimicrobial effects.
Nursing Process Phase: analysis; client need: safe and effective care environment; concern area: medical/surgical

37. **Correct Answer: C.** Used in glaucoma to help increase the drainage of the aqueous humor and reduce intraocular pressure.

Rationales for Other Answer Choices: A. These medications cause dilation of the pupil. **B.** These medications increase blood pressure. **D.** These medications increase urine output.
Nursing Process Phase: planning; client need: safe and effective care environment; concern area: medical/surgical

38. **Correct Answer: D.** Always seek further information about what the medication caused (e.g., an allergic reaction? side effects?)

Rationales for Other Answer Choices: A. This is paternalism—no longer an acceptable practice. **B.** This medication should not be taken until more information is obtained. **C.** Clients have the right to refuse medications.
Nursing Process Phase: implementation; client need: safe and effective care environment; concern area: psychiatric nursing

39. **Correct Answer: A.** This practice should be avoided because it increases the incidence of gastrointestinal (GI) discomfort and diarrhea.

Rationales for Other Answer Choices: B. Will help prevent aspiration of the feeding. **C.** Important while client is on tube feedings. **D.** This practice helps prevent infections.
Nursing Process Phase: planning; client need: safe and effective care environment; concern area: medical/surgical

40. **Correct Answer: D.** D50W is a concentrated glucose solution to which protein solutions, electrolytes, and vitamins are added to make TPN.

Rationales for Other Answer Choices: A. A common isotonic IV solution. **B.** A commonly used IV solution compatible with most medications. **C.** A common isotonic IV solution.
Nursing Process Phase: planning; client need: safe and effective care environment; concern area: medical/surgical

41. **Correct Answer: A.** TPN is extremely hypertonic and tends to cause vein irritation if run through a smaller vein where there is little hemodilution.

Rationales for Other Answer Choices: B. This is a true statement but has nothing to do with the osmotic nature of the solution. **C.** This is a true statement but has nothing to do with the osmotic nature of the solution. **D.** This is a necessary measure to prevent infections.
Nursing Process Phase: implementation; client need: safe and effective care environment; concern area: medical/surgical

42. **Correct Answer: B.** Diabetes insipidus is caused by a malfunctioning posterior pituitary and decreased antidiuretic hormone (ADH) secretion. It causes the client to lose large amounts of water and electrolytes.

Rationales for Other Answer Choices: A. Should be on a reduced-potassium diet. **C.** No interaction with aspirin and potassium except to irritate the gastric lining. **D.** Only clients with chronic diarrhea lose potassium.
Nursing Process Phase: analysis; client need: safe and effective care environment; concern area: medical/surgical

43. **Correct Answer: A.** Normal potassium level is 3.5 to 5.5 mEq/L. A potassium below 3 is dangerous and may cause cardiac arrest.

Rationales for Other Answer Choices: B. Level is too low. **C.** Route is correct. **D.** This is a standard dose for this medication and should not cause any vein irritation.
Nursing Process Phase: implementation; client need: safe and effective care environment; concern area: medical/surgical

44. **Correct Answer: B.** Standard Isocal has 1 cal/mL.

Rationales for Other Answer Choices: A. Only half the amount needed. **C.** Twice the amount needed. **D.** Untrue statement.
Nursing Process Phase: planning; client need: safe and effective care environment; concern area: medical/surgical

45. **Correct Answer: D.** This is a hypotonic solution that will be absorbed into and rehydrate the tissues.

Rationales for Other Answer Choices: A. Isotonic solution; not best for rapid rehydration. **B.** Isotonic solution; not best for rapid rehydration. **C.** Isotonic solution; not best for rapid rehydration.
Nursing Process Phase: implementation; client need: safe and effective care environment; concern area: medical/surgical

46. **Correct Answer: D.** Cancer treatment is considered successful only when all the cancer cells have been killed.

Rationales for Other Answer Choices: A. Not 100%. **B.** Not 100%. **C.** Not 100%.
Nursing Process Phase: implementation; client need: psychosocial integrity; concern area: medical/surgical

47. **Correct Answer: C.** Cancer cells grow without restraint in a haphazard manner.

Rationales for Other Answer Choices: A. True; mutant cells are usually removed by the immune system so that they cannot reproduce and form cancer. **B.** True; reproduction of cells is not perfect, but these cells are destroyed by the immune system. **D.** True; when the immune system is suppressed, mutant and abnormal cells can reproduce and grow.
Nursing Process Phase: evaluation; client need: health promotion and maintenance; concern area: medical/surgical

48. **Correct Answer: B.** Medications with a high first-order kinetics will kill 95% or more of all the existing cancer cells the first time it is given. The second time it is given, it will kill 95% or more of the remaining cancer cells, and so forth.

Rationales for Other Answer Choices: A. Does not explain the term—does not have any connection with how rapidly it is given. **C.** No relationship to the MOA of the drug. **D.** Untrue statement—medication is equally effective each time it is given.
Nursing Process Phase: implementation; client need: health promotion and maintenance; concern area: medical/surgical

49. **Correct Answer: C.** Paradoxical reactions are opposite of the normally expected effects or side effects.

Rationales for Other Answer Choices: A. Normally expected side effects of this medication. **B.** Normally expected side effects of this medication. **D.** Normally expected side effects of this medication.
Nursing Process Phase: assessment; client need: safe and effective care environment; concern area: medical/surgical

50. **Correct Answer: D.** The GI system adjusts to the presence of the feeding continuously and can produce gastric secretions at a rate that will promote absorption.

Rationales for Other Answer Choices: A. Incidence is the same or increased with continuous feeding. **B.** Incidence is the same for both. **C.** Is not similar to normal feeding, which is usually intermittent.
Nursing Process Phase: planning; client need: safe and effective care environment; concern area: medical/surgical

1. A client is to receive ampicillin 1 GM IV in 50 mL D5W to run over 15 minutes. At what rate should the nurse set the volumetric pump?
   A. 200 mL/h
   B. 37 gtt/min
   C. 25 mL/h
   D. 100 mL/h

2. Which of the following would be the most serious side effects for a client receiving isoniazid (INH)?
   A. Nausea and vomiting
   B. Urinary retention
   C. Liver failure
   D. Intracranial hemorrhage

3. Which of the following statements by a client would indicate that the nurse's teaching about potassium chloride (KCL) was effective?
   A. "If I get dizzy, I should stop taking the medication."
   B. "I need to take the medication with meals."
   C. "I must avoid fresh fruits and vegetables when I am taking this medication."
   D. "I have to decrease my fluid intake while on this medication."

4. Which of the following clients would the nurse question if a narcotic analgesic medication was ordered?
   A. A 68-year-old client with rheumatoid arthritis
   B. A 42-year-old three-day postoperative gall bladder client
   C. An 8-year-old burn client
   D. A 22-year-old car accident client with head injury

5. The physician orders meperidine (Demerol) 100 mg IM q 4 h prn for a 30-year-old client with a fractured leg. The best response by the nurse to this order is to
   A. Give the medication as ordered
   B. Hold the medication and notify the physician that the dose is too large
   C. Hold the medication and notify the physician that the dose is too small
   D. Give half the dose now to see what effect it has

6. The most serious side effect the nurse needs to monitor in a client who is receiving meperidine (Demerol) is?
   A. Pain relief
   B. Constipation
   C. Urinary retention
   D. Respiratory depression

7. Reye's syndrome is often associated with children who have viral diseases and have received
   A. acetaminophen (Tylenol)
   B. chloral hydrate (Noctec)
   C. aspirin
   D. meperidine (Demerol)

8. A client receiving chloral hydrate (Noctec) most likely has:
   A. A viral infection
   B. A bacterial infection
   C. Acute anxiety
   D. Difficulty sleeping

9. The physician orders temazepam (Restoril) 250 mg PO HS prn. The best response by the nurse to this order is to:
   A. Give the medication as ordered.
   B. Hold the medication and notify the physician that the dose is too large.
   C. Hold the medication and notify the physician that the dose is too small.
   D. Give half the dose now to see what effect it has.

10. A nurse is to give heparin 4500 U IV to a client. The drug comes 10,000 U mL. How much is given?
    A. 4.5 mL
    B. 1 mL
    C. 1.5 mL
    D. 0.45 mL

11. Aminophylline 250 mg in 500 mL D5W is ordered at a rate of 15 mg/h. How fast should this medication run?
    A. 10 mL/h
    B. 15 mL/h
    C. 25 mL/h
    D. 30 mL/h

12. In a hurry to get to surgery for his next operation, a surgeon wrote the following order: "Oxazepam (Serax) 10 mg PO q 4 h prn headache." What would be an appropriate response to this order?
    A. Question the order because the medication is inappropriate for the condition.
    B. Give the medication as ordered because the client has a severe headache at this time.
    C. Give the medication IV instead of PO because it works better that way.
    D. Notify the physician that the dose is incorrect.

13. Which of the following dosage orders for the medication oxazepam (Serax) would the nurse not question?
   A. 10 mg PO tid
   B. 1 GM IV, q 4 h
   C. 0.25 mg IM q 6 h
   D. 7.5 mg PO qd

14. A class of diseases that are caused by sudden abnormal electrical activity in the brain is called:
   A. Convulsions
   B. Seizures
   C. Epilepsy
   D. Congestive heart failure (CHF)

15. Phenytoin (Dilantin) 100 mg IV push has been ordered as a "stat" dose for a client who is having a seizure. The medication vial is labeled "100 mg per 2 mL." The nurse should give the drug:
   A. IM instead because it cannot be given IV
   B. Slowly over a 4-minute period with normal saline (NS)
   C. As fast as she can push it in because speed is of importance
   D. In 50 mL D5W and slowly let it drip into the vein

16. If a medication is known to be nephrotoxic, the most important nursing action which should be implemented before starting therapy with this medication is:
   A. Obtain a blood urea nitrogen (BUN) and creatinine.
   B. Obtain a thorough visual assessment of the client.
   C. Explain to the client that his/her eighth cranial nerve will be severely damaged by the medication.
   D. Obtain a baseline audiogram.

17. A client is receiving levodopa (Dopar). He most likely has:
   A. Acute anxiety
   B. Severe depression
   C. Idiopathic epilepsy
   D. Parkinson's disease

18. The nurse should be most concerned if a client develops which of the following side effects while on levodopa (Dopar)?
   A. Nausea and vomiting
   B. Blurred vision
   C. Tachycardia
   D. Edema

19. A client is receiving orphenadrine citrate (Norgesic) for which of the following conditions?
   A. Gastroesophageal reflux
   B. Congestive heart failure
   C. Back sprain
   D. Urinary retention

20. A child with attention deficit hyperactivity disorder would most likely be receiving which medication?
    A. phenytoin (Dilantin)
    B. methylphenidate (Ritalin)
    C. dexamethasone (Decadron)
    D. cimetidine (Tagamet)

21. A client is diagnosed as having idiopathic epilepsy. He is taking phenytoin (Dilantin). He should be advised that he:
    A. Needs renal function studies approximately every other week
    B. Should ingest his usual amount of alcohol daily
    C. Should brush and floss his teeth frequently
    D. May notice swelling of his feet and ankles, but this is a normal side effect of the medication

22. The nurse teaches the client that a synergistic interaction is likely if which of the following medications are taken together?
    A. alcohol and diazepam (Valium)
    B. tetracycline and magnesium hydroxide (Maalox)
    C. cimetidine (Tagamet) and prochlorperazine (Compazine)
    D. vincristine (Oncovin) and penicillin

23. A 32-year-old male client is admitted to the unit. During the initial assessment, the nurse notes that he has gingival hyperplasia. Although he does not remember the names of the medications he is taking at home, it is very likely that one of the medications is:
    A. oxazepam (Serax)
    B. phenytoin (Dilantin)
    C. diazepam (Valium)
    D. chlordiazepoxide (Librium)

24. Which of the following nursing implications would be the most important for a client receiving amphetamine (Dexedrine)?
    A. Give the last dose at bedtime.
    B. Monitor the patient's blood pressure.
    C. Monitor the patient for depression.
    D. Give medication on an empty stomach.

25. Which of the following would be an appropriate dose for a client receiving dopamine (Intropin)?
    A. 12 μg/kg/min IV
    B. 150 mg/h IV
    C. 2500 U SC q 12 h
    D. 0.25 mg PO qd

26. Which of the following are appropriate routes for the administration of epinephrine (Adrenalin)?
    A. IV, IM, PO
    B. IV, PO, inhalation
    C. IV, SC, inhalation
    D. SC, IM, PO

27. For which of the following conditions would a client most likely be receiving isoproterenol (Isuprel)?
    A. Asthma
    B. Tachycardia
    C. Diarrhea
    D. Anxiety

28. In teaching her client about prednisone, the nurse should include the fact that the primary effect of naturally occurring glucocorticoids on the body is to:
    A. Regulate carbohydrate and fat metabolism
    B. Stimulate the sympathetic nervous system
    C. Regulate electrolyte and fluid balance
    D. Regulate the growth of the sex organs

29. A client is receiving metoprolol (Lopressor) for which of the following medications?
    A. Bronchospasm
    B. Seizures
    C. High blood pressure
    D. Lupus

30. Diazepam (Valium) 15 mg qid PO was ordered for a 25-year-old client this morning. When the nurse goes in to give him his second dose of this medication, she notes that he is highly agitated, very loud, and seems disoriented. What is the most appropriate action by the nurse at this time?
    A. Get him up in a chair and when he calms down, give him the medication.
    B. Give him the medication as ordered because it is a scheduled medication and will help calm him.
    C. Give him half the dose of the medication because the dose is very large for a patient his age.
    D. Hold the medication and notify the physician of the reasons why it was held.

31. Which of the following side effects should the nurse monitor for the client who just received atropine IV?
    A. Moon face, hirsutism
    B. Tachycardia, dry mouth
    C. Edema of the extremities, bradycardia
    D. Constricted pupils, diarrhea

32. Which of the following medications would the nurse expect to be used for the client who has a gastric ulcer?
    A. atropine
    B. benztropine (Cogentin)
    C. trihexyphenidyl (Artane)
    D. dicyclomine (Bentyl)

33. What do atropine, benztropine (Cogentin), trihexyphenidyl (Artane), and dicyclomine (Bentyl) all have in common?
    A. All are used in gastrointestinal (GI) disorders.
    B. All are classified as anticholinergics.
    C. All are given only PO.
    D. All are classified as analgesics.

34. A client is ordered to receive dexamethasone (Decadron) 25 mg IV q 4 hours. The best response by the nurse to this order is to:
- **A.** Give the medication as ordered
- **B.** Hold the medication and notify the physician that the dose is too large
- **C.** Hold the medication and notify the physician that the dose is too small
- **D.** Give half the dose now to see what effect it has

35. A client is being given carbamazepine (Tegretol) for a recently diagnosed seizure disorder. He asks the nurse, "How long will I have to be on this medication before it cures me?" The best answer to the question would be:
- **A.** "Most clients are cured in 24 to 72 hours."
- **B.** "You had better ask your doctor about that. Nurses can't give out that information."
- **C.** "This medication will not cure you; it only controls the symptoms of the disease."
- **D.** "It's really hard to say. Every client's response to the medication is so different."

36. Which of the following clients would most likely be receiving methylprednisone (Solu-Medrol)?
- **A.** A client with wide-angle glaucoma
- **B.** A client with hypertension
- **C.** A client with type 2 diabetes
- **D.** A client with an autoimmune disorder

37. When giving methylprednisolone (Solu-Medrol), the nurse would most likely be giving it by which route?
- **A.** Inhalation
- **B.** PO
- **C.** IV
- **D.** SL

38. A client is ordered to receive levothyroxine (Synthroid) 0.05 mg PO q A.M. The best response by the nurse to this order is:
- **A.** Give the medication as ordered.
- **B.** Hold the medication and notify the physician that the dose is too large.
- **C.** Hold the medication and notify the physician that the dose is too small.
- **D.** Give half the dose now to see what effect it has.

39. A client is receiving propylthiouracil (Propacil) for which condition?
- **A.** Graves' disease
- **B.** Cushing's syndrome
- **C.** Cretinism
- **D.** Myxedema

40. A client mistakenly receives a dose of insulin twice as large as was ordered. Symptoms he most likely will experience are:
- **A.** Deep slow respirations, dry skin
- **B.** Low blood pressure, increased urine output
- **C.** Diaphoresis, disorientation
- **D.** Edema, tachycardia

41. In teaching a newly diagnosed type 1 diabetic client about insulin, the nurse should include the fact that the peak action of NPH insulin will occur:
   A. 1 to 2 hours after administration
   B. 3 to 4 hours after administration
   C. 6 to 8 hours after administration
   D. 10 to 12 hours after administration

42. A physician orders chlorpropamide (Diabinase) 50 mg PO bid for a client. The nurse's best response to this order is to:
   A. Give the medication as ordered
   B. Hold the medication and notify the physician that the dose is too large
   C. Hold the medication and notify the physician that the dose is too small
   D. Hold the medication and notify the physician that the route is incorrect

43. To which of the following clients would the nurse be administering glyburide (Micronase)?
   A. Type 1 diabetic client
   B. Type 2 diabetic client
   C. Head trauma victim
   D. Cardiac client

44. The nurse would know that the teaching about exercise for diabetic clients had been successful if the client stated that:
   A. "Moderate exercise is dangerous due to cardiovascular disease diabetic clients all have."
   B. "Moderate exercise increases the need for insulin."
   C. "Moderate exercise decreases the need for food."
   D. "Moderate exercise decreases the need for insulin."

45. A nurse would know that the teaching about ampicillin (Omnipen) was successful if the client states:
   A. "When I feel better, I can stop taking the medication."
   B. "I need to take the medication with meals."
   C. "I must avoid fresh fruits and vegetables when I am taking this medication."
   D. "I have to increase my fluid intake while on this medication."

46. A child is burned over 20% of his body in an accident at home. The physician orders silver sulfadiazine (Silvadine). The nurse knows that this medication:
   A. Must be taken with a full glass of water to prevent GI irritation.
   B. Is effective only if given IV push.
   C. Should be applied liberally to the burned skin areas.
   D. Can cause sedation and respiratory depression.

47. A physician orders amoxicillin (Amoxil) 0.5 mg PO q 8 h for a client. The best response to this order by the nurse is to:
   A. Give the medication as ordered
   B. Hold the medication and notify the physician that the dose is too large
   C. Hold the medication and notify the physician that the dose is too small
   D. Hold the medication and notify the physician that the route is incorrect

48. A nursing student has just given a client 10 g of ceftazidime (Fortaz). Which of the following might the student expect from the client?
   A. Immediate improvement of the infection
   B. Development of renal failure
   C. Immediate development of a superinfection
   D. Decreased blood pressure and heart rate

49. While the client is receiving IV gentamicin (Garamycin), the nurse would monitor for:
   A. Elevated blood sugar
   B. Sodium retention
   C. Aplastic anemia
   D. Renal failure

50. Teaching for clients who are receiving tetracycline (Sumycin) should include instructions on how to:
   A. Avoid taking with milk or antacids
   B. Stay in the direct sunlight as much as possible to increase the production of natural vitamin D
   C. Eat fresh fruits to prevent constipation
   D. Reduce fluid intake to prevent renal failure

1. **Correct Answer: A.** $\dfrac{\text{volume to infuse}}{\text{time (h)}} = \dfrac{50 \text{ mL}}{0.25} = 200$

Rationales for Other Answer Choices: B, C, D are incorrect.
Nursing Process Phase: implementation; client need: safe and effective care environment; concern area: medical/surgical

2. **Correct Answer: C.** Liver failure may lead to death.

Rationales for Other Answer Choices: A. Distressing but not serious. **B.** Not a common side effect of this medication. **D.** Not a side effect of this medication.
Nursing Process Phase: planning; client need: safe and effective care environment; concern area: medical/surgical

3. **Correct Answer: B.** Medication is irritating to the lining of the stomach and should be taken with food or liquids.

Rationales for Other Answer Choices: A. Client needs to notify the physician. **C.** Client should eat fresh fruits and vegetables in normal amounts. **D.** Fluid has little effect on the medication.
Nursing Process Phase: evaluation; client need: health promotion and maintenance; concern area: medical/surgical

4. **Correct Answer: D.** Narcotics mask the symptoms of increased intracranial pressure and should not be used with head trauma.

Rationales for Other Answer Choices: A. Narcotics can be used for severe arthritic pain. **B.** Postoperative pain control is an appropriate use. **C.** Age and size of child will indicate a smaller dose.
Nursing Process Phase: implementation; client need: safe and effective care environment; concern area: medical/surgical

5. **Correct Answer: A.** This is in the usual dosage range (25–100 mg).

Rationales for Other Answer Choices: B. Dose is appropriate. **C.** Dose is appropriate. **D.** Not an acceptable practice by nurses.
Nursing Process Phase: implementation; client need: safe and effective care environment; concern area: medical/surgical

6. **Correct Answer: D.** This side effect may lead to death.

Rationales for Other Answer Choices: A. Pain relief is a desired effect. **B.** Common but not serious side effect. **C.** Common but generally not serious.
Nursing Process Phase: assessment; client need: safe and effective care environment; concern area: medical/surgical

7. **Correct Answer: C.** Varicella (chicken pox) is the most common virus, but as many as 14 other viruses have been linked to the disorder.

Rationales for Other Answer Choices: A. The medication of choice in children. **B.** Adult medication used for sleep. **D.** Not associated with Reye's syndrome.
Nursing Process Phase: planning; client need: safe and effective care environment; concern area: pediatrics

8. Correct Answer: D. This is a hypnotic drug that is used to induce sleep in adults.

Rationales for Other Answer Choices: A. No antiviral effects. **B.** No antibacterial effects. **C.** May reduce anxiety as a side effect, but not the primary use.
Nursing Process Phase: analysis; client need: safe and effective care environment; concern area: medical/surgical

9. Correct Answer: B. Usual dosage range is 15–30 mg PO HS prn.

Rationales for Other Answer Choices: A. Dose is too large. **C.** Dose is too large. **D.** Not an acceptable practice—½ dose is still too large.
Nursing Process Phase: implementation; client need: safe and effective care environment; concern area: medical/surgical

10. Correct Answer: D. $10,000 : 1 :: 4500 : x$
$$10,000\,x = 4500$$
$$x = 0.45$$

Rationales for Other Answer Choices: A, B, and **C** are incorrect.
Nursing Process Phase: planning; client need: safe and effective care environment; concern area: medical/surgical

11. Correct Answer: D.   concentration $= \dfrac{250}{500} = 0.5$ mg/mL
$$\text{rate} = 0.5 : 1 :: 15 : x$$
$$0.5x = 15$$
$$x = 30$$

Rationales for Other Answer Choices: A, B, and **C** are incorrect.
Nursing Process Phase: implementation; client need: safe and effective care environment; concern area: medical/surgical

12. Correct Answer: A. This is an antianxiety medication, not an analgesic.

Rationales for Other Answer Choices: B. Inappropriate use of this medication. **C.** No IV form of the medication. **D.** Dose is correct.
Nursing Process Phase: implementation; client need: safe and effective care environment; concern area: medical/surgical

13. Correct Answer: A. Usual dosage range is 10–30 mg tid or qid.

Rationales for Other Answer Choices: B. Dosage is too large—antibiotic type dose. **C.** Dose is too small—loading dose for lanoxin. **D.** Dose is too small—dose for coumadin.
Nursing Process Phase: implementation; client need: safe and effective care environment; concern area: medical/surgical

14. Correct Answer: C. This defines the disorder.

Rationales for Other Answer Choices: A. A symptom of epilepsy. **B.** Another word for convulsion—a symptom of the disease. **D.** CHF marked by fluid volume excess, not convulsions.

Nursing Process Phase: analysis; client need: safe and effective care environment; concern area: medical/surgical

15. **Correct Answer: B.** This drug can be given IV, but slowly (1 mL/2 min) and only with normal saline.

Rationales for Other Answer Choices: A. Can be given IV; is poorly absorbed IM. **C.** Giving it rapidly may damage the vein. **D.** Cannot be given in D5W because it precipitates.
Nursing Process Phase: implementation; client need: safe and effective care environment; concern area: medical/surgical

16. **Correct Answer: A.** This action will indicate if there is any current renal damage, and serve as baseline values for later tests.

Rationales for Other Answer Choices: B. This action is important for all clients but not specific to this medication. **C.** This damage is caused by ototoxic medications. **D.** This action should be taken with ototoxic medications.
Nursing Process Phase: implementation; client need: safe and effective care environment; concern area: medical/surgical

17. **Correct Answer: D.** This drug helps replenish the depleted dopamine stores found in clients with this disorder.

Rationales for Other Answer Choices: A. May increase anxiety and nervousness. **B.** Not an approved medication for depression. **C.** Not used for this disorder.
Nursing Process Phase: analysis; client need: safe and effective care environment; concern area: medical/surgical

18. **Correct Answer: C.** Cardiac side effects are the most serious and may lead to ventricular tachycardia (VT) and death.

Rationales for Other Answer Choices: A. Not as serious. **B.** Common but less serious side effect. **D.** Not a common side effect of this medication.
Nursing Process Phase: assessment; client need: health promotion and maintenance; concern area: medical/surgical

19. **Correct Answer: C.** This is a muscle relaxant often used for strains and sprains of major muscles.

Rationales for Other Answer Choices: A. Not used to treat this disorder. **B.** Muscle relaxants not effective in treating CHF. **D.** Has no effect on this problem.
Nursing Process Phase: analysis; client need: safe and effective care environment; concern area: medical/surgical

20. **Correct Answer: B.** Most commonly used medication for this disorder.

Rationales for Other Answer Choices: A. Used for seizure disorders. **C.** Steroid medication used for many disorders but not for attention deficit hyperactivity disorder (ADHD). **D.** Used for peptic ulcers and upper GI problems.
Nursing Process Phase: planning; client need: safe and effective care environment; concern area: pediatrics

21. **Correct Answer: C.** Gingival hyperplasia is the most common side effect of this medication. Good oral care is a must.

Rationales for Other Answer Choices: A. Not necessary—low toxicity to kidneys. **B.** Should avoid all alcohol while on this medication. **D.** This is not a side effect of this medication.
Nursing Process Phase: implementation; client need: safe and effective care environment; concern area: medical/surgical

22. **Correct Answer: A.** A synergistic interaction produces an effect greater than the sum of the effects of the medications.

Rationales for Other Answer Choices: B. These would have an antagonistic effect. **C.** These would have an additive effect. **D.** The effect of these two would be indifference.
Nursing Process Phase: implementation; client need: health promotion and maintenance; concern area: medical/surgical

23. **Correct Answer: B.** Common side effect of this medication.

Rationales for Other Answer Choices: A. Not a side effect. **C.** Not a side effect. **D.** Not a side effect.
Nursing Process Phase: assessment; client need: health promotion and maintenance; concern area: medical/surgical

24. **Correct Answer: B.** Elevation of BP is a common and sometimes dangerous side effect of this medication.

Rationales for Other Answer Choices: A. May keep the client awake at night; give last dose in the afternoon. **C.** Depression occurs as a withdrawal symptom when the medication is stopped suddenly. **D.** Best if taken with food.
Nursing Process Phase: implementation; client need: safe and effective care environment; concern area: medical/surgical

25. **Correct Answer: A.** This medication is usually ordered based on the client's body weight. Range can be anywhere from 5 µg/kg/min–50 µg/kg/min, depending on client's condition and use.

Rationales for Other Answer Choices: B. Not administered this way. **C.** Does not come in units. **D.** No PO form of the medication.
Nursing Process Phase: planning. client need: safe and effective care environment; concern area: medical/surgical

26. **Correct Answer: C.** No PO forms of this medication.

Rationales for Other Answer Choices: A. No PO form, usually not given IM because of vasoconstriction. **B.** No PO form. **D.** No PO form; not given IM.
Nursing Process Phase: planning; client need: safe and effective care environment; concern area: medical/surgical

27. **Correct Answer: A.** This is a potent bronchodilator and cardiac stimulant. Other uses include bradycardia and heart block.

Rationales for Other Answer Choices: B. Side effect of this medication. **C.** Side effect of this medication. **D.** Side effect of this medication.
Nursing Process Phase: analysis; client need: safe and effective care environment; concern area: medical/surgical

28. **Correct Answer: A.**   This is the role that the glucocorticoids normally fulfill in the body of the client with normally functioning adrenal glands.

Rationales for Other Answer Choices: B. Do not have this mechanism of action (MOA). **C.** This is the MOA of mineralocorticoids. **D.** MOA of growth hormone made in the pituitary gland.
Nursing Process Phase: planning; client need: health promotion and maintenance; concern area: medical/surgical

29. **Correct Answer: C.**   This is a beta-blocker that is frequently used for control of moderate hypertension.

Rationales for Other Answer Choices: A. Should not be used by clients with respiratory disorders. **B.** Not appropriate for this disorder. **D.** Not used for this disease.
Nursing Process Phase: analysis; client need: safe and effective care environment; concern area: medical/surgical

30. **Correct Answer: D.**   This would seem to be an idiosyncratic reaction, and the medication should not be given again.

Rationales for Other Answer Choices: A. Medication should not be given again. **B.** May make him even more agitated. **C.** Changing doses is not an acceptable practice by nurses.
Nursing Process Phase: implementation; client need: safe and effective care environment; concern area: psychiatric nursing

31. **Correct Answer: B.**   These are common anticholinergic side effects of this medication.

Rationales for Other Answer Choices: A. Side effects of glucocorticoids. **C.** Side effects of calcium channel blockers, beta-blockers. **D.** This medication dilates pupils and is used to treat diarrhea.
Nursing Process Phase: assessment; client need: safe and effective care environment; concern area: medical/surgical

32. **Correct Answer: D.**   This anticholinergic medication is often combined with other medications to reduce the acid secreted by the gastric mucosa.

Rationales for Other Answer Choices: A. Not commonly used for gastric ulcers. **B.** Used for Parkinson's disease. **C.** Used for Parkinson's disease.
Nursing Process Phase: planning; client need: safe and effective care environment; concern area: medical/surgical

33. **Correct Answer: B.**   They are all anticholinergic medications used for different disorders.

Rationales for Other Answer Choices: A. Only Bentyl is used for GI disorders. **C.** Can be given PO, IM, IV. **D.** Do not have any direct effect on pain.
Nursing Process Phase: planning; client need: safe and effective care environment; concern area: medical/surgical

34. **Correct Answer: B.**   Usual dosage is 4 mg q 8 h. Often a large dose (like 25 mg) is given as a loading dose once.

Rationales for Other Answer Choices: A. Dose is too large for a scheduled medication.   **C.** Dose is too large.   **D.** Not an acceptable practice by nurses.
Nursing Process Phase: implementation; client need: safe and effective care environment; concern area: medical/surgical

35. Correct Answer: C.   Antiseizure medications only control the seizures; they do not cure the disorder.

Rationales for Other Answer Choices: A. Untrue; does not cure the disorder.   **B.** Nurses should know the answer to the question.   **D.** Untrue; does not cure the disorder.
Nursing Process Phase: implementation; client need: psychosocial integrity; concern area: medical/surgical

36. Correct Answer: D.   The most widely used medication for autoimmune disorders such as lupus, glomerulonephritis, and so forth.

Rationales for Other Answer Choices: A. Should not be used in this disorder—tends to increase intraocular pressure.   **B.** Tends to increase blood pressure due to fluid retention.   **C.** Raises the blood sugar levels and makes diabetes difficult to control.
Nursing Process Phase: analysis; client need: safe and effective care environment; concern area: medical/surgical

37. Correct Answer: C.   The "solu" part of the brand name means that it is in an injectable form.

Rationales for Other Answer Choices: A. Not given by this route.   **B.** There are oral forms of methylprednisolone, but not this one.   **D.** No SL forms of this medication.
Nursing Process Phase: planning; client need: safe and effective care environment; concern area: medical/surgical

38. Correct Answer: A.   Usual dosage range 0.05–0.1 mg.

Rationales for Other Answer Choices: B. Dosage is correct.   **C.** Dosage is correct.   **D.** Not an acceptable practice by nurses.
Nursing Process Phase: implementation; client need: safe and effective care environment; concern area: medical/surgical

39. Correct Answer: A.   This medication is used to treat hyperthyroidism, also known as Graves' disease.

Rationales for Other Answer Choices: B. Cushing's, caused by hypersecretion of the adrenal glands is treated with surgery.   **C.** Hypothyroidism in children is treated with thyroid supplements.   **D.** Hypothyroidism in adults is treated with thyroid supplements.
Nursing Process Phase: analysis; client need: safe and effective care environment; concern area: medical/surgical

40. Correct Answer: C.   These are common symptoms associated with hypoglycemia.

Rationales for Other Answer Choices: A. Symptoms of diabetic ketoacidosis (DKA).   **B.** Symptoms of Addison's disease.   **D.** Symptoms of CHF.

Nursing Process Phase: assessment; client need: safe and effective care environment; concern area: medical/surgical

41. **Correct Answer: C.** This is an intermediate-acting insulin that peaks in these time ranges—most likely the period of an insulin reaction.

Rationales for Other Answer Choices: A. Peak for short-acting insulin. **B.** There are no insulins with this peak time. **D.** Peak for long-acting insulins.
Nursing Process Phase: planning; client need: health promotion and maintenance; concern area: medical/surgical

42. **Correct Answer: C.** This first-generation oral hypoglycemic has a usual dosage range of 500 mg to 2 g/d, depending on the client and the response to the medication. It is often given in divided doses.

Rationales for Other Answer Choices: A. Dosage is too small. **B.** Dosage is too small. **D.** Dosage is too small.
Nursing Process Phase: implementation; client need: safe and effective care environment; concern area: medical/surgical

43. **Correct Answer: B.** This is a potent second-generation oral hypoglycemic used for type 2 diabetic clients to simulate insulin production.

Rationales for Other Answer Choices: A. Not effective on type 1 diabetic clients; there is no insulin production. **C.** Not an appropriate use for this medication. **D.** No cardiovascular effects for this medication.
Nursing Process Phase: analysis; client need: safe and effective care environment; concern area: medical/surgical

44. **Correct Answer: D.** Moderate exercise lowers the blood sugar and decreases the need for insulin.

Rationales for Other Answer Choices: A. Not all diabetic clients have cardiovascular disease; exercise may help decrease its effects. **B.** Decreases the need for insulin. **C.** Increases the need for food intake if the insulin dose remains the same.
Nursing Process Phase: evaluation; client need: health promotion and maintenance; concern area: medical/surgical

45. **Correct Answer: D.** Fluid intake should always be increased while taking antibiotics; it helps prevent nephrotoxicity.

Rationales for Other Answer Choices: A. Should complete the course of treatment to prevent resistant bacteria. **B.** Works best on an empty stomach. **C.** No particular effect on diet.
Nursing Process Phase: evaluation; client need: safe and effective care environment; concern area: medical/surgical

46. **Correct Answer: C.** This is a commonly used antimicrobial ointment used on burn injuries.

Rationales for Other Answer Choices: A. Not taken PO. **B.** No IV form. **D.** Does not have these side effects.
Nursing Process Phase: planning; client need: safe and effective care environment; concern area: pediatrics

47. Correct Answer: C. Usual dosage for this medication is 500–1000 mg q 8 h.

Rationales for Other Answer Choices: A. Dose is too small. **B.** Dose is too small. **D.** Can be given only by the oral route.
Nursing Process Phase: planning; client need: safe and effective care environment; concern area: medical/surgical

48. Correct Answer: B. This dosage is 10 times the usual dose. These medications in high doses are nephrotoxic.

Rationales for Other Answer Choices: A. Infection should improve over several days if the client lives. **C.** A likely side effect, but it may take several days or weeks. **D.** Not a common side effect of this medication.
Nursing Process Phase: assessment; client need: safe and effective care environment; concern area: medical/surgical

49. Correct Answer: D. This is a serious and relatively common side effect of this medication. Check intake and output (I&O), BUN, and creatine.

Rationales for Other Answer Choices: A. Side effect of steroid medications. **B.** Side effect of steroid medications. **C.** Side effect of cancer medications and chloramphenicol.
Nursing Process Phase: assessment; client need: safe and effective care environment; concern area: medical/surgical

50. Correct Answer: A. These inactivate tetracycline medications.

Rationales for Other Answer Choices: B. Need to avoid sunlight because of photosensitivity. **C.** One side effect is diarrhea. **D.** Fluid intake should be increased.
Nursing Process Phase: planning; client need: safe and effective care environment; concern area: medical/surgical

TEST 4

1. The physician orders primidone (Mysoline) for a 28-year-old male client. The nurse would suspect that the client has:
   A. Severe migraine headaches
   B. Seizure disorder
   C. Peptic ulcers
   D. Anxiety disorder

2. The nurse teaches a client that the best time for her to take sulfamethoxazole/trimethoprim (Septra) is:
   A. With meals
   B. 1 hour before or 2 hours after meals
   C. qid and HS
   D. 9 q A.M.

3. A client is receiving rifampin (Rifandin) for which of the following conditions?
   A. Acute asthma attack
   B. Angina pectoris
   C. Tuberculosis
   D. Chronic low blood pressure

4. Which group of clients would the nurse need to monitor closely while taking rifandin (Rifampin)?
   A. Clients with a history of liver disease
   B. Clients with a history of hyperthyroidism
   C. Clients with a history of narcolepsy
   D. Clients with a history of encephalitis

5. The nurse would know that her teaching concerning rifandin (Rifampin) was successful if the client states:
   A. "The longer I take this medication the worse the side effects will become."
   B. "I need to take the medication with antacids."
   C. "I must take this medication daily for 6 months."
   D. "I have to decrease my fluid intake while on this medication."

6. The nurse should anticipate which of the following from a client who is receiving a medication that stimulates the sympathetic nervous system?
   A. Tachycardia and hypertension
   B. Pupillary dilation and tachypnea
   C. Increased peristalsis and sphincter tone relaxation
   D. CNS suppression and urinary retention

7. A child receiving nystatin (Mycostatin) most likely has a:
   A. Viral infection
   B. Bacterial infection
   C. Fungal infection
   D. Nosocomial infection

8. The nurse recognizes that metronidazole (Flagyl) is effective against:
   A. Protozoal and gram-negative infections
   B. Aerobic and gram-positive infections
   C. Viral and bacterial infections
   D. All central nervous system (CNS) and urinary tract infections

9. Which of the following medications would the nurse anticipate administering to a 10-year-old client with a pinworm infection?
   A. theophylline (Aminophylline)
   B. metronidazole (Flagyl)
   C. mebendazole (Vermox)
   D. chloramphenicol (Chloromycetin)

10. Medications such as meperidine (Demerol) that are used medically and have a high potential for abuse are classified as:
    A. Schedule I
    B. Schedule II
    C. Schedule III
    D. Schedule IV

11. A nursing student is preparing to give a client a dose of isoniazid (INH). The client says to the student, "This pill is yellow; the one I usually take is green." The best response of the student to this comment would be to:
    A. Encourage the client to take the pill, explaining that different drug companies make the same pills in different colors.
    B. Encourage the client to take the pill, explaining that it is very important to never stop taking the medication suddenly.
    C. Consult with another student who is in the room about whether or not the client should take the medication.
    D. Hold the medication, and recheck the dosage with the medex.

12. A physician orders metaproterenol (Alupent) for a client. The nurse would anticipate administering this medication in what way?
    A. IV
    B. IM
    C. Inhalation
    D. Rectal suppository

13. Which of the following side effects would a client likely experience after receiving a dose of metaproterenol (Alupent)?
    A. Tachycardia, shaking
    B. Bleeding peptic ulcer, vomiting
    C. Moderate hypotension, dizziness
    D. Edema, moon face

14. After giving a client levodopa (Dopar), the nurse would monitor the client for which of the following?
    A. Bradycardia
    B. Glaucoma
    C. Postural hypotension
    D. Excessive urination and dehydration

15. The physician orders diphenhydramine (Benadryl) 125 mg IV q 4 h prn for a client. The best response to this order by the nurse is to:
    A. Give the medication as ordered
    B. Hold the medication and notify the physician that the dose is too large
    C. Hold the medication and notify the physician that the dose is too small
    D. Hold the medication and notify the physician that the route is incorrect

16. Which of the following assessments would indicate to a nurse that a client was experiencing a usual side effect of the medication phenylephrine (Neo-Synephrine)?
    A. Crackles and rhonchi
    B. Tachycardia
    C. Jaundice
    D. Drowsiness and somnolence

17. The nurse would anticipate that the physician would order acetylcystine (Mucomyst) for a client with which of the following conditions?
    A. Chronic bronchitis
    B. Cardiac arrest
    C. Hypertensive crisis
    D. Hypothyroidism

18. A client with Parkinson's syndrome asks the nurse, "Why am I taking thrihexyphenioyl (Artane)?" The best response by the nurse would be:
    A. It counteracts the side effects of the levodopa.
    B. It prevents depression from developing.
    C. It controls the symptoms of drooling and muscle rigidity.
    D. It helps the client relax so he or she can sleep.

19. A client is displaying the symptoms of anorexia, depression, bradycardia, and headache. Most likely, he or she is receiving which of the following medications?
    A. atropine
    B. epinephrine
    C. digoxin (Lanoxin)
    D. levodopa (Dopar)

20. Which of the following would the nurse expect to see in the client who was receiving a sympatholytic medication?
    A. Tachycardia
    B. Hypotension
    C. Anxiety
    D. Dilated pupils

21. When administering a calcium channel blocker, the nurse recognizes that these medications are used primarily to:
    A. Control postoperative pain
    B. Increase the heart rate
    C. Induce sleep
    D. Control angina

22. The nurse would administer methyldopa (Aldomet) PO to a client who had:
    A. Angina
    B. Insomnia
    C. Hypertension
    D. Gastric ulcer

23. Which of the following doses ordered for methyldopa (Aldomet) to be given to an adult client would the nurse administer without question?
    A. 20 mg PO qd
    B. 150 mg PO bid
    C. 250 mg PO tid
    D. 1000 mg PO qid

24. Which of the following home-care measures would be most appropriate for the nurse to teach a client to perform who is taking nadolol (Corgard)?
    A. Home pregnancy test
    B. Blood pressure
    C. Blood glucose monitoring
    D. Urine for glucose and acetone

25. An important nursing implication for a client receiving furosemide (Lasix) is to:
    A. Give the IV medication rapidly to maximize effect
    B. Encourage the patient to drink extra fluids to replace losses
    C. Encourage a diet high in fresh fruits and vegetables
    D. Limit the patient's exercise

26. It would be most important for the nurse to monitor the client receiving mannitol (Osmitrol) for which of the following?
    A. Circulatory overload
    B. Disorientation
    C. Bradycardia
    D. Skin rashes

27. Which of the following statements made by a client taking warfarin (Coumadin) would indicate that additional teaching would be required before discharge?
    A. "This medication will dissolve the clot in my leg."
    B. "I should avoid eating cabbage and broccoli."
    C. "I should avoid rubbing my leg when it hurts."
    D. "If I notice any bleeding, I should call the physician."

28. A physician has just ordered heparin 10,000 U/h IV for a client with a pulmonary embolus. The best response by the nurse to this order is to:
    A. Give the medication as ordered
    B. Hold the medication and notify the physician that the dose is too large
    C. Hold the medication and notify the physician that the dose is too small
    D. Hold the medication and notify the physician that the route is incorrect

29. In assessing the effectiveness of heparin therapy, the nurse would evaluate which laboratory test?
    A. Partial thromboplastin time (PTT)
    B. Prothrombin time (PT)
    C. Glutamate pyruvate transaminase (GPT)
    D. Platelets

30. To which of the following clients would the nurse administer streptokinase (Streptase) without questioning the order?
    A. Meningitis
    B. Acute myocardial infarction
    C. Unstable angina pectoris
    D. Hypothyroidism

31. The physician wrote an order for methylphenidate HCL (Ritalin) 10 mg PO bid for a child with attention deficit hyperactivity disorder (ADHD). The best response by the nurse to this order is to:
    A. Question the order because the dosage is too large
    B. Give the medication as ordered
    C. Give the medication IV instead of PO because it works better that way
    D. Hold the medication and verify the use with the physician before giving

32. The nurse teaches an adult client with lupus who is taking large doses of prednisone to avoid eating:
    A. Fresh fruits and raw vegetables
    B. Cold cuts and hot dogs
    C. Canned peaches and beans
    D. White bread and cooked rice

33. The most important factor to teach a client who is to take sucralfate (Carafate) at home is to:
    A. Eat extra fresh fruits and drink extra fluids
    B. Suck on hard candy to control dry mouth
    C. Take the medication until the stomach pain is gone
    D. Avoid taking aspirin

34. The nurse anticipates a negative inotropic effect after giving which of the following medications?
    A. atropine sulfate
    B. aminophylline (Theophylline)
    C. propranolol (Inderal)
    D. digoxin (Lanoxin)

35. A client asks the nurse about the classification of the medication docusate calcium (Surfak). The best response by the nurse is that this medication is classified as a:
    A. Calcium channel blocker
    B. Laxative
    C. Positive inotropic
    D. Antibiotic

36. Which of the following client statements indicates that a client who is taking bisacodyl (Dulcolax) requires further teaching?
    A. "I must not take these pills with milk."
    B. "I might experience cramping after taking the medication."
    C. "If I have trouble swallowing the pills, I can chew them."
    D. "I should increase my fluid intake."

37. Rantidine (Zantac) is to be given IV. Of the following dosages, which would the nurse give without questioning?
    A. 1 g IV q 8 h
    B. 50 mg IVPB q 6 h
    C. 300 mg IVPB q 4 h
    D. 0.5 mg IVPB q 2 h

38. A disoriented, combative client with liver failure would most likely be receiving which of the following medications?
    A. diazepam (Valium)
    B. meperidine (Demerol)
    C. lactulose (Chronulac)
    D. dopamine (Intropin)

39. To which of the following clients would the nurse anticipate giving metoclopramide (Reglan)?
    A. A client with liver failure
    B. A client who is unresponsive
    C. A client with chronic renal failure
    D. A client who has diabetic gastric stasis

40. A client asks the nurse why there are so many side effects from the chemotherapy he is taking for his cancer. The best response by the nurse is:
    A. "These medications have systemic effects."
    B. "Chemotherapy works against disseminated diseases."
    C. "The medication kills both normal body cells and cancer cells."
    D. "Chemotherapy attacks malignant cells during their vulnerable period of growth."

41. Which of the following is an appropriate measure for the nurse to teach a client who is receiving anticancer medications?
    A. Avoid brushing your teeth to prevent gum bleeding.
    B. Stay in the direct sunlight as much as possible to increase the production of natural vitamin D.
    C. Avoid eating for 6 hours after medication to prevent nausea.
    D. Increase daily fluid intake to 2–3 L.

42. The most important nursing measure when administering vincristine (Oncovan) is to:
    A. Monitor the client's blood pressure every 15 minutes
    B. Keep the client in the recumbent position
    C. Monitor the IV site closely for infiltration
    D. Give it with milk, food, or an antacid

43. Pilocarpine (Isopto Carpine) would most likely be used to treat a client with:
   A. Congestive heart failure
   B. Wide-angle glaucoma
   C. Metastatic breast cancer
   D. Chronic constipation

44. The nurse must monitor a client who is taking glucocorticoids for the development of:
   A. Dehydration
   B. Hypotension
   C. Peripheral edema
   D. Graves' disease

45. A client receiving acetazolamide (Diamox) should be monitored for:
   A. Photosensitivity
   B. Constipation
   C. Renal failure
   D. Hyponatremia

46. A client is to receive timolol maleate (Timoptic). The best way for the nurse to administer this medication is:
   A. IV push slowly over 2 to 4 minutes
   B. IVPB diluted in at least 50 mL of saline
   C. PO followed by a full glass of water
   D. 1 to 2 drops in each eye

47. A client receiving cefoxitin (Mefoxin) is probably suffering from:
   A. Cancer of the prostate
   B. Glaucoma
   C. Peptic ulcer disease
   D. Severe bladder infection

48. Which of the following foods are generally not allowed in the diets of clients who have peptic ulcer disease?
   A. Colas, coffee, and tea
   B. Milk, yogurt, and cheeses
   C. Raw fruits, pancakes, and grapefruit juice
   D. Cornflakes, bananas, and avocados

49. A client is to receive isosorbide (Isordil). The condition he is most likely being treated for is:
   A. Essential hypertension
   B. Stable angina
   C. Inflammatory bowel disease
   D. Liver failure

50. A client is taking warfarin (Coumadin). He is most likely suffering from:
   A. Glaucoma
   B. Irritable bowel syndrome
   C. Thrombophlebitis
   D. Unstable angina

1. **Correct Answer: B.** This medication is used to control grand mal, focal, and psychomotor seizures.

Rationales for Other Answer Choices: A. Not an appropriate use. **C.** Not an appropriate use. **D.** Not an appropriate use.
Nursing Process Phase: analysis; client need: safe and effective care environment; concern area: medical/surgical

2. **Correct Answer: B.** This medication works best on an empty stomach.

Rationales for Other Answer Choices: A. Food interferes with absorption. **C.** Generally not given 5 times per day. **D.** Need at least 2 doses per day.
Nursing Process Phase: planning; client need: health promotion and maintenance; concern area: medical/surgical

3. **Correct Answer: C.** This is a primary medication for the treatment of tuberculosis.

Rationales for Other Answer Choices: A. Not used to treat this disorder. **B.** Has no effects on this disorder. **D.** Does not affect blood pressure.
Nursing Process Phase: analysis; client need: safe and effective care environment; concern area: medical/surgical

4. **Correct Answer: A.** This medication is hepatotoxic and can worsen existing liver disease.

Rationales for Other Answer Choices: B. Does not directly affect thyroid function. **C.** Has no effect on sleep disorders. **D.** Not used to treat infections of the CNS.
Nursing Process Phase: planning; client need: safe and effective care environment; concern area: medical/surgical

5. **Correct Answer: C.** This medication needs to be taken without interruption for 6 to 12 months.

Rationales for Other Answer Choices: A. Side effects tend to be more severe early in therapy but improve later. **B.** Antacids and food tend to decrease effectiveness—best taken on an empty stomach. **D.** Should increase fluid to 2–3 L/d.
Nursing Process Phase: evaluation; client need: health promotion and maintenance; concern area: medical/surgical

6. **Correct Answer: A.** These conditions are normal consequences of sympathetic stimulation.

Rationales for Other Answer Choices: B. Produces pupillary constriction. **C.** Tends to decrease these parasympathetic functions. **D.** Stimulates CNS and does not produce retention.
Nursing Process Phase: assessment; client need: safe and effective care environment; concern area: medical/surgical

7. **Correct Answer: C.** This is an antifungal medication.

Rationales for Other Answer Choices: A. Has no effect on viruses. **B.** Has no effect on bacteria. **D.** A nosocomial infection is hospital-acquired and usually bacterial in nature.
Nursing Process Phase: analysis; client need: safe and effective care environment; concern area: pediatrics

8. **Correct Answer: A.** These are the primary uses for this potent antiprotozoal medication.

Rationales for Other Answer Choices: B. Not as effective against these infections as other groups of medications. **C.** Not effective against viral infections. **D.** Only effective against these infections if the organisms are appropriate.
Nursing Process Phase: planning; client need: safe and effective care environment; concern area: medical/surgical

9. **Correct Answer: C.** This medication is used for several different types of worm infestations, including pinworms.

Rationales for Other Answer Choices: A. Not effective against worm infestations. **B.** Little effect on worm infestations. **D.** Not primary medication used for worm infestations.
Nursing Process Phase: implementation; client need: safe and effective care environment; concern area: pediatrics

10. **Correct Answer: B.** This schedule defines the group and includes most of the narcotic medications used for pain control.

Rationales for Other Answer Choices: A. These medications are highly addictive and have no medical use. **C.** These medications have lower potential for abuse and often include sleeping aids, sedatives, and so forth. **D.** These medications have a reduced potential for abuse and include tranquilizers, and combination medications.
Nursing Process Phase: planning; client need: safe and effective care environment; concern area: medical/surgical

11. **Correct Answer: D.** Always double-check if a client questions a medication.

Rationales for Other Answer Choices: A. This may be true, but it may also be the wrong medication. Check first. **B.** This is a true statement, but is it the correct medication in the correct dose? **C.** Avoid this action—other students would likely not know more.
Nursing Process Phase: implementation; client need: safe and effective care environment; concern area: therapeutic communication

12. **Correct Answer: C.** A potent bronchodilator most often given by hand-held nebulizer (HHN) or other respiratory treatment.

Rationales for Other Answer Choices: A. Not a common route of administration. **B.** Not a common route of administration. **D.** Not available in this form.
Nursing Process Phase: planning; client need: safe and effective care environment; concern area: medical/surgical

13. **Correct Answer: A.** This medication stimulates beta receptors to dilate the bronchioli but also stimulates the CV system.

Rationales for Other Answer Choices: B. Not common side effects of this medication. **C.** More likely to cause hypertension. **D.** Side effects of steroid medications.
Nursing Process Phase: assessment; client need: safe and effective care environment; concern area: medical/surgical

14. Correct Answer: C. Common side effect that may lead to injuries from falls.

Rationales for Other Answer Choices: A. Causes tachycardia. **B.** May complicate glaucoma but does not cause it. **D.** Not side effects of this medication.
Nursing Process Phase: assessment; client need: safe and effective care environment; concern area: medical/surgical

15. Correct Answer: B. The usual adult dose is 25–50 mg.

Rationales for Other Answer Choices: A. Dose is too large. **C.** Dose is too large. **D.** Can be given IV, IM, or PO.
Nursing Process Phase: implementation; client need: safe and effective care environment; concern area: medical/surgical

16. Correct Answer: B. This alpha-adrenergic stimulant produces vasoconstriction in the swollen mucous membranes but tends to stimulate the cardiovascular (CV) system also.

Rationales for Other Answer Choices: A. Symptoms of congestive heart failure (CHF); medication may help with this disorder. **C.** Symptom of liver failure; not associated with this medication. **D.** Tends to produce nervousness and insomnia.
Nursing Process Phase: assessment; client need: safe and effective care environment; concern area: medical/surgical

17. Correct Answer: A. This is a mucolytic that is commonly used for respiratory disorders that produce excessive amounts of mucus.

Rationales for Other Answer Choices: B. Not an appropriate medication for this problem. **C.** Not used for this disorder. **D.** Not effective against this disorder.
Nursing Process Phase: analysis; client need: safe and effective care environment; concern area: medical/surgical

18. Correct Answer: C. It is an anticholinergic used to control these symptoms.

Rationales for Other Answer Choices: A. Does not do this. **B.** Has no effect on depression. **D.** Does not normally produce relaxation.
Nursing Process Phase: implementation; client need: psychosocial integrity; concern area: medical/surgical

19. Correct Answer: C. These are symptoms of lanoxin toxicity.

Rationales for Other Answer Choices: A. Tends to produce tachycardia. **B.** Has tachycardia as a common side effect. **D.** Produces tachycardia.
Nursing Process Phase: assessment; client need: safe and effective care environment; concern area: medical/surgical

20. Correct Answer: B. These medications block the effects of the sympathetic system, causing hypotension, bradycardia, constricted pupils.

Rationales for Other Answer Choices: A. Causes bradycardia.   **C.** Often produces sedation.   **D.** Causes constricted pupils.
Nursing Process Phase: assessment; client need: health promotion and maintenance; concern area: medical/surgical

21. **Correct Answer: D.**   These negative inotropic, negative chronotropic medications reduce the workload of the heart and its oxygen use, thus reducing chest pain.

Rationales for Other Answer Choices: A. Not effective for this condition.   **B.** They slow the heart rate.   **C.** Not effective for inducing sleep.
Nursing Process Phase: planning; client need: safe and effective care environment; concern area: medical/surgical

22. **Correct Answer: C.**   This is an alpha-adrenergic stimulant that dilates blood vessels, thereby lowering blood pressure.

Rationales for Other Answer Choices: A. Not a primary use of this medication.
B. Not effective for this disorder.   **D.** No effect on gastric acid secretions.
Nursing Process Phase: analysis; client need: safe and effective care environment; concern area: medical/surgical

23. **Correct Answer: C.**   Usual dosage range for adults: 250–500 mg tid.

Rationales for Other Answer Choices: A. Dose too small.   **B.** Dose too small.
D. Dose too large.
Nursing Process Phase: planning; client need: safe and effective care environment; concern area: medical/surgical

24. **Correct Answer: B.**   This medication is used to treat hypertension. Monitoring the blood pressure at home would help determine effectiveness.

Rationales for Other Answer Choices: A. Medication has no effect on fertility.
C. Not used for the control of blood sugar.   **D.** Does not affect these measurements.
Nursing Process Phase: planning; client need: health promotion and maintenance; concern area: medical/surgical

25. **Correct Answer: C.**   This potent diuretic causes potassium loss, which can be replaced by eating foods high in potassium.

Rationales for Other Answer Choices: A. Should be given slowly IV.   **B.** If used for CHF, fluids should be restricted.   **D.** No particular contraindication for exercise.
Nursing Process Phase: planning; client need: safe and effective care environment; concern area: medical/surgical

26. **Correct Answer: A.**   This osmotic diuretic draws fluid from the tissues into the vascular system; clients in CHF may develop fluid overload as a result.

Rationales for Other Answer Choices: B. May increase orientation with increased intracranial pressure (IICP).   **C.** Not a common side effect.   **D.** Not a common side effect.
Nursing Process Phase: assessment; client need: safe and effective care environment; concern area: medical/surgical

27. **Correct Answer: A.**   The medication does *not* dissolve clots; it prevents clots from getting larger so that the body's own antithrombin enzymes can break it down.

Rationales for Other Answer Choices: B. These foods contain vitamin K which tends to counteract the effect of this medication.   **C.** Rubbing the leg may dislodge the clot.   **D.** Excessive bleeding is a common side effect of this medication—may indicate high PT.
Nursing Process Phase: evaluation; client need: health promotion and maintenance; concern area: medical/surgical

28. **Correct Answer: B.**   Average therapeutic dose is 800 to 1500 U/h. A client receiving this large a dose is at high risk for bleeding.

Rationales for Other Answer Choices: A. Dose is too large.   **C.** Dose is too large.   **D.** Can be given IV or SC.
Nursing Process Phase: implementation; client need: safe and effective care environment; concern area: medical/surgical

29. **Correct Answer: A.**   PTT is the appropriate test to monitor therapeutic effect of heparin.

Rationales for Other Answer Choices: B. Used for Coumadin therapy.   **C.** Liver enzyme not affected by heparin.   **D.** Not affected by heparin therapy.
Nursing Process Phase: planning; client need: safe and effective care environment; concern area: medical/surgical

30. **Correct Answer: B.**   This potent antithrombolytic medication is used to dissolve the clots in the coronary arteries that cause MI.

Rationales for Other Answer Choices: A. Medication has no antimicrobial effect.   **C.** Not indicated for long-term control of this disorder.   **D.** Medication has no direct effect on the thyroid gland.
Nursing Process Phase: planning; client need: safe and effective care environment; concern area: medical/surgical

31. **Correct Answer: B.**   This is the correct dose and use of this medication.

Rationales for Other Answer Choices: A. Dose is correct.   **C.** No IV form of the medication.   **D.** Primary medication for attention deficit hyperactivity disorder.
Nursing Process Phase: implementation; client need: psychosocial integrity; concern area: pediatrics

32. **Correct Answer: A.**   Due to the immunosuppressive effects of this medication, the client is more susceptible to infections. These foods tend to have higher levels of bacteria than cooked foods.

Rationales for Other Answer Choices: B. These foods may have high levels of sodium that will increase the fluid retention often associated with the medication, but this is not as serious as infections.   **C.** These foods are appropriate.   **D.** These foods are appropriate.
Nursing Process Phase: implementation; client need: health promotion and maintenance; concern area: medical/surgical

33. **Correct Answer: A.**   These measures will help prevent the constipation often associated with use of this medication.

Rationales for Other Answer Choices: B. Appropriate, but lower priority. **C.** Medication should be taken for full course of treatment. **D.** Appropriate, but lower priority.
Nursing Process Phase: planning; client need: health promotion and maintenance; concern area: medical/surgical

34. **Correct Answer: C.** Beta-blockers decrease the force of contraction (negative inotropic).

Rationales for Other Answer Choices: A. Neutral inotropic effect. **B.** Positive inotropic effect. **D.** Positive inotropic effect.
Nursing Process Phase: planning; client need: safe and effective care environment; concern area: medical/surgical

35. **Correct Answer: B.** This medication is used for mild to moderate constipation.

Rationales for Other Answer Choices: A. Does not affect calcium in the cell. **C.** Has no effect on cardiac contractions. **D.** No antimicrobial effects with this medication.
Nursing Process Phase: implementation; client need: safe and effective care environment; concern area: medical/surgical

36. **Correct Answer: C.** They should never be chewed or crushed.

Rationales for Other Answer Choices: A. Should not be taken with milk or antacids. **B.** Common side effect when taking this medication. **D.** Will increase the effectiveness of the medication.
Nursing Process Phase: evaluation; client need: safe and effective care environment; concern area: medical/surgical

37. **Correct Answer: B.** Usual dose for adults.

Rationales for Other Answer Choices: A. Dose is much too large. **C.** Dose for Tagamet. **D.** Dose is too large.
Nursing Process Phase: planning; client need: safe and effective care environment; concern area: medical/surgical

38. **Correct Answer: C.** These are symptoms of hepatic encephalopathy, which has lactulose as one of the key components of the treatment regimen.

Rationales for Other Answer Choices: A. This medication is hepatotoxic and should be avoided in liver failure. **B.** Not indicated in this client. **D.** Sympathetic stimulant medication used in severe CHF.
Nursing Process Phase: planning; client need: safe and effective care environment; concern area: psychiatric nursing

39. **Correct Answer: D.** This medication increases peristalsis in the intestines and is often used for this condition.

Rationales for Other Answer Choices: A. Inappropriate for this condition. **B.** Has no CNS effects. **C.** Has no effect on renal function.
Nursing Process Phase: analysis; client need: safe and effective care environment; concern area: medical/surgical

40.   **Correct Answer: C.**   These medications kill the fastest growing cells first (one of the characteristics of cancer cells) but also damage and kill normal body cells.

Rationales for Other Answer Choices: A. True statement but is included in **C.   B.** True statement but does not answer the question.   **D.** True statement but does not answer the question.
Nursing Process Phase: implementation; client need: health promotion and maintenance; concern area: therapeutic communication

41.   **Correct Answer: D.**   This measure will help decrease renal toxicity and prevent renal failure.

Rationales for Other Answer Choices: A. Good oral care is important; use a soft toothbrush.   **B.** Most cause photosensitivity; avoid sunlight.   **C.** Eating low-fat, high-carbohydrate foods may help decrease nausea.
Nursing Process Phase: implementation; client need: safe and effective care environment; concern area: medical/surgical

42.   **Correct Answer: C.**   This is a vesicant medication that may cause extensive tissue damage if it infiltrates.

Rationales for Other Answer Choices: A. Not required for this medication.   **B.** Does not produce postural hypotension.   **D.** Medication is given IV.
Nursing Process Phase: implementation; client need: safe and effective care environment; concern area: medical/surgical

43.   **Correct Answer: B.**   Commonly used miotic medication that helps reduce intraocular pressure.

Rationales for Other Answer Choices: A. Not effective for this disorder.   **C.** No effect on cancer.   **D.** No effect on constipation.
Nursing Process Phase: analysis; client need: safe and effective care environment; concern area: medical/surgical

44.   **Correct Answer: C.**   This medication causes sodium and fluid retention, which often leads to edema.

Rationales for Other Answer Choices: A. Not associated with use of these medications.   **B.** Tends to increase blood pressure.   **D.** No direct effect on the thyroid gland.
Nursing Process Phase: assessment; client need: safe and effective care environment; concern area: medical/surgical

45.   **Correct Answer: D.**   This is a potent diuretic medication used to lower intraocular pressure, but it also causes fluid and electrolyte loss.

Rationales for Other Answer Choices: A. Not a side effect of this medication.   **B.** Not a side effect of this medication.   **C.** Very low incidence of this complication.
Nursing Process Phase: assessment; client need: safe and effective care environment; concern area: medical/surgical

46.   **Correct Answer: D.**   This is available only as an eyedrop.

Rationales for Other Answer Choices: A. Not available IV.   **B.** Not available IVPB.   **C.** Not taken PO.

Nursing Process Phase: implementation; client need: safe and effective care environment; concern area: medical/surgical

47. **Correct Answer: D.** This is a second-generation cephalosporin used to treat moderate to severe infections.

Rationales for Other Answer Choices: A. Has no antineoplastic effects. **B.** Not effective against this disorder. **C.** Not effective against this disorder.
Nursing Process Phase: analysis; client need: safe and effective care environment; concern area: medical/surgical

48. **Correct Answer: A.** Clients with ulcers should avoid caffeine.

Rationales for Other Answer Choices: B. Appropriate foods for this disorder. **C.** Appropriate foods for this disorder. **D.** Appropriate foods for this disorder.
Nursing Process Phase: planning; client need: safe and effective care environment; concern area: medical/surgical

49. **Correct Answer: B.** This long-acting nitrate is used for the control of stable angina.

Rationales for Other Answer Choices: A. May lower the BP as a side effect but is not the primary use of this medication. **C.** No effect on the GI system. **D.** Not appropriate for this disorder.
Nursing Process Phase: analysis; client need: safe and effective care environment; concern area: medical/surgical

50. **Correct Answer: C.** Oral anticoagulant used to treat clot disorders.

Rationales for Other Answer Choices: A. Inappropriate for this disorder. **B.** No gastrointestinal (GI) effects. **D.** Not used for this condition.
Nursing Process Phase: analysis; client need: safe and effective care environment; concern area: medical/surgical

1. The physician orders a dose of 80 mg of garamycin (Gentamicin) for a patient with peritonitis. The medication comes in ampules of 100 mg in 5 mL of fluid. How many mL should the client receive?
   A. 4 mL
   B. 8 mL
   C. 10 mL
   D. 40 mL

2. Which of the following medication combinations would a client with a transplanted kidney likely be receiving?
   A. Garamycin, prednisone, imuran
   B. Aminophylline, garamycin, prednisone
   C. Prednisone, imuran, cyclosporine
   D. Imuran, garamycin, cyclosporine

3. Which of the following medications would a client who developed frequent premature ventricular contractions (PVCs) most likely be given immediately?
   A. cyclosporine (Sandimmune) PO
   B. epinephrine IV
   C. lidocaine IV
   D. digoxin (lanoxin) IM

4. A medication is classified as an anticholinergic agent. The nurse knows that the effects that are produced:
   A. Cause bradycardia
   B. Are similar to those produced by sympathetic stimulants
   C. Have a high potential for addiction and abuse
   D. Mimic the effects of parasympathetic stimulation

5. A client develops a bradycardia of 34 beats per minute (BPM). If all of the following medications are available IV, which one should the nurse give first?
   A. epinephrine (Adrenalin)
   B. verapamil (Calan)
   C. atropine sulfate
   D. procainamide (Pronestyl)

6. A client is taking propranolol (Inderal). Which side effects of this medication would the nurse expect the client to develop?
   A. Paralysis of his lower extremities
   B. Tachycardia
   C. Second-degree, type II heart block
   D. Disorientation and weakness

7. A post-MI client is taking 2.5 mg of warfarin (Coumadin) daily. The nurse would know that her teaching about this medication was effective if the client states:
   A. "I need to eat extra cabbage and broccoli to keep my potassium at normal."
   B. "I have to use a straight-blade razor when I shave."
   C. "I should brush my teeth with a soft-bristle toothbrush."
   D. "I need to take one baby aspirin each morning."

8. Silver sulfadiazine is the topical antibiotic of choice for most burn wounds because it:
   A. Is rapidly absorbed by blood
   B. Is effective against bacterial growth with few side effects
   C. Is a carbonic anhydrase inhibitor
   D. Maintains adequate pH of the newly forming skin buds

9. For a client with deep second-degree burns over 40% of his or her body, the physician has ordered 3600 mL of intravenous fluid to be given during the first 8 hours. At what rate should the IV run if the client is on a volumetric pump?
   A. 240 mL/h
   B. 450 mL/h
   C. 480 mL/h
   D. 60 gtt/min

10. A client with renal failure is taking 6 calcium carbonate tablets with each meal per the physician's advice. The nurse explains that the primary reason for taking these tablets is to:
    A. Relieve gastric irritation from a low-protein diet
    B. Bind phosphates in the intestinal tract
    C. Prevent metabolic acidosis
    D. Relieve heart burn and gas

11. The nurse recognizes that a medication that depresses the sympathetic branch of the autonomic nervous system would most likely:
    A. Produce a tachycardia
    B. Produce a bradycardia
    C. Produce ventricular tachycardia
    D. Have no effect on cardiac function

12. If a nurse were to treat a client with a ventricular escape rhythm, which of the following medications are the best ones to use?
    A. Lidocaine and pronestyl
    B. Inderal and calan
    C. Quinidine and lanoxin
    D. Atropine and epinephrine

13. The nurse will know that instruction concerning the medication nitroglycerine has been successful if the client states:
    A. "I need to take this medication even when I begin to feel like my old self."
    B. "If I develop a headache, I need to notify my doctor."
    C. "When I take the medicine, I should be lying or sitting down."
    D. "If I lose my appetite or start vomiting, I need to call the doctor."

14. A client has all of the following medications ordered prn. The most appropriate medication for the nurse to give in response to a client who has just gone into atrial tachycardia is:
    A. Epinephrine IV
    B. Verapamil (Calan) IV
    C. Atropine sulfate IV
    D. Furosemide (Lasix) PO

15. A client is to receive furosemide (Lasix) 60 mg IV push stat. The medication comes in a vial labeled 100 mg in 10 mL. How long should it take the nurse to administer this medication?
    A. 100 mL/h
    B. 2 minutes
    C. 6 minutes
    D. 34 gtt/min

16. The nurse recognizes that clients who have overdosed on narcotic drugs are at risk for the development of acute respiratory failure (ARF) because:
    A. Narcotics produce respiratory alkalosis.
    B. Narcotics affect enzyme activity and pH.
    C. Confusion and disorientation affect the patient's ability to breathe consciously.
    D. Suppression of the medulla oblongata produces hypoventilation.

17. A client is receiving theophylline (Aminophylline) IV for severe chronic obstructive pulmonary disease (COPD). Which of the following would the nurse observe the client for after administration of this medication?
    A. Drowsiness and lethargy
    B. Constipation and bradycardia
    C. Insomnia and tachycardia
    D. Edema and wet lung sounds

18. The nurse will know that his or her teaching concerning the medication verapamil (Calan) has been successful when the client voices which of the following statements?
    A. "I can stop taking this medication when I begin to feel like my old self."
    B. "If I begin to feel dizzy, weak, or have swelling in my ankles, I need to notify my doctor."
    C. "If I miss a dose, I need to double up on the next dose."
    D. "I must take this medication with meals so that it doesn't upset my stomach."

19. A client is started on a heparin drip. The heparin is mixed 20,000 units in 500 mL of D5W. It is to run at 1000 U/h. At what rate should the volumetric pump be set to deliver this dosage of medication?
  A. 60 mL/h
  B. 25 mL/h
  C. 10 mL/h
  D. 16 mL/h

20. All of the following would be appropriate uses for isoproterenal (Isuprel) except:
  A. Asthma
  B. Heart block
  C. Chronic bronchitis
  D. Supraventricular tachycardia

21. Which would be an inappropriate medication for a client diagnosed with asthma?
  A. propranolol (Inderal)
  B. acetaminophen (Tylenol)
  C. isoproterenol (Isuprel)
  D. epinephrine (Adrenalin)

22. The physician orders a combination medication containing dicyclomide (Bentyl) for a client. What condition does this patient most likely have?
  A. Elevated blood pressure
  B. Slow heart rate
  C. Seizure disorder
  D. Peptic ulcer

23. Which of the following toxic effects should a nurse monitor for a child who is receiving phenytoin (Dilantin)?
  A. Stevens-Johnson syndrome
  B. Folate deficiency
  C. Leukopenic aplastic anemia
  D. Granulocytosis and nephrosis

24. A medication whose primary use is to produce relaxation is referred to as a(n):
  A. Analgesic
  B. Hypnotic
  C. Sedative
  D. Antipyretic

25. While teaching a client with Parkinson's disease about the home use of levodopa, the nurse should include which of the following statements:
  A. "You must limit your intake of foods that contain pyridoxine."
  B. "You must limit your intake of foods that contain vitamin K."
  C. "You must limit your intake of foods that contain iron."
  D. "You must limit your intake of foods that contain calcium."

26. The nurse would need to include in the care plan "monitor the serum glucose levels" of a client who was receiving which of the following medications?
  A. norepinephrine (Levophed)
  B. dobutamine (Dobutrex)
  C. propanolol (Inderal)
  D. epinephrine (Adrenalin)

27. A client with obstructive pulmonary disease is receiving all of the following medications. After the administration of which of the following would the nurse monitor the client for bronchospasms?
    A. verapamil (Isoptin)
    B. amrinone (Incor)
    C. epinephrine
    D. propranolol (Inderal)

28. While reviewing a 76-year-old client's medication list at home, a home-health-care nurse notes the following medications. Which one would most likely elevate the serum digoxin level?
    A. Potassium chloride
    B. Synthroid
    C. Quinidine
    D. Theophylline

29. A hospitalized child with a congenital heart defect exhibits disorientation, lethargy, and seizures. The nurse assesses that he may be having a toxic reaction to:
    A. digoxin (Lanoxin)
    B. lidocaine (Xylocaine)
    C. quinidine sulfate (Quinidex)
    D. nitroglycerine (NTG)

30. While teaching a client about home use of SL nitroglycerine (NTG), the nurse should include mention of which of the following in his teaching plan?
    A. A stinging, burning sensation when placed under the tongue
    B. Temporary blurring of vision for 5 minutes after taking
    C. Prolonged use will cause generalized urticaria
    D. Urinary frequency is a common side effect

31. The nurse notes that the IV of a client who is receiving dopamine (Intropine) has infiltrated. Which of the following medications should the nurse administer directly into the infiltration site?
    A. phentolamine (Regitine)
    B. epinephrine
    C. phenylephrine (Neo-Synephrine)
    D. sodium bicarbonate

32. The nurse notes on the care plan of a child with serious burn injuries to give all medications IV because this route:
    A. Delays absorption to promote extended therapeutic effect
    B. Facilitates absorption, whereas absorption from the muscles is unpredictable
    C. Allows the nurse to discontinue the medication immediately if an allergic reaction occurs
    D. Avoids producing the additional pain that occurs from IM or SC injections

33. Which of the following medications used for treatment of burn injuries best penetrates the eschar?
   A. mafenide acetate (Sulfamylon)
   B. silver sulfadiazine (Silvadine)
   C. neomycin sulfate (Neosporin)
   D. providone iodine (Betadine)

34. A 76-year-old male client is being taught about safety measures in relation to his home medications prior to discharge. The nurse should include in the teaching plan that in order to prevent falls that may occur when taking furosemide (Lasix) 80 mg PO bid, the client should take the medication:
   A. Upon arising and no later than 6 P.M.
   B. Every 12 hours at 9 A.M. and 9 P.M.
   C. With a full glass of water to prevent dehydration
   D. At noon and HS

35. While passing 0900 scheduled medications, the nurse finds the client in the bathroom. The client says to the nurse through the door, "Leave my pills by my bed; I'll take them when I come out." Which of the following would be the most appropriate action for the nurse to take?
   A. Leave the medications at the bedside with a note for the client to take them as soon as possible.
   B. Return the medications to the client's medication drawer, and chart "medications refused."
   C. Take the medications away, but return in 10 minutes to administer them.
   D. Wait in the room until the client comes out of the bathroom.

36. A client boasts that he can take his pills "dry." The nurse knows that the minimal amount of liquid required for all oral medications is at least:
   A. 15 mL
   B. 45 mL
   C. 100 mL
   D. No liquid is required if the client can swallow the pills without it

37. Which of the following statements made by a client would indicate to the nurse that the teaching plan to reduce the risks associated with furosemide (Lasix) therapy had been successful?
   A. "I'll make sure to rise slowly and sit for a few minutes after I lie down."
   B. "I must walk at least 2 blocks every day to increase my activity tolerance."
   C. "I can drink only 4 glasses of water a day."
   D. "I'll avoid taking aspirin while I'm on the Lasix."

38. A client who is being treated for mild ulcerative colitis is receiving all the following medications. Which of them should the home-health-care nurse question?
   A. methylprednisolone sodium succinate (Solu-Medrol)
   B. loperamide (Imodium)
   C. psyllium (Metamucil)
   D. 6-mercaptopurine

39. Which of the following laboratory results from a client who is receiving IV heparin therapy would the nurse report to the physician immediately?
  A. PTT: 92 seconds
  B. Hemoglobin: 15.2 g/dL
  C. Platelet count: 164,000
  D. PT: 16 seconds

40. A nurse who was instructing a client prior to discharge about the home use of warfarin (Coumadin) would know that additional teaching was required if the client stated:
  A. "I should shave with an electric razor until after I am taken off this medication."
  B. "I need to tell my dentist that I am on this medication before he works on me."
  C. "I will continue taking my usual dose of aspirin for my arthritis after I get home."
  D. "I should get and wear an ID bracelet that indicates that I am taking an anticoagulant."

41. A 58-year-old female client with COPD is admitted to the hospital in severe distress. After 2 days on IV aminophylline, a theophylline level is drawn. Which of the following results would indicate to the nurse that the correct dose was being administered?
  A. 4 µg/mL
  B. 14 µg/mL
  C. 25 µg/mL
  D. 31 µg/mL

42. In attempting to administer oral medications to a client from a Hispanic culture, the nurse is unable to have him drink either ice water or any of the fruit juices on the unit. What would be the best action by the nurse in response to this situation?
  A. Reinforce the necessity to increase fluid intake when taking oral medications.
  B. Try using hot coffee or hot tea instead of the cold fluids.
  C. Obtain an order to administer the medications IV or IM instead of PO.
  D. Explore with the client what fluids he would prefer.

43. If a 52-year-old male client has or does all of the following, which would the nurse recognize as a factor that will require an alteration in his daily dose of theophylline?
  A. He is allergic to morphine sulfate.
  B. He has a history of arthritis.
  C. He operates dangerous machinery.
  D. He is being treated for an ulcer with cimetidine.

44. The most important nursing consideration when giving aspirin to a client is to:
  A. Always give the medication before the pain starts.
  B. Monitor for effectiveness.
  C. Give with a full glass of water or food.
  D. Never give IM injections, because of bleeding tendencies.

45. Which of the following statements by a client who is being instructed to use beclomethasone dipropionate (Vanceril) inhalation device at home would indicate to the nurse an understanding of the teaching concerning the prevention of oral fungal infections?
  - **A.** "I should rinse the plastic holder that aerolizes the drug with hydrogen peroxide every other day."
  - **B.** "I should rinse my mouth and gargle with warm water after each use of the inhaler."
  - **C.** "I need to take calcium carbonate just before the treatment to neutralize the acid in my mouth."
  - **D.** "I should rinse my mouth before each use to lessen the growth of bacteria."

46. The nurse will know that further teaching about cimetidine (Tagamet) is required if the client states:
  - **A.** "I can take the medication on an empty stomach or with food."
  - **B.** "Smoking doesn't change the effectiveness of the medication."
  - **C.** "I shouldn't stop taking it suddenly."
  - **D.** "I should avoid alcohol while taking the medication."

47. Ranitidine (Zantac) differs from cimetidine (Tagamet) in that:
  - **A.** Ranitidine is less potent than cimetidine and requires a larger dose.
  - **B.** Ranitidine works on a different mechanism than cimetidine.
  - **C.** Ranitidine is more potent than cimetidine and requires a smaller dose.
  - **D.** There is no difference between the medications.

48. The magnesium sulfate ($MgSO_4$) blood level of a client receiving $MgSo_4$ for pregnancy-induced hypertension (PIH) is 4.7 $\mu g/mL$. The nurse should:
  - **A.** Increase the rate of infusion of the medication
  - **B.** Give calcium gluconate
  - **C.** Begin an infusion of naloxone (Narcan)
  - **D.** Continue the medication at its present rate

49. The physician orders 1 mg of the medication sucralfate (Carafate) for a client with a peptic ulcer, four times a day. The nurse would know that:
  - **A.** The dose is correct for the condition.
  - **B.** The dose is much too large and may be lethal.
  - **C.** The dose is too small to be effective.
  - **D.** The physician ordered the wrong medication.

50. An important factor for the nurse to keep in mind when administering sucralfate (Carafate) is:
  - **A.** It works best if it is taken with food.
  - **B.** It works best if taken on an empty stomach.
  - **C.** The blood pressure (BP) and pulse must be taken before the medication can be given.
  - **D.** Diarrhea is the most common side effect.

ANSWERS/RATIONALES

1. **Correct Answer: A.** $100 : 5 :: 80 : x$

   $$100x = 400$$
   $$x = 4$$

Rationales for Other Answer Choices: B, C, and **D** are incorrect.
Nursing Process Phase: planning; client need: safe and effective care environment; concern area: medical/surgical

2. **Correct Answer: C.** This is a commonly used combination of medications to suppress the immune system and prevent rejection of organs.

Rationales for Other Answer Choices: A. Garamycin is a nephrotoxic antibiotic. **B.** Aminophylline is a bronchodilator. **D.** Garamycin is a nephrotoxic antibiotic.
Nursing Process Phase: planning; client need: safe and effective care environment; concern area: medical/surgical

3. **Correct Answer: C.** Most commonly used of the antidysrhythmics to control ventricular ectopic beats, such as PVCs.

Rationales for Other Answer Choices: A. Antirejection medication. **B.** Emergency medication used in cardiac arrest, asthma. **D.** Positive inotropic medication used in congestive heart failure (CHF).
Nursing Process Phase: planning; client need: safe and effective care environment; concern area: medical/surgical

4. **Correct Answer: B.** Anticholinergics block the parasympathetic system and allow the sympathetic system to take over.

Rationales for Other Answer Choices: A. Produce tachycardia. **C.** Low abuse potential **D.** Have the opposite effect.
Nursing Process Phase: planning; client need: safe and effective care environment; concern area: medical/surgical

5. **Correct Answer: C.** Atropine is a parasympathetic blocker that allows the heart rate to increase.

Rationales for Other Answer Choices: A. Would be a second-line medication if the atropine did not work. **B.** Tends to slow the pulse down—not appropriate. **D.** Antidysrhymic used for ventricular dysrhythmias.
Nursing Process Phase: implementation; client need: safe and effective care environment; concern area: medical/surgical

6. **Correct Answer: C.** Beta-blockers such as propranolol may produce slow heart rates and A-V blocks caused by the effect on the A-V node.

Rationales for Other Answer Choices: A. Not associated with this medication. **B.** Not associated with this medication. **D.** Very rare side effects of beta blockers.
Nursing Process Phase: assessment; client need: safe and effective care environment; concern area: medical/surgical

7. **Correct Answer: C.** A soft toothbrush would prevent bleeding from the gums—a common side effect.

Rationales for Other Answer Choices: A. These foods contain vitamin K and decrease the effectiveness of the medication. **B.** Should use an electric razor to prevent cuts and bleeding. **D.** Should avoid ASA—may cause increased bleeding.
Nursing Process Phase: evaluation; client need: health promotion and maintenance; concern area: medical/surgical

8. **Correct Answer: B.** Has a soothing effect on burns and helps control infections.

Rationales for Other Answer Choices: A. Has very limited absorption into the system. **C.** Not its category. **D.** Untrue statement.
Nursing Process Phase: planning; client need: safe and effective care environment; concern area: medical/surgical

9. **Correct Answer: B.** $\frac{3600}{8} = 450$

Rationales for Other Answer Choices: A, C, and **D** are incorrect.
Nursing Process Phase: implementation; client need: safe and effective care environment; concern area: medical/surgical

10. **Correct Answer: B.** The calcium binds with the phosphate to help lower the usually high serum phosphate levels in renal failure clients and help prevent osteoporosis.

Rationales for Other Answer Choices: A. Not used for this purpose. **C.** Does not help prevent this. **D.** Not the primary use for clients in renal failure.
Nursing Process Phase: implementation; client need: safe and effective care environment; concern area: medical/surgical

11. **Correct Answer: B.** Suppression of the sympathetic branch slows the heart rate and decreases the force of contraction.

Rationales for Other Answer Choices: A. Caused by suppression of the parasympathetic branch. **C.** Not associated with these medications. **D.** Untrue; slows the heart rate.
Nursing Process Phase: planning; client need: safe and effective care environment; concern area: medical/surgical

12. **Correct Answer: D.** Both these medications will increase the heart rate.

Rationales for Other Answer Choices: A. These should never be given to a client with a ventricular escape rhythm—will suppress the ventricular focus. **B.** Tend to slow the heart rate but have little ventricular effects. **C.** Tend to slow the heart rate but have little ventricular effects.
Nursing Process Phase: implementation; client need: safe and effective care environment; concern area: medical/surgical

13. **Correct Answer: C.** A common side effect is postural hypotension caused by the vasodilating effects. Client may fall if standing.

Rationales for Other Answer Choices: A. Is taken prn for chest pain. **B.** Common side effect—no need to notify MD. **D.** Not side effects of this medication.

Nursing Process Phase: evaluation; client need: health promotion and maintenance; concern area: medical/surgical

14. **Correct Answer: B.** This calcium channel blocker is commonly used to treat fast atrial dysrhythmias, such as AT.

Rationales for Other Answer Choices: A. Would increase the heart rate. **C.** Used for slow dysrhythmias. **D.** Diuretic—not used for this problem.
Nursing Process Phase: implementation; client need: safe and effective care environment; concern area: medical/surgical

15. **Correct Answer: C.** Like many IV push medications, this can be given at 1 mL/min.

Rationales for Other Answer Choices: A. Too slow rate. **B.** Too fast rate—may cause ototoxicity. **D.** Not an appropriate measure for this medication.
Nursing Process Phase: planning; client need: safe and effective care environment; concern area: medical/surgical

16. **Correct Answer: D.** The respiratory centers are located here and, when suppressed, produce hypoventilation, resulting in low oxygen levels and high carbon dioxide levels.

Rationales for Other Answer Choices: A. Produce respiratory acidosis secondary to hypoventilation. **B.** Not a direct effect of narcotics. **C.** Not a true statement—breathing is involuntary.
Nursing Process Phase: planning; client need: safe and effective care environment; concern area: medical/surgical

17. **Correct Answer: C.** Stimulates not only the beta$_2$ receptors in the bronchiolus, producing bronchodilation, but also the beta$_1$ and alpha-receptors in the heart and central nervous system (CNS), producing these common side effects.

Rationales for Other Answer Choices: A. Not side effects of this medication. **B.** Would have diarrhea and tachycardia. **D.** Symptoms of CHF.
Nursing Process Phase: assessment; client need: safe and effective care environment; concern area: medical/surgical

18. **Correct Answer: B.** These are side effects of the medication that may indicate the development of CHF or heart block.

Rationales for Other Answer Choices: A. Need to take the medication—never stop taking it suddenly. **C.** Should take the missed dose as soon as possible, but never double the dose. **D.** Works best on an empty stomach.
Nursing Process Phase: evaluation; client need: health promotion and maintenance; concern area: medical/surgical

19. **Correct Answer: B.** concentration: $\dfrac{20000}{500} = 40$ U/mL

dose: $\dfrac{1000}{40} = 25$ mL/h

Rationales for Other Answer Choices: A, C, and **D** are incorrect calculations.
Nursing Process Phase: implementation; client need: safe and effective care environment; concern area: medical/surgical

20. Correct Answer: D. Would tend to increase the heart rate so would be inappropriate for this condition.

Rationales for Other Answer Choices: A. Produces bronchodilation. **B.** Increases the heart rate. **C.** Produces bronchodilation.
Nursing Process Phase: implementation; client need: safe and effective care environment; concern area: medical/surgical

21. Correct Answer: A. This medication blocks the beta receptors in the lungs and constricts the bronchioli.

Rationales for Other Answer Choices: B. No effect on respiratory system. **C.** Produces bronchodilation—appropriate for asthma. **D.** Used in severe asthma attacks for bronchodilation.
Nursing Process Phase: planning; client need: safe and effective care environment; concern area: medical/surgical

22. Correct Answer: D. This anticholinergic medication is used to block the production of acid in the stomach in clients with ulcers.

Rationales for Other Answer Choices: A. No primary effect on blood pressure. **B.** May increase the rate slightly, but that is not its primary use. **C.** Not used for this condition.
Nursing Process Phase: analysis; client need: safe and effective care environment; concern area: medical/surgical

23. Correct Answer: A. Common condition with phenytoin toxicity.

Rationales for Other Answer Choices: B. Is a side effect but not a toxic effect. **C.** Toxic effect of carbamazepine (Tegretol). **D.** Toxic effects of trimethadione (Tridione).
Nursing Process Phase: evaluation; client need: safe and effective care environment; concern area: pediatrics

24. Correct Answer: C. Defines sedative.

Rationales for Other Answer Choices: A. Relieves pain. **B.** Produces sleep. **D.** Reduces fever states.
Nursing Process Phase: planning; client need: safe and effective care environment; concern area: psychiatric nursing

25. Correct Answer: A. Pyridoxine (vitamin B_6) is a cofactor in the peripheral decarboxylation of levodopa to dopamine. Symptoms of the disease become worse when clients ingest large amounts of pyridoxine and levodopa.

Rationales for Other Answer Choices: B. No effect on levodopa conversion. **C.** No effect on levodopa conversion. **D.** No effect on levodopa conversion.
Nursing Process Phase: planning; client need: safe and effective care environment; concern area: medical/surgical

26. Correct Answer: D. Epinephrine increases serum glucose levels and inhibits insulin release.

Rationales for Other Answer Choices: A. Primary side effects: vasoconstriction and CNS stimulation. **B.** Primary side effects: increased heart rate and blood pressure. **C.** Primary side effects: bradycardia and hypotension.
Nursing Process Phase: planning; client need: health promotion and maintenance; concern area: medical/surgical

27. Correct Answer: D. Beta-blocking agents cause bronchoconstriction and increased airway resistance.

Rationales for Other Answer Choices: A. May cause nasal or chest congestion, wheezing, and shortness of breath. **B.** Has no respiratory side effects. **C.** Causes bronchodilation and decreases respiratory resistance.
Nursing Process Phase: evaluation; client need: safe and effective care environment; concern area: medical/surgical

28. Correct Answer: C. Increases digoxin levels markedly by preventing its excretion.

Rationales for Other Answer Choices: A. May help prevent digoxin toxicity by preventing hypokalemia. **B.** Thyroid supplements lower digoxin levels. **D.** Has no known effect on digoxin levels.
Nursing Process Phase: analysis; client need: safe and effective care environment; concern area: medical/surgical

29. Correct Answer: B. These are toxic effects of this medication—also heart block, headache, tremors.

Rationales for Other Answer Choices: A. Toxic effects are headache, hypotension, A-V blocks, green or yellow halos. **C.** Toxic effects are heart block, liver failure, thrombocytopenia, and respiratory arrest. **D.** Side effects are hypotension, headache, flushing.
Nursing Process Phase: assessment; client need: safe and effective care environment; concern area: pediatrics

30. Correct Answer: A. This is to be expected when fresh, potent NTG is placed under the tongue.

Rationales for Other Answer Choices: B. Not an expected effect of this medication. **C.** Prolonged use may make the NTG less effective. **D.** Has no effect on urine production.
Nursing Process Phase: planning; client need: health promotion and maintenance; concern area: medical/surgical

31. Correct Answer: A. This medication will cause vasodilation in the area and help prevent ischemia and necrosis of the local tissue.

Rationales for Other Answer Choices: B. This medication will increase the vasoconstriction of the tissues and increase necrosis. **C.** This medication will increase the vasoconstriction of the tissues and increase necrosis. **D.** This medication is incompatible with dopamine and highly irritating to tissues.
Nursing Process Phase: implementation; client need: health promotion and maintenance; concern area: medical/surgical

32. Correct Answer: B. Fluid is sequestered in the muscle tissues of clients with burns. Medications given IM are absorbed unpredictably or not at all.

Rationales for Other Answer Choices: A. IV is the fastest route of absorption. **C.** Medications given IV cannot be reclaimed. **D.** Not the primary rationale for IV route.
Nursing Process Phase: planning; client need: safe and effective care environment; concern area: pediatrics

33. **Correct Answer: A.** Although somewhat toxic, this bacteriostatic agent is effective against gram-positive and gram-negative organisms and best penetrates the dead skin (eschar).

Rationales for Other Answer Choices: B. Penetrates eschar poorly. **C.** No penetration of eschar. **D.** No penetration of eschar.
Nursing Process Phase: implementation; client need: safe and effective care environment; concern area: medical/surgical

34. **Correct Answer: A.** These times allow for adequate spacing of the medication and limit the client's need to void at night, a time when he is more likely to fall.

Rationales for Other Answer Choices: B. Time spacing is good, but late-night dose may necessitate need to get up during the night. **C.** Does not reduce the risk for falls. **D.** Late-night dose may require him to get up during the night.
Nursing Process Phase: planning; client need: safe and effective care environment; concern area: medical/surgical

35. **Correct Answer: C.** This would be the best action to ensure that the client received his medications.

Rationales for Other Answer Choices: A. Legally, medications should not be left at the bedside without a written order. **B.** Inappropriate—the client did not refuse to take the medications. **D.** This is an alternative action, but most busy nurses do not have the time to wait around in clients' rooms.
Nursing Process Phase: implementation; client need: safe and effective care environment; concern area: medical/surgical

36. **Correct Answer: C.** Research has shown that at least 100 mL of fluid is needed for oral medications to enter the stomach. The liquid also helps the medication dissolve and absorb.

Rationales for Other Answer Choices: A. Amount is too small. **B.** Amount is too small. **D.** Pills taken "dry" may lodge in the esophagus and cause esophageal ulcers or irritation.
Nursing Process Phase: assessment; client need: safe and effective care environment; concern area: medical/surgical

37. **Correct Answer: A.** These actions help prevent postural hypotension and falls.

Rationales for Other Answer Choices: B. Although a good way to increase cardiac output, the action itself does not prevent falls. **C.** Unless contraindicated, the client should drink 2 to 3 liters of water per day. **D.** Aspirin has no effect on this medication.
Nursing Process Phase: evaluation; client need: safe and effective care environment; concern area: medical/surgical

38. **Correct Answer: D.** This is a powerful immunosuppressant that is used only in the most severe cases of ulcerative colitis.

Rationales for Other Answer Choices: A. Commonly used to suppress the inflammation of the disease.　**B.** Used to control the diarrhea associated with the disease.　**C.** Helps regulate the stools and increases their bulk.
Nursing Process Phase: analysis; client need: safe and effective care environment; concern area: medical/surgical

39. **Correct Answer: A.**　PTT normal is 35 to 45 seconds, therapeutic is considered 2 to 2½ times normal.

Rationales for Other Answer Choices: B. This is in the normal range.　**C.** This is in the normal range.　**D.** This is a normal PT—used for warfarin (Coumadin).
Nursing Process Phase: implementation; client need: safe and effective care environment; concern area: medical/surgical

40. **Correct Answer: C.**　Aspirin potentiates the effects of oral anticoagulants. The client needs to discuss possible alternative treatments for arthritis with the physician.

Rationales for Other Answer Choices: A. Appropriate action—prevents accidental cuts.　**B.** Appropriate action—all other health-care providers should know.　**D.** Appropriate action—lets emergency personnel know why a client may be bleeding excessively.
Nursing Process Phase: evaluation; client need: health promotion and maintenance; concern area: medical/surgical

41. **Correct Answer: B.**　Therapeutic range is 10 to 20 μg/mL.

Rationales for Other Answer Choices: A. Subtherapeutic.　**C** and **D** are too high—may indicate toxicity.
Nursing Process Phase: analysis; client need: safe and effective care environment; concern area: medical/surgical

42. **Correct Answer: D.**　Some clients from a Hispanic background have a classification system for diseases as either "hot" or "cold." The disease must be treated by balancing the disease with the opposite temperature.

Rationales for Other Answer Choices: A. Will have little positive effect if the liquid is wrong for the disease.　**B.** May be effective, but the actual temperature may have little to do with it. The type of liquid is more important.　**C.** This is an inappropriate measure at this time.
Nursing Process Phase: implementation; client need: psychosocial integrity; concern area: medical/surgical

43. **Correct Answer: D.**　Cimetidine interferes with the excretion of theophylline and may produce toxic blood levels. Dose should be lowered.

Rationales for Other Answer Choices: A. No cross-allergies with theophylline.　**B.** Not affected by theophylline.　**C.** May actually make him more alert.
Nursing Process Phase: planning; client need: safe and effective care environment; concern area: medical/surgical

44. **Correct Answer: C.**　Gastric irritation, a major side effect of ASA, can be prevented if taken with food or liquid.

Rationales for Other Answer Choices: A. Works better if taken before the pain becomes severe, but not a necessity. **B.** A nursing consideration, but of lower priority. **D.** Does increase bleeding tendencies, but IM injections can still be given.
Nursing Process Phase: planning; client need: health promotion and maintenance; concern area: medical/surgical

45. **Correct Answer: B.** This will help reduce the droplets of glucocorticoid in the mouth after use and help prevent the growth of fungus and yeasts.

Rationales for Other Answer Choices: A. Should be rinsed with warm water once a day. **C.** Will have no effect on the growth of organisms. **D.** Bacteria do not cause fungal infections.
Nursing Process Phase: evaluation; client need: health promotion and maintenance; concern area: medical/surgical

46. **Correct Answer: B.** Smoking decreases the effectiveness of the H_2 inhibitors. Clients should stop smoking when taking these medications.

Rationales for Other Answer Choices: A. True statement. **C.** True statement—causes a rebound effect if stopped suddenly. **D.** Alcohol and other CNS drugs affect cimetidine.
Nursing Process Phase: evaluation; client need: health promotion and maintenance; concern area: medical/surgical

47. **Correct Answer: C.** Clients that switch from cimetidine to rantidine need to be aware of the smaller dosages.

Rationales for Other Answer Choices: A. Ranitidine is more potent. **B.** Both are H_2 inhibitors. **D.** Ranitidine is more potent.
Nursing Process Phase: planning; client need: health promotion and maintenance; concern area: medical/surgical

48. **Correct Answer: B.** This blood level is well above the low toxic range of 2. Calcium gluconate is the antidote for $MgSO_4$ toxicity.

Rationales for Other Answer Choices: A. Would make the client only more toxic. **C.** Not an antidote for $MgSO_4$. **D.** Would make the toxicity worse.
Nursing Process Phase: analysis; client need: health promotion and maintenance; concern area: maternity

49. **Correct Answer: C.** Normal dose is 1 g.

Rationales for Other Answer Choices: A. Dose is too small. **B.** Dose is too small. **D.** Right medication, wrong dose.
Nursing Process Phase: planning; client need: safe and effective care environment; concern area: medical/surgical

50. **Correct Answer: B.** Cytoprotective agents coat the mucous membranes best when the stomach is empty.

Rationales for Other Answer Choices: A. False statement. **C.** Has no effect on cardiac output or BP. **D.** Constipation is a common side effect.
Nursing Process Phase: planning; client need: health promotion and maintenance; concern area: medical/surgical

1. In planning care for a client with severe pregnancy-induced hypertension (PIH) receiving magnesium sulfate (MgSO$_4$), one of the nurse's implementations is, "Place in a quiet, darkened room" because:
   A. The medication makes the client restless.
   B. The client has photophobia as a side effect of MgSO$_4$.
   C. Noise and bright lights may trigger a seizure.
   D. Clients on MgSO$_4$ are easily annoyed by noise and lights.

2. A 32-year-old male accountant is diagnosed with inflammatory bowel syndrome (Crohn's disease). Which of the following medications would most likely be included in his treatment regimen?
   A. Psyllium (Metamucil)
   B. Diphenoxylate (Lomotil)
   C. Dimenhydrinate (Dramamine)
   D. Lactulose

3. In accordance with an established local protocol, a 17-year-old high school student is given 0.2 mL of 1/1000 solution of epinephrine SC by the school nurse for a severe asthma attack. Which of the following would indicate to the nurse that the treatment had been effective?
   A. Pulse rate of 128 beats per minute (BPM).
   B. The student is able to expectorate 50 mL of thick mucus.
   C. Respiratory rate of 14 with decreased inspiratory effort.
   D. Increased alertness and slight tremors of hands.

4. By which route should a nurse administer ribavirin to a 16-month-old child who has respiratory syncytial virus (RSV)?
   A. Oral
   B. IM
   C. IV
   D. Aerosol

5. Common side effects that a client should be monitored for while receiving prochlorperazine (Compazine) include:
   A. Diarrhea, urinary retention, and tachycardia
   B. Drowsiness, respiratory depression, and hypotension
   C. Alopecia, bleeding, and bone marrow suppression
   D. Bradycardia, renal failure, and anxiety

6. A 22-year-old nursing student gets motion sickness when she flies. She takes dimenhydrinate (Dramamine) for this condition. An important factor she needs to remember in relation to this medication is:
   A. It works best when taken with alcoholic beverages.
   B. It should be taken only after the symptoms begin.
   C. It should be taken 30 to 60 minutes before flying.
   D. Constipation is a common side effect.

7. Which of the following statements made by a client who is to take theophylline (Theo-Dur) at home for his chronic obstructive pulmonary disease (COPD) would indicate to the nurse that teaching had been successful?
   A. "I will call my physician if my heart races or if I get dizzy or restless."
   B. "I have to stop smoking because I can become theophylline toxic from its effects."
   C. "For best effectiveness, I must take the medicine on an empty stomach."
   D. "I should not take the medication if my pulse is below 60 BPM."

8. A client who is 8 months pregnant is diagnosed with pyelonephritis. The nurse anticipates that the physician will prescribe:
   A. Oxytocin
   B. Magnesium sulfate
   C. Ampicillin
   D. Tetracycline

9. A nursing student who gets motion sickness is taking dimenhydrinate (Dramamine) 200 mg PO q 4 h while flying to Mexico on vacation. A fellow student who is flying with her should recommend that:
   A. She increase the dosage to every 2 hours.
   B. She increase the dosage to 300 mg every 4 hours.
   C. She continue to take the medication as she is.
   D. She decrease the dosage to 50 mg every 4 hours.

10. A client is to receive insulin by continuous IV drip. The nurse would mix which of the following insulins with normal saline?
    A. Humalin N
    B. NPH
    C. Humalin R
    D. Lente

11. The nurse is to administer furosemide (Lasix) oral solution 0.5 mL stat to an infant in congestive heart failure (CHF). If the medication comes 10 mg/mL, how much should the nurse give?
    A. 5 mg
    B. 0.05 mg
    C. 0.005 mg
    D. 20 mg

12. A client with chest pain develops multiform premature ventricular contractions while in the ER. If all of the following medications are ordered prn, which should the nurse administer first?
    A. Furosemide (Lasix) 40 mg IV
    B. Nitroglycerin gr 1/150 SL
    C. Lidocaine 100 mg IVP
    D. Digoxin (Lanoxin) 0.25 mg IV

13. A client who is taking isoniazid and rifampin for tuberculosis asks the nurse why he must also take vitamin B_6? The best response by the nurse is, "Vitamin B_6 helps:
    A. Increase the activity of isoniazid."
    B. Decrease the peripheral neuropathy caused by the isoniazid."
    C. Increase the half-life of rifampin."
    D. Maintain a satisfactory nutritional status."

14. Which of the following actions by the nurse would best prevent the development of drug resistance in a client who has tuberculosis?
    A. Monitor liver function studies every month.
    B. Assess the client for peripheral neuropathy every week.
    C. Evaluate effectiveness of respiratory isolation.
    D. Monitor home compliance with medication therapy.

15. The nurse would recognize if the sodium polystyrene sulfonate (Kayexalate) she had given to a 6-year-old client in renal failure was effective by a(an):
    A. Increase in the serum magnesium
    B. Decrease in the serum HCO_3
    C. Increase in the serum calcium
    D. Decrease in the serum potassium

16. The nurse is to give phenytoin (Dilantin) IV for an unconscious client with a seizure disorder. With which of the following IV solutions should the nurse administer this medication?
    A. Ringer's lactate
    B. D5W
    C. D5 and normal saline
    D. Normal saline

17. In assessing a client who was receiving gentamicin for a severe incisional infection, the nurse would closely monitor his:
    A. Serum creatinine
    B. Serum sodium
    C. Serum calcium
    D. Serum potassium

18. Lactulose (Chronulac) exerts its effect by:
    A. Stimulating the pancreas to increase the production of insulin
    B. Slowing the propulsive movements in the intestines
    C. Stimulating the production of mucus in the small and large intestinal linings
    D. Pulling water into the intestinal lumen

19. Which response would the nurse expect to find in a postoperative client who was given metoclopramide (Reglan) 1 hour ago?
    A. Increased gastric secretions in the nasogastric (NG) tube
    B. Increased peristalsis
    C. Decreased disorientation
    D. Decreased drowsiness

20. The physician orders lactulose liquid 30 g PO qid for a client. The best response by the nurse to this order is to:
    A. Give the medication as ordered.
    B. Hold the medication, and check the dosage with the physician.
    C. Change the medication times to AC and HS.
    D. Hold the medication, and have the physician change it to bid.

21. A client who is taking chlorpromazine for several months for schizophrenia wants to attend a picnic on the 4th of July with the other residents. The nurse would be most concerned about which of the medication's side effects?
    A. Hypotension
    B. Photosensitivity
    C. Increased appetite
    D. Constipation

22. Which of the following would be the most appropriate instructions for a nurse to give to the parents of a child who was receiving chemotherapy, concerning the development of alopecia?
    A. Children are much less concerned about the loss of hair than adults are.
    B. The loss will be barely noticeable because the hair comes out gradually.
    C. Girls should choose a wig similar to their hair color and style before the hair begins to fall out.
    D. Both the parents and the child will soon get accustomed to the hair loss, and it will no longer bother them.

23. Which of the following teaching plans would be best for a client who was recently started on lithium carbonate because she was exhibiting signs of mania? She is 34 years old and has no known physical problems.
    A. Regular diet, including foods such as bacon, ham, tomato juice, and salted peanuts
    B. Fluid restrictions no more than 1000 mL/d; avoid coke and diet sodas
    C. Low-protein, low-sodium, low-fat diet high in calories to meet increased energy demands
    D. If nausea, vomiting, or diarrhea occur, she should stop the medication immediately.

24. A client is to receive ampicilin (Omnipen) IVPB 2 g in 50 mL D5W. At what rate would the nurse set the volumetric pump to administer this medication in 30 minutes? The IV tubing has a drip factor of 10.
    A. 50 mL/h
    B. 100 mL/h
    C. 54 gtt/min
    D. 200 mL/h

25. Which of the following medications would be most appropriate to give to a hospitalized alcoholic client who was becoming increasingly irritable and agitated and displaying tremors of the hands?
    A. An opiate
    B. A benzodiazepine
    C. A tricyclic antidepressant
    D. A phenothiazine

26. A 21-year-old female client who was treated two months ago with trimethoprim-sulfamethoxazole (Bactrim DS) on an outpatient basis for a urinary tract infection is admitted with pyelonephritis. In obtaining her history, which of these statements made to the nurse by the client would be a reason she developed pyelonephritis?
  A. "I usually drink 6 to 8 glasses of water per day."
  B. "I have been getting bladder infections since I was a child."
  C. "I took the Bactrim until the burning and pain went away, then I saved the rest for the next time."
  D. "I just got over a really bad case of flu and sore throat."

27. An alcoholic client who is completing the inpatient segment of a substance abuse program was started on disulfiram (Antabuse). Which of the following teaching points should the nurse include in her discharge instructions?
  A. If you drink alcohol while you are taking this medication, you will have nausea, vomiting, and elevated blood pressure.
  B. It is best that this medication be started as late in the program as possible.
  C. This medication works by densensitizing you to alcohol.
  D. You may experience the effects of this medication if you drink alcohol as much as 2 weeks after you stop taking it.

28. A postmenopausal client who has developed major depression is started on fluoxetine (Prozac) therapy. Which is the most important point for the nurse to include in the discharge instructions?
  A. You can take your daily dose of fluoxetine either in the morning or evening.
  B. There are no restrictions on driving or other hazardous activities because this medication is nonsedating.
  C. You may develop a rash or itching when you first start taking the medication, but it will go away later.
  D. It is safe to take over-the-counter or other prescription medications because there are few drug interactions with fluoxetine.

29. A client diagnosed with bipolar disorder is started on lithium carbonate for control of the symptoms. Which of the following would be the most important factor to teach the client in order to prevent lithium toxicity?
  A. Eat a regular diet, but keep sodium intake to less than 3 g/d.
  B. Take the lithium between meals to increase the absorption rate.
  C. If diarrhea, vomiting, or diaphoresis develop, and you are unable to take fluids, withhold the medication.
  D. If a fever develops, take acetaminophen (Tylenol) instead of aspirin.

30. Medications that would decrease the effectiveness of laxatives and cathartics include:
  A. Anticholinergics
  B. Cholinergics
  C. Central nervous system (CNS) stimulants
  D. Glucocorticoids

31. Which of these statements by a client would indicate that the nurse's instructions concerning the home use of sublingual nitroglycerin tablets have been successful?
    A. "I should call my physician if I develop a headache after taking these."
    B. "I need to keep the tablets in the refrigerator when not in use."
    C. "If I take three of these and the pain does not go away, I should call my physician."
    D. "I can only take these pills with water, not soda or milk."

32. A 28-year-old client is receiving once weekly chemotherapy in the outpatient oncology unit. What would be the best method for the nurse to administer antiemetics to this client?
    A. Start the antiemetics when the client becomes nauseated and continue for 24 hours after.
    B. Administer the antiemetics before the chemotherapy is started and continue for 24 hours after.
    C. Administer antiemetics one at a time to avoid compounding the side effects.
    D. Administer the antiemetics at set intervals throughout the entire course of chemotherapy.

33. An important nursing implication that the nurse should keep in mind when giving a client metoclopramide (Reglan) includes:
    A. Increasing the fluid intake to 3000 to 5000 mL/d
    B. Taking the medication on an empty stomach
    C. Monitoring his pulse and blood pressure (BP)
    D. Avoid giving the medication with cholinergics

34. While performing her morning assessments, a nurse discovered a manic-depressive client who was receiving lithium therapy in a confused mental state. He was also vomiting, twitching, and displaying coarse hand tremors. Which of the following should the nurse do first?
    A. Administer the next dose of lithium early, then call her evaluation to the physician.
    B. Hold the next dose of lithium, and call her observations to the physician.
    C. Make the client NPO to decrease the excretion of the lithium, and monitor his condition.
    D. Call the laboratory to draw a lithium level in 30 minutes, and notify the physician of the client's condition.

35. If a nurse finds all of the following in a 34-year-old female client who is receiving vincristine (Oncovan), which should the nurse be most concerned about?
    A. Respiratory rate of 16/min
    B. Pulse rate of 62 BPM
    C. Sore, stiff muscles
    D. Sore throat

36. A client with manic-depressive disorder who is started on lithium and another psychotropic medication asks the nurse why he must take two medications. The best answer by the nurse is:
    A. "Your condition is so unstable that you need the extra medication to control your activity."
    B. "We always give two medications to clients who have your condition."
    C. "It may take up to 2 weeks for the lithium to become effective. The second medication is faster acting."
    D. "Don't worry about your medications now; it's more important that you do not injure yourself."

37. Glucocorticoids are primarily responsible for the regulation of:
    A. Carbohydrate and protein metabolism
    B. Secondary sexual development
    C. Electrolyte and fluid balance
    D. Function of the cardiovascular system

38. A client diagnosed with alcoholism asks the nurse why he is receiving neomycin (Mycifradin) every 6 hours. The nurse explains that neomycin:
    A. Is an antibiotic that will help prevent the tuberculosis that many alcoholics have
    B. Acts as an antacid and helps prevent gastric ulcers often seen in alcoholics
    C. Decreases the number of nitrogen-forming bacteria in the intestines and prevents ammonia intoxication
    D. Irritates the lower intestine to aid in the evacuation of protein substances

39. The nurse is monitoring a 15-year-old client with type 1 diabetes who has an admission blood sugar of 452. Before beginning an insulin drip, the nurse would be most concerned if the client's serum:
    A. Chloride level was 90 mEq/L
    B. Sodium level was 136 mEq/L
    C. Potassium level was 3.1 mEq/L
    D. Potassium level was 6.3 mEq/L

40. Which assessment would lead the nurse to conclude that a client who was receiving magnesium sulfate was developing toxicity?
    A. A 3 + patellar tendon reflex
    B. Respiratory rate of 10
    C. Urine output 40 mL/h
    D. Urine 2 + positive for protein

41. A client is admitted to the medical/surgical unit after overdosing on phenelzine sulfate (Nardil). Which of the following diets would the nurse anticipate being prescribed for this client?
    A. High-carbohydrate, low-cholesterol
    B. High-protein, high-carbohydrate
    C. Regular, 1 g sodium
    D. As tolerated, tyramine-free

42. After 7 hours in restraints and a total of 30 mg of haloperidol in divided doses, a client complains of stiffness in his neck and his tongue "pulling to one side." If all of the following medications are available prn for this client, which should the nurse give to relieve the client's complaints?
    A. Lorazepam (Ativan)
    B. Benztropine (Cogentin)
    C. Thiothixene (Navane)
    D. Flurazepan (Dalmane)

43. What would be the primary reason that a 66-year-old automobile accident victim with a possible skull fracture would be given dexamethasone (Decadron)?
    A. It suppresses the immune response and therefore will prevent any infections from the injuries.
    B. It will reduce the swelling of the brain and prevent increased intracranial pressure.
    C. It disrupts the formation of histamine and will prevent any allergic reactions to medications.
    D. It will increase protein and carbohydrate metabolism so that healing of injured tissues will occur at an increased rate.

44. A client is started on alteplase tissue plasminogen activator (t-PA)/heparin therapy after experiencing an acute myocardial infarction. Which assessment should cause the nurse the most concern?
    A. BP 158/92
    B. Blood in the urine
    C. Pulse rate 102
    D. Partial thromboplastin time (PTT) 62 seconds

45. A 78-year-old nursing-home client is being treated with trimethoprim-sulfamethoxazole (Bactrim) IV for sepsis. For which of the following assessments should the nurse stop the medication and call the physician?
    A. Nausea 1 h post administration
    B. Increasing disorientation to place and time
    C. Rash on hands and face
    D. Urine output of 35 mL/h

46. After a renal transplant, a client is started on cyclosporin (Sandimmune). The nurse will know the discharge instructions about this medication have been successful if the client states:
    A. "I need to make sure I don't develop low blood pressure while I'm taking the medication."
    B. "I need to come into the physician's office once a month to have blood drawn to see how my kidney is working."
    C. "When I really start feeling better and I don't have any temperature, I can stop taking the medication."
    D. "I can go to church or the shopping mall as soon as my stitches are taken out."

47. A client is receiving terbutaline sulfate (Brethine) to stop her premature labor. In planning care for this client, the nurse recognizes that terbutaline sulfate exerts its action because of its:
   A. Sedative effects
   B. Anticonvulsive effects
   C. Beta-adrenergic effects
   D. Anticholinergic effects

48. Which of the following actions would be most appropriate for a nurse to implement in caring for a 5-year-old child on the pediatric unit who is receiving liquid oral iron supplements?
   A. Give the iron preparation once a week on Mondays to maintain consistency.
   B. Dilute the medication in a cup of tea with milk to disguise the taste.
   C. Give the medication three times a day because it has a low toxicity level.
   D. Brush the child's teeth after giving the oral liquid.

49. Which of the following assessments made by the nurse would indicate the effectiveness of low-dose nitroglycerin IV and furosemide (Lasix) IV therapy for a client in left-sided congestive heart failure?
   A. BP of 130/900, up from 100/50
   B. Serum potassium of 5.0 mEq/L
   C. Pulmonary capillary wedge pressure of 10 mm Hg, down from 22 mm Hg
   D. A decrease in premature ventricular ectopic beats

50. A 24-year-old female client is brought into the ER with an overdose of heroin. Which of the following interventions is of highest priority for the nurse to implement at this time?
   A. Assess the breath sounds for indications of developing pulmonary edema.
   B. Evaluate the size and reaction of the pupils.
   C. Call for a stat psychiatric consult because it seems to be an attempted suicide.
   D. Check for diminished or absent deep tendon reflexes.

ANSWERS/RATIONALES

1. **Correct Answer: C.** Convulsions are a severe complication of PIH and can be limited with rest on a quiet dark room.

Rationales for Other Answer Choices: A. Will likely be anxious with the condition but not necessarily restless. Dark room would not help. **B.** Photophobia is not associated. **D.** Not more so than other clients.
Nursing Process Phase: planning; client need: safe and effective care environment; concern area: maternity

2. **Correct Answer: B.** Persistent diarrhea is a common complication of this disorder. Lomotil will decrease it.

Rationales for Other Answer Choices: A. Laxative—used for constipation. **C.** Antiemetic. **D.** Laxative—used with liver failure.
Nursing Process Phase: planning; client need: physiological integrity; concern area: medical/surgical

3. **Correct Answer: C.** The respiratory rate is in normal limits and the decreased respiratory effort indicates dilation of bronchi.

Rationales for Other Answer Choices: A. Increased heart rate is a side effect of this medication. **B.** Increased mucus is not a primary action of epinephrine. **D.** Side effects of epinephrine do not indicate its effectiveness.
Nursing Process Phase: evaluation; client need: physiological integrity; concern area: pediatrics

4. **Correct Answer: D.** An aerosol particle generator unit aerosolizes this medication for quick absorption by oxygen hood, croup tent, or aerosol mask.

Rationales for Other Answer Choices: A. No oral form of this medication. **B.** Not approved for IM. **C.** Not approved for IV.
Nursing Process Phase: implementation; client need: physiological integrity; concern area: pediatrics

5. **Correct Answer: B.** Common side effects of this medication.

Rationales for Other Answer Choices: A. Side effects of anticholinergics. **C.** Side effects of chemotherapy. **D.** Nonspecific side effects.
Nursing Process Phase: assessment; client need: health promotion and maintenance; concern area: medical/surgical

6. **Correct Answer: C.** This medication is more effective if taken *before* the person becomes nauseated.

Rationales for Other Answer Choices: A. Alcohol should be avoided. **B.** Untrue statement. **D.** Drowsiness is the most common side effect.
Nursing Process Phase: planning; client need: physiological integrity; concern area: medical/surgical

7. **Correct Answer: A.** These are signs of theophylline toxicity.

Rationales for Other Answer Choices: B. Although it is a good idea to stop smoking, the effect is to lower the theophylline levels. **C.** Should be taken with food because of irritation to the gastrointestinal (GI) tract. **D.** Increases the pulse rate; this is appropriate for someone on lanoxin.
Nursing Process Phase: evaluation; client need: health promotion and maintenance; concern area: medical/surgical

8. **Correct Answer: C.** This is from the penicillin group and has no known teratogenic effects that may lead to birth defects.

Rationales for Other Answer Choices: A. Used to induce labor. **B.** Used to control PIH and premature labor. **D.** Not as safe as penicillin during pregnancy—may turn the baby's teeth yellow.
Nursing Process Phase: planning; client need: health promotion and maintenance; concern area: maternity

9. **Correct Answer: D.** This is the normal dose for this medication.

Rationales for Other Answer Choices: A. The dose is already excessive. **B.** The dose is already excessive. **C.** The dose needs to be decreased.
Nursing Process Phase: analysis; client need: health promotion and maintenance; concern area: medical/surgical

10. **Correct Answer: C.** This is a regular (short-acting) insulin, the only type that can be given IV.

Rationales for Other Answer Choices: A. Humalin N is an intermediate-acting insulin and cannot be administered IV. **B.** NPH is an intermediate-acting insulin and cannot be administered IV. **D.** Lente is an intermediate-acting insulin and cannot be administered IV.
Nursing Process Phase: implementation; client need: safe and effective care environment; concern area: medical/surgical

11. **Correct Answer: A.** 1 mg = 0.1 mL

$$0.5 \text{ mL} = \frac{1.0 \text{ mg}}{0.1 \text{ mL}} = 5 \text{ mg}$$

Rationales for Other Answer Choices: B, C, and **D** are miscalculations.
Nursing Process Phase: implementation; client need: safe and effective care environment; concern area: pediatrics

12. **Correct Answer: C.** Suppresses the irritable areas in the ventricles to control ventricular ectopic beats.

Rationales for Other Answer Choices: A. Diuretic used for CHF. **B.** Vasodilator used for chest pain. **D.** Cardiac glycoside used for CHF.
Nursing Process Phase: implementation; client need: safe and effective care environment; concern area: pediatrics

13. **Correct Answer: B.** Common side effect of isoniazid (INH) is peripheral neuropathy (tingling, numbness, loss of sensation). Vitamin B_6 helps reduce these.

Rationales for Other Answer Choices: A. Does not increase the activity of INH. **C.** Does not increase the half-life of rifampin. **D.** By itself, has little effect on nutritional status.
Nursing Process Phase: implementation; client need: health promotion and maintenance; concern area: medical/surgical

14. **Correct Answer: D.** Failure to take the medications for even a few days can lead to mutation of organisms and the development of resistance.

Rationales for Other Answer Choices: A. Important action but does not prevent resistance. **B.** Important action but does not prevent resistance. **C.** Important action but does not prevent resistance.
Nursing Process Phase: implementation; client need: safe and effective care environment; concern area: medical/surgical

15. **Correct Answer: D.** This medication is an ion exchange resin that exchanges sodium ions for potassium ions. It is used in clients who have hyperkalemia.

Rationales for Other Answer Choices: A. Not affected by the medication. **B.** Not affected by the medication. **C.** Not affected by the medication.
Nursing Process Phase: evaluation; client need: health promotion and maintenance; concern area: pediatrics

16. **Correct Answer: D.** Phenytoin is only compatible with normal saline.

Rationales for Other Answer Choices: A. Will cause medication to precipitate. **B.** Causes medication to precipitate. **C.** Causes medication to precipitate.
Nursing Process Phase: implementation; client need: safe and effective care environment; concern area: medical/surgical

17. **Correct Answer: A.** Nephrotoxicity and renal failure are serious side effects of this medication, first indicated by increasing creatinine.

Rationales for Other Answer Choices: B. Not affected by the medication. **C.** Not affected by the medication. **D.** May increase after the client is in renal failure but is not the earliest indicator.
Nursing Process Phase: assessment; client need: safe and effective care environment; concern area: medical/surgical

18. **Correct Answer: D.** Disaccharide cathartics like lactulose pull water into the intestine to soften the stool.

Rationales for Other Answer Choices: A. mechanism of action (MOA) of second-generation oral hypoglycemics. **B.** MOA of anticholinergics. **C.** MOA of some cathartics.
Nursing Process Phase: planning; client need: physiological integrity; concern area: medical/surgical

19. **Correct Answer: B.** Helps to increase peristalsis and gastric emptying in postoperative clients.

Rationales for Other Answer Choices: A. Does not stimulate gastric secretions. **C.** Has no direct effect on orientation. **D.** Tends to increase drowsiness as a side effect.

Nursing Process Phase: evaluation; client need: physiological integrity; concern area: medical/surgical

20. Correct Answer: A. This is the appropriate dose for this medication.

Rationales for Other Answer Choices: B. Not necessary—correct dose. **C.** Timing of this medication has little effect. **D.** Incorrect frequency.
Nursing Process Phase: implementation; client need: safe and effective care environment; concern area: medical/surgical

21. Correct Answer: B. This is a hot time of the summer, and the client may burn easily when out in the sun.

Rationales for Other Answer Choices: A. An occasional side effect that usually occurs early in treatment. **C.** An occasional side effect but not serious for this client. **D.** Should not affect the client on the picnic.
Nursing Process Phase: evaluation; client need: safe and effective care environment; concern area: psychiatric nursing

22. Correct Answer: C. A wig that looks like the child's own hair will help prevent depression and promote adjustment to later hair loss.

Rationales for Other Answer Choices: A. Children may be even more sensitive to body-image changes, particularly in the teen years. **B.** Hair usually falls out in clumps with chemotherapy and the loss is very noticeable. **D.** Although they may get used to the child without hair, it is still a traumatic experience and a constant reminder of the child's illness.
Nursing Process Phase: planning; client need: psychosocial integrity; concern area: pediatrics

23. Correct Answer: A. This would be an appropriate diet for a healthy client taking lithium. Adequate sodium is necessary because the lithium may cause sodium depletion.

Rationales for Other Answer Choices: B. Client should drink 2000–3000 mL/d. **C.** This is a renal failure diet; sodium intake needs to be adequate. **D.** Although these may be signs of lithium toxicity, her blood levels should be evaluated before stopping the medication.
Nursing Process Phase: planning; client need: psychosocial integrity; concern area: psychiatric nursing

24. Correct Answer: B.
$$\frac{\text{volume to be delivered}}{\text{infusion time (h)}} = \text{mL/h}$$
$$\frac{50 \text{ mL}}{0.5 \text{ h}} = 100 \text{ mL/h}$$

Rationales for Other Answer Choices: A, C, D are incorrect.
Nursing Process Phase: planning; client need: physiological integrity; concern area: medical/surgical

25. Correct Answer: B. These medications, such as Librium, have a sedative effect and are often used to control the withdrawal symptoms of alcohol that the client is displaying.

Rationales for Other Answer Choices: A. Opiates are not used for alcohol withdrawal. **C.** Antidepressants may be dangerous to this client. **D.** Although phenothiazines can be used, they are more effective in treatment of psychotic disorders.
Nursing Process Phase: analysis; client need: safe and effective care environment; concern area: psychiatric nursing

26. **Correct Answer: C.** The most common cause of pyelonephritis is improper treatment of bladder infections. Even after the client feels better, the entire course of antibiotic needs to be taken.

Rationales for Other Answer Choices: A. This will help prevent pyelonephritis. **B.** Not a cause if the infections are treated properly—she may need some personal hygiene instructions. **D.** Not a cause of pyelonephritis.
Nursing Process Phase: analysis; client need: health promotion and maintenance; concern area: medical/surgical

27. **Correct Answer: D.** Disulfiram has a long half-life, and clients have been known to develop symptoms as much as 2 weeks after they discontinue the medication.

Rationales for Other Answer Choices: A. Does cause nausea and vomiting but not hypertension. **B.** Is more successful when used early in the treatment. **C.** It is a type of aversion therapy, not desensitization.
Nursing Process Phase: planning; client need: safe and effective care environment; concern area: psychiatric nursing

28. **Correct Answer: C.** Some of the less serious side effects, such as rash and itching, occur when this medication is first taken, but they are easily controlled with antihistamines or corticosteroids.

Rationales for Other Answer Choices: A. The dose should be taken in the morning; afternoon doses may cause insomnia. **B.** This medication is less sedating than many other psychotropic medications, but some clients experience dizziness or drowsiness when first started on the medication. **D.** It interacts with many other medications. Always check with the physician before taking anything.
Nursing Process Phase: implementation; client need: psychosocial integrity; concern area: psychiatric nursing

29. **Correct Answer: C.** If the client becomes dehydrated, the lithium levels may increase to a toxic range.

Rationales for Other Answer Choices: A. A normal diet with 2 to 3 g of sodium will help prevent toxicity. **B.** Should be taken with food because of its irritating effect on the stomach. **D.** Should check with the physician about any over-the-counter medications taken with lithium.
Nursing Process Phase: implementation; client need: psychosocial integrity; concern area: psychiatric nursing

30. **Correct Answer: A.** Anticholinergics decrease GI motility and would make cathartics less effective.

Rationales for Other Answer Choices: B. Cholinergics stimulate GI motility. **C.** CNS stimulants tend to stimulate GI motility. **D.** Glucocorticoids have no effect on laxatives.

Nursing Process Phase: planning; client need: safe and effective care environment; concern area: medical/surgical

31. Correct Answer: C. If the pain is not relieved, it may be an MI instead of simple angina.

Rationales for Other Answer Choices: A. This is a common side effect; there is no need to call physician. **B.** While they should be kept cool and in a dark bottle, there is no need to refrigerate them; she needs to carry them with her. **D.** Mucous membranes must be moist for best effect, but these tablets should not be swallowed.
Nursing Process Phase: evaluation; client need: health promotion and maintenance; concern area: medical/surgical

32. Correct Answer: B. If a client is known to become nauseated with chemotherapy, the medication should be given before and continued after therapy until the chemotherapy blood levels decrease.

Rationales for Other Answer Choices: A. Waiting until after the nausea begins may make controlling it more difficult. **C.** If several are being used, they should be given at the same time for best effect. **D.** These intervals may not coincide with the chemotherapy administration.
Nursing Process Phase: planning; client need: physiological integrity; concern area: medical/surgical

33. Correct Answer: B. This medication works best on an empty stomach.

Rationales for Other Answer Choices: A. Fluid has no effect on this medication. **C.** Medication does not affect cardiac output. **D.** Cholinergics have no effect on this medication.
Nursing Process Phase: planning; client need: safe and effective care environment; concern area: medical/surgical

34. Correct Answer: B. These are obvious symptoms of lithium toxicity. Further directions from the physician are needed to treat the toxicity.

Rationales for Other Answer Choices: A. Giving the next dose would make the client more toxic. **C.** Increased fluids may help lower the lithium level and reduce the toxicity. **D.** The lithium level must be drawn immediately.
Nursing Process Phase: implementation; client need: psychosocial integrity; concern area: psychiatric nursing

35. Correct Answer: D. Vincristine is an anticancer medication that lowers the WBCs and makes the client more susceptible to infections. A sore throat may indicate infection.

Rationales for Other Answer Choices: A. Normal respiratory rate. **B.** Normal pulse rate. **C.** Not side effects associated with this medication—more associated with bed rest.
Nursing Process Phase: assessment; client need: safe and effective care environment; concern area: medical/surgical

36. Correct Answer: C. It often takes 1 to 2 weeks for lithium levels to reach therapeutic levels. Another medication may be used early in the therapy, then stopped later.

Rationales for Other Answer Choices: A. Not a true or therapeutic statement. **B.** Not a true statement. **D.** This is a paternalistic statement and does not answer the client's question.
Nursing Process Phase: implementation; client need: psychosocial integrity; concern area: psychiatric nursing

37. **Correct Answer: A.** The "gluco" in glucocorticoids is a tipoff to its mode of action.

Rationales for Other Answer Choices: B. Estrogen does this. **C.** Mineralocorticoids do this. **D.** This is not a primary function of glucocorticoids.
Nursing Process Phase: analysis; client need: health promotion and maintenance; concern area: medical/surgical

38. **Correct Answer: C.** Neomycin is an aminoglycoside antibiotic that kills off the intestinal flora, reducing protein digestion, lowering ammonia levels, and preventing hepatic coma.

Rationales for Other Answer Choices: A. Not an approved medication for treating tuberculosis (TB). **B.** Has no antacid effects. **D.** May indirectly cause diarrhea as a side effect—alcoholic patients are often given lactulose to promote excretion of protein from GI tract.
Nursing Process Phase: implementation; client need: physiological integrity; concern area: medical/surgical

39. **Correct Answer: C.** Insulin brings not only glucose into the cell but also potassium. A pretreatment level below normal (normal 3.5–5.5) may lead to severe hypokalemia.

Rationales for Other Answer Choices: A. Normal is 98–106. These are a little low but should come up with the administration of normal saline. **B.** Normal is 135 to 145. Acceptable. **D.** Elevated K is often found in diabetics in DKA because of dehydration; will lower with insulin treatment.
Nursing Process Phase: assessment; client need: safe and effective care environment; concern area: pediatrics.

40. **Correct Answer: B.** The CNS depressant effects of the medication often suppress the respiratory centers. Respiratory rates less than 16 are considered dangerous.

Rationales for Other Answer Choices: A. This may indicate ineffectiveness of the medication; normal reflexes are 2 +. **C.** This is a normal urine output. **D.** Proteinuria indicates the onset of preeclampsia.
Nursing Process Phase: assessment; client need: health promotion and maintenance; concern area: maternity nursing

41. **Correct Answer: D.** Nardil is a MAO inhibitor, and even though the client may not be currently taking the medication, he should avoid tyramine foods for at least 3 weeks after the medication is stopped.

Rationales for Other Answer Choices: A. No need for increased carbs or decreased fats. **B.** Many protein foods contain tyramine. **C.** No indication for a low-sodium diet.

Nursing Process Phase: planning; client need: psychosocial integrity; concern area: psychiatric nursing

42. **Correct Answer: B.** This is an anticholinergic medication used to decrease the extrapyramidal symptoms the client is showing and which are often associated with antipsychotic medications like haloperidol.

Rationales for Other Answer Choices: A. Antianxiety medication; it has no effect on the basal ganglia where the symptoms originate. **C.** Antipsychotic that may increase the symptoms. **D.** Hypnotic that will produce sleep but not control the symptoms.
Nursing Process Phase: implementation; client need: psychosocial integrity; concern area: psychiatric nursing.

43. **Correct Answer: B.** The anti-inflammatory effects of steroid medications like Decadron will help reduce brain swelling.

Rationales for Other Answer Choices: A. Incorrect answer; suppression of the immune system increases potential for infections. **C.** Minor effect of the medication—not the primary reason. **D.** Untrue statement.
Nursing Process Phase: planning; client need: safe and effective care environment; concern area: medical/surgical

44. **Correct Answer: B.** Bleeding is a common and serious complication of t-PA therapy; may produce an excessively high PTT.

Rationales for Other Answer Choices: A. BP usually decreases with this therapy. **C.** A little elevated, but may be due to stress response or disease process. **D.** Above normal but within the therapeutic range of two times normal (normal 25–35 seconds).
Nursing Process Phase: assessment; client need: safe and effective care environment; concern area: medical/surgical

45. **Correct Answer: C.** A rash may indicate a developing allergy to the medication which could produce anaphylaxis.

Rationales for Other Answer Choices: A. Nausea after administration may or may not be due to the medication. **B.** Not a known side effect of the medication. **D.** This is an acceptable urine output.
Nursing Process Phase: implementation; client need: safe and effective care environment; concern area: medical/surgical

46. **Correct Answer: B.** Although this medication is used to suppress rejection, it can interfere with renal and liver functions. Blood urea nitrogen (BUN) and creatinine should be checked once a month for the first 3 months, then every 6 months.

Rationales for Other Answer Choices: A. A common side effect is hypertension. **C.** Client should never stop taking this medication without the physician's approval. **D.** Because of the suppressed immune system, the client should avoid activities or places that would bring him in contact with large numbers of people.
Nursing Process Phase: evaluation; client need: health promotion and maintenance; concern area: medical/surgical

47. **Correct Answer: C.** This medication blocks beta-adrenergic receptors and causes relaxation of the uterus.

Rationales for Other Answer Choices: A. Has no sedative effects, actually causes restlessness. **B.** Has no anticonvulsive effects. **D.** Anticholinergic effects include tachycardia, dry mouth, and constipation.
Nursing Process Phase: planning; client need: health promotion and maintenance; concern area: maternity nursing

48. **Correct Answer: D.** Oral liquid iron preparations can stain the teeth in children. They should be given with a straw, and the teeth should be brushed after.

Rationales for Other Answer Choices: A. These supplements should be given daily. **B.** Tea makes iron insoluble and lowers hemoglobin and hematocrit (H & H)—should be given with an acid substance, such as orange juice. **C.** Iron is highly toxic and a leading cause of poisoning in children; should be given once a day.
Nursing Process Phase: implementation; client need: safe and effective care environment; concern area: pediatrics

49. **Correct Answer: C.** Nitroglycerin (NTG) is a vasodilator that reduces preload and afterload. Lasix is a diuretic that rids the body of extra fluid, producing a normal PCWP between 8 and 12 mm Hg.

Rationales for Other Answer Choices: A. These medications tend to lower blood pressure. **B.** This is normal, but diuretics tend to lower the potassium. It would be expected to be lower. **D.** Neither of these medications has any antidysrhythmic effects, although an indirect result of lower PCWP may be a decrease in all types of dysrhythmias.
Nursing Process Phase: evaluation; client need: safe and effective care environment; concern area: medical/surgical

50. **Correct Answer: A.** Pulmonary edema is a common and deadly complication of narcotic overdoses. It needs to be detected and treated early.

Rationales for Other Answer Choices: B. Important but of lower priority. **C.** Would not be needed until the client was stabilized. **D.** Important but of lower priority.
Nursing Process Phase: analysis; client need: safe and effective care environment; concern area: psychiatric nursing

1. The most important factor for the nurse to consider in caring for a hospitalized client receiving prednisone is the client's:
   A. Increased susceptibility to infections
   B. Depression and suicidal tendencies
   C. Need for extra glucose and fluids
   D. Tendency to excrete potassium and sodium

2. A client has just returned from surgery for a carotid endarterectomy. Which of the following postoperative orders would the nurse anticipate in the plan of care?
   A. Nifedipine (Procardia) 10 mg SL for BP 145/90
   B. Furosemide (Lasix) 20 mg IV for urine output less than 30 mL/h
   C. Magnesium salicylate for pain and inflammation
   D. Nitroglycerin gr 1/150 for chest pain

3. In assessing a recently hospitalized 72-year-old client 1 hour after receiving hydralazine (Apresoline) 20 mg PO, the nurse notes that his blood pressure is 68/42. He has been taking this medication for several years at home without difficulty. Which of the following factors most likely attributed to the hypotension?
   A. Dose is excessive for this medication.
   B. Total intake for the past 48 hours is 2000 mL.
   C. Serum potassium was 5.8 mEq/L.
   D. Heart rate was 145 BPM.

4. A client tells the home–health-care nurse, "My physician told me to stop taking one of my medications because it lowers my red blood cells, but I can't remember which one." If the client is on all of the following medications, which one should be discontinued?
   A. prednisone (Deltasone)
   B. timolol maleate (Blocadren)
   C. gentamicin (Garamycin)
   D. phenytoin (Dilantin)

5. The nurse will know that teaching concerning the toxic effects of sodium salicylate for treatment of juvenile rheumatoid arthritis was successful if the child's parents state:
   A. "I will notify the physician if my child develops tinnitus and nausea."
   B. "I will notify the physician if my child develops dermatitis and blurred vision."
   C. "I will notify the physician if my child develops lethargy and acetone odor to the breath."
   D. "I will notify the physician if my child develops fever of 101 and chills."

6. Which of the following would be an accurate statement for the nurse to include in teaching the parents of a 7-year-old client just diagnosed with type 1 diabetes mellitus about the function of insulin?
   A. "Insulin helps the transport of glucose into the body cells and its storage in the liver as glycogen."
   B. "Insulin increases glyconeogenesis and helps in its use for energy."
   C. "Insulin promotes glycogenolysis and catabolism."
   D. "Insulin decreases anabolism and hypoglycemia."

7. A 9-year-old child develops gingival hyperplasia secondary to phenytoin (Dilantin) administration for a seizure disorder. What alternate method for cleaning the teeth should the nurse instruct the mother to use when even a soft toothbrush causes excessive bleeding and pain?
   A. Water pick
   B. Rinse with water
   C. Foam swab with hydrogen peroxide
   D. Coat teeth and gums with baking soda solution

8. Prior to beginning lithium therapy on a 35-year-old female client with bipolar disorder, the nurse should evaluate which of the following diagnostic tests?
   A. Hemoglobin, hematocrit, and white blood cell (WBC) count
   B. Electrolytes, blood urea nitrogen (BUN), and creatinine
   C. Fasting blood sugar and glucose tolerance test
   D. Electroencephalogram, brain scan, and head magnetic resonance imaging (MRI)

9. In providing care for a client with major depression who is scheduled for electroconvulsive therapy, which of the following ordered medications would the nurse administer just prior to the treatment?
   A. thioridazine (Mellaril) and benztropine
   B. Succinylcholine chloride (Anectine) and atropine sulfate
   C. potassium chloride and magnesium gluconate
   D. carbamazepine (Tegretol) and trihexyphenidyl (Artane)

10. A 24-year-old female client who is being discharged from the hospital after treatment for a pulmonary emboli asks the nurse why she must take warfarin (Coumadin) at home for 6 months. The best response by the nurse is:
    A. "This medication will dissolve any clots that may be left in your lungs."
    B. "It prevents the conversion of prothrombin to thrombin and will prevent further clot development."
    C. "If you do not take it as scheduled, you will develop a larger clot than before and die."
    D. "It inhibits the synthesis of vitamin K and reduces your chances for developing another clot."

11. The serum lithium level of an inpatient client who has been taking lithium 300 mg PO bid for the past 3 weeks is 1 mEq/L. The best action by the nurse at this time is to:
    A. Call the results to the physician immediately.
    B. Hold the morning dose and monitor for toxicity.
    C. Administer the morning dose as ordered.
    D. Give a stat dose of calcium gluconate.

12. A client with severe chest pain secondary to a myocardial infarction (MI) asks the nurse why he is being given this medication. The most accurate statement by the nurse in response to this question is:
   A. "It helps relieve pain, and increases the level of consciousness."
   B. "It helps relieve pain, and increases the rate and depth of respirations for better oxygenation."
   C. "It helps relieve pain, and increases peripheral vasodilation."
   D. "It helps relieve pain, and increases fluid excretion through the skin."

13. As part of a preoperative medication, a child is to receive atropine 0.15 mg (1/400 gr IM). If the medication comes in a vial labeled "Atropine 0.4 mg (1/150 gr)/mL," how much should the nurse draw up in the syringe?
   A. 0.06 mL
   B. 0.38 mL
   C. 2.7 mL
   D. 3.8 mL

14. Three days after a hysterectomy, a client develops an incisional infection with *Pseudomonas aeruginosa*. In planning care for this client, the nurse would anticipate the use of which of the following medications?
   A. cefoperazone (Cefobid)
   B. clindamycin (Cleocin)
   C. dicloxacillin (Dycill)
   D. erythromycin (Erythrocin)

15. A client is admitted to the obstetrics unit at 27 weeks gestation with ruptured membranes. In planning care for this client, the nurse would anticipate the use of which of the following medications?
   A. magnesium sulfate (MgSO$_4$)
   B. betamethasone
   C. Exosurf
   D. ritodrine

16. All of the following are possible side effects of glucocorticoid medications, except:
   A. Peptic ulcers and gastrointestinal (GI) bleeding
   B. Hypoglycemia and central nervous system (CNS) stimulation
   C. Delayed wound healing and immunosuppression
   D. Increased appetite and muscle wasting

17. A 56-year-old male client is receiving chemotherapy with methotrexate and 5-fluorouracil (5-FU) for cancer of the prostate. In planning care for this client, the nurse would expect which of the following to be administered adjunct to the chemotherapy?
   A. Premarin
   B. folic acid
   C. testosterone
   D. Theragram M

18. A client diagnosed with moderate anxiety is started on a short-acting benzodiazepine. In evaluating the effect of this medication, the nurse would observe the client for:
    A. Euphoria and restlessness 1 hour after administration
    B. Calmer and more controlled after the first 24 hours
    C. Unsteadiness while ambulating that may lead to falls
    D. Sleepy and difficult to arouse 2 hours after administration

19. The most important nursing measure to be considered before giving a penicillin class medication IVPB to a client for the first time would be to:
    A. Double-check the dose and route of the medication.
    B. Give the client an injection of epinephrine SC.
    C. Ask the client if he or she has ever had an allergic reaction to penicillin.
    D. Give the medication within 2 hours of mixing and on an empty stomach.

20. What is the most important assessment the nurse needs to make prior to beginning chemotherapy on a 6-year-old child who has leukemia?
    A. Developmental stage
    B. Tendency for nausea and vomiting
    C. Presence of a central intravenous line
    D. Fluid and electrolyte status

21. A 22-month-old baby being treated with cefaclor (Ceclor) for a urinary tract infection (UTI) develops white patches in her mouth that cannot be removed and is very fussy when she eats. The child probably has:
    A. A superinfection with *Candida albicans*
    B. Allergic reaction to the medication manifested by the development of stomatitis
    C. A herpes type 1 simplex virus post antibiotic therapy
    D. An idiosyncratic reaction to the medication

22. What would be the most appropriate action by the nurse when the theophylline level of a hospitalized 8-year-old client with severe asthma comes back 16 μg/mL?
    A. Institute seizure precautions.
    B. Monitor the BP and pulse every hour.
    C. Give the next scheduled dose of aminophylline as ordered.
    D. Notify the physician of the level stat, and hold the next dose of medication.

23. A 4-year-old client who has finished a course of chemotherapy for a Wilm's tumor is to receive filgrastim (Neupogen) daily for 5 days. If the filgrastim therapy is effective, the nurse would note:
    A. Decreased immunoglobulin level
    B. Increased white blood cell count
    C. Decreased tumor cell levels
    D. Increased platelet count

24. A 21-year-old client has been taking cephalexin (Keflex) 500 mg tid PO for an infected cut on her arm. On her eighth day of a ten-day course of treatment she begins experiencing nausea, "bloating," diarrhea, and generalized GI discomfort. The best course of action would be to:
    A. Stop taking the medication immediately because this indicates the development of gastric ulcers secondary to the medication.
    B. Cut the dosage of the medication in half.
    C. Call the physician because this is an allergic reaction to the medication.
    D. Continue to take the medication as ordered.

25. A 2-month-old infant with a ventricular septal defect is started on furosemide (Lasix) therapy. Which of the following should the nurse teach the mother as the most important assessment of the effectiveness of this therapy?
    A. Resting pulse rate
    B. Daily weights
    C. Specific gravity of urine
    D. 24-hour urine output

26. As compared with the penicillins and cephalosporins, the aminoglycosides are more effective against:
    A. Upper respiratory infections
    B. Gram-negative organisms
    C. Gram-positive organisms
    D. Aerobic organisms

27. Which of the following would indicate to the nurse that a client who was receiving clozapine (Clozaril) was developing a serious side effect of the medication?
    A. Fasting glucose of 45 mg/dL
    B. BP of 212/132
    C. WBC count of 2200
    D. Heart rate of 52 BPM

28. Postmyocardial infarction, a client in the intensive care unit develops congestive heart failure. His laboratory values include:
    BUN 19 mg/dL
    Creatinine 2.4 mg/dL
    Glucose 101 mg/dL
    Potassium 2.7 mEq/L
    Sodium 155 mEq/L
    In planning care for this client, the nurse would anticipate administering which of the following?
    A. bumeyanide (Bumex)
    B. glucose (Glutosa)
    C. spironolactone (Aldactone)
    D. furosemide (Lasix)

29. A 56-year-old client with type 1 diabetes is brought into the emergency room with dry mouth and mucous membranes, low urine output for the past 24 hours, and serum potassium of 6.2 mEq/L. If all of the following IV solutions are available to the registered nurse (RN), which should she use for this client?
    A. 0.45% normal saline
    B. dextrose 10% in water
    C. Ringer's lactate
    D. dextrose 5% and 0.45% normal saline

30. Post thyroidectomy, a client asks the nurse why she must take a thyroid hormone supplement. The best answer by the nurse would be:
    A. "Thyroid hormones promote hyperkinesis to prevent you from feeling so tired all the time."
    B. "Thyroid hormones increase cholinergic activity in the body to prevent you from feeling cold."
    C. "Thyroid hormones improve calorigensis and increase metabolic rate to maintain normal metabolism."
    D. "Thyroid hormones reduce protein, fat, and carbohydrate metabolism to keep your weight under control."

31. A 32-year-old client with insulin-dependent diabetes mellitus says to the nurse, "I think I am having an insulin reaction." Which of the following assessments of the client by the nurse would verify this statement?
    A. Skin warm and dry, flushed face, and thirsty
    B. Polyuria, polydipsia, and polyphagia
    C. BP 98/52; glucose 342 mg/dL, poor skin turgor
    D. Skin cool and moist, disorientation, and weakness

32. The physician orders gentamicin (Garamycin) 50 mg IVPB now. The medication comes from the pharmacy labeled "80 mg in 2 mL." How much will the nurse draw up for administration?
    A. 12.5 mL
    B. 0.8 mL
    C. 1.6 mL
    D. 1.25 mL

33. Which of the following is the most serious of the side effects of the aminoglycosides?
    A. Ototoxicity
    B. Photosensitivity
    C. Syncope
    D. Nephrotoxicity

34. A condition in which the bone marrow fails to produce adequate numbers of blood elements, often resulting in granulocytopenia and thrombocytopenia, caused by the use of certain medications, is called:
    A. Hemophilia
    B. Aplastic anemia
    C. Pheochromocytoma
    D. Pernicious anemia

35. A postoperative client with nausea is given prochlorperazine (Compazine) 1 hour before his noon meal. One hour after lunch, the client has a respiratory rate of 7, oxygen saturation of 88% by pulse oximeter, and is lethargic. The first action by the nurse is to:
   A. Start oxygen at 4 L/min by nasal cannula.
   B. Obtain a manual ventilator (Ambu-Bag) and begin ventilating the client at 12 breaths per minute.
   C. Arouse the client and have him take several deep breaths.
   D. Replace the pulse oximeter lead and re-evaluate the oxygen saturation.

36. Which of the following medications would be most useful for the treatment of a child with meningitis?
   A. sulfadiazine (Microsulfon)
   B. gentamicin (Garamycin)
   C. ampicillin (Omnipen)
   D. ceftazidine (Fortaz)

37. An unconscious 12-year-old child with type 1 diabetes is admitted to the hospital with an insulin reaction. If the physician orders all of the following, which should the nurse question?
   A. glucagon 0.5 mg IM
   B. dextrose 50% 25 mL IV push
   C. insulin (regular) 5 U IV
   D. epinephrine 1 : 1000 0.25 mL IV

38. The nurse would know that her teaching plan for a client with pernicious anemia had been successful if the client states:
   A. "My vitamin B_{12} injections must be continued for the rest of my life."
   B. "My vitamin B_{12} injections can be stopped when my symptoms go away."
   C. "My vitamin B_{12} injections can be changed to oral vitamin B_{12} when it reaches a therapeutic blood level."
   D. "My vitamin B_{12} injections must be taken every 6 months."

39. A postoperative client with a total-hip replacement states to the nurse about his patient-controlled analgesia (PCA) pump, "This pump doesn't help my pain at all." What should be the nurse's first response to this statement?
   A. Notify the physician that the ordered dose of medication is not sufficient for pain control.
   B. Push the "Flush" button on the PCA to make sure the IV is not infiltrated.
   C. Press the dose delivery button to give the client a stat dose of medication.
   D. Assess the client's understanding of the PCA.

40. A client develops a UTI. The physician prescribes sulfamethoxazole/trimethoprim (Bactrim) 1000 mg bid PO for 10 days. An important element to be included in the instructions for this client is:
   A. Drink 2000 to 3000 mL of water per day and stay out of the direct sunlight.
   B. Weigh daily to detect for any renal failure.
   C. Avoid sexual activity until the infection clears.
   D. Stop taking the medication when the burning on urination goes away.

41. When a client asks, "Why is the physician prescribing danazol (Danocrine) for my endometriosis?" the best answer by the nurse is:

A. "Danazol decreases the secretion of follicle-stimulating hormone (FSH) and luteinizing hormone (LH)."

B. "Danazol increases the production of estrogen."

C. "Danazol causes the body to release an LH surge."

D. "Danazol increases the activity of the ovaries."

42. A nursing student's purified protein derivative (PPD) skin test has converted from negative to positive, but she has no other symptoms. Assuming that there are no contraindications, she will most likely be prescribed which of the following medications for prophylaxis of this disease?

A. nystatin (Mycostatin)

B. chloramphenicol (Chloromycetin)

C. rifampin (Rifandin)

D. metronidazole (Flagyl)

43. The mother of a 2-year-old child tells the ER nurse that she thinks the child has just eaten between 10 and 15 children's Tylenol tablets. The protocol for acetaminophen overdose includes activated charcoal lavage followed by Mucomyst (N-acetylcysteine) per nasogastric (NG) tube. What should the nurse do first?

A. Teach the parents about medication safety in the home.

B. Place a large-bore NG tube.

C. Calm the mother and child.

D. Ask the mother when the child ate last.

44. The mother of a 2-year-old child who is being treated for an acetaminophen overdose asks the nurse why they are giving the child Mucomyst (N-acetylcysteine). The best response by the nurse is:

A. "Mucomyst is a mucolytic medication that will help prevent respiratory arrest by breaking up thick mucus."

B. "Mucomyst helps maintain a normal pulse rate and blood pressure until the acetaminophen is cleared by the kidneys."

C. "Mucomyst helps reduce liver damage by altering hepatic metabolism and restoring glutathione levels."

D. "Mucomyst increases the excretion of the acetaminophen through the GI tract."

45. In assessing a client who was taking haloperidol (Haldol) 2 mg PO tid, the nurse would anticipate finding:

A. Jaundice and an elevated blood pressure

B. Muscular rigidity and drooling

C. Increased thirst and diaphoresis

D. Marked nausea and vomiting

46. If a client with Graves' disease who is taking propranolol (Inderal) develops all of the following symptoms, which would the nurse report to the physician as a side effect of the medication?

A. Diaphoresis

B. Hypertension

C. Bradycardia

D. Exophthalmos

47. The nurse would know that the teaching of a client with Graves' disease who is to receive I^{131} was successful if the client states:
   A. "For the next three days, I need to drink 2 to 3 quarts of fluid a day."
   B. "I can go visit my pregnant sister as soon as I leave here today."
   C. "I shouldn't have any pain or discomfort in my neck."
   D. "I'll have to stay in the hospital for a few days after you give me the medication."

48. Pyridoxine (vitamin B_6) is given concurrently with INH to prevent:
   A. Liver dysfunction
   B. Peripheral neuritis
   C. Ototoxicity
   D. Damage to visual acuity and color vision

49. A postoperative client who also is a known IV drug abuser frequently asks for his prn IV narcotic pain medication. The most therapeutic measure by the nurse for this client is to:
   A. Give only oral pain medications to decrease his dependence on IV drugs.
   B. Call the physician for an order for a nonnarcotic pain medication so that the client can withdraw from the narcotics.
   C. Medicate the client as ordered if his vital signs are stable and there are no complications.
   D. Discuss the client's drug addiction problems with him so that he will request the medication less often.

50. A 66-year-old client taking benztropine (Cogentin) for Parkinson's disease should be monitored for:
   A. Tardive dyskinesia
   B. Bradycardia
   C. Hypotension
   D. Constipation

ANSWERS/RATIONALES

1. **Correct Answer: A.** Clients on steroids are at high risk for infection. One needs to be careful when assigning rooms.

Rationales for Other Answer Choices: B. Lower priority. **C.** Not needed; clients have hyperglycemia and edema. **D.** Tend to retain these.
Nursing Process Phase: planning; client need: safe and effective care environment; concern area: medical/surgical

2. **Correct Answer: A.** This calcium channel blocker will lower the blood pressure to a safe point to prevent rupture of the graft site.

Rationales for Other Answer Choices: B. Low urine output better managed postoperatively by increasing the IV rate. **C.** Other medications are safer for this complication. **D.** Chest pain not an expected postoperative complication.
Nursing Process Phase: planning; client need: physiological integrity; concern area: medical/surgical

3. **Correct Answer: B.** This medication is a vasodilator. If the client does not have an adequate fluid intake, hypotension will result.

Rationales for Other Answer Choices: A. Normal dosage range is 5 to 25 mg. **C.** Potassium has no effect on this medication. **D.** Increased heart rate is a reflex response that accompanies hypotension.
Nursing Process Phase: analysis; client need: safe and effective care environment; concern area: medical/surgical

4. **Correct Answer: D.** Dilantin can cause decreased blood cell counts and aplastic anemia. Another antiseizure medication should be started before stopping the Dilantin to prevent a rebound effect.

Rationales for Other Answer Choices: A. Prednisone reduces the WBCs but may actually promote the production of red blood cells (RBCs). **B.** This beta-blocker has not been associated with anemia. **C.** Aminoglycosides are renal toxic.
Nursing Process Phase: implementation; client need: safe and effective care environment; concern area: medical/surgical

5. **Correct Answer: A.** These are common symptoms of the toxic effects of aspirin.

Rationales for Other Answer Choices: B. Not associated with aspirin. **C.** Symptoms of diabetic ketoacidosis (DKA). **D.** Symptoms of infection.
Nursing Process Phase: evaluation; client need: health promotion and maintenance; concern area: pediatrics

6. **Correct Answer: A.** These are important functions of insulin in the body.

Rationales for Other Answer Choices: B. This is a function of epinephrine in the stress response. **C.** Insulin is an anabolic hormone that promotes the rebuilding of protein. **D.** Insulin does just the opposite.

Nursing Process Phase: implementation; client need: physiological integrity; concern area: pediatrics

7. Correct Answer: A. A water pick set on low provides teeth cleaning and gingival stimulation.

Rationales for Other Answer Choices: B. May not be adequate for cleaning or gingival stimulation. **C.** Hydrogen peroxide may cause pain. **D.** Not a good cleaning method—unpleasant taste of baking soda.
Nursing Process Phase: planning; client need: health promotion and maintenance; concern area: pediatrics

8. Correct Answer: B. Lithium affects electrolytes, particularly sodium, and is excreted through the kidneys. Any abnormalities in these results may indicate problems in lithium therapy.

Rationales for Other Answer Choices: A. Important tests for all clients but not particularly significant for clients on lithium. **C.** Used when diabetes is suspected. **D.** Do not help evaluate renal function.
Nursing Process Phase: assessment; client need: safe and effective care environment; concern area: psychiatric nursing

9. Correct Answer: B. Anectine is an anesthetic agent used to provide muscle relaxation, and atropine is an anticholinergic used to dry secretions and prevent aspiration.

Rationales for Other Answer Choices: A. Mellaril is used for schizophrenia, and benztropine is an antianxiety agent. **C.** Potassium is used in clients who are hypokalemic, and magnesium is used for clients who have low Mg levels. **D.** Tegretol is an antiseizure medication, and Artane is used in Parkinson's disease.
Nursing Process Phase: implementation; client need: safe and effective care environment; concern area: psychiatric nursing

10. Correct Answer: D. This is the action and use for this medication.

Rationales for Other Answer Choices: A. Anticoagulants do not dissolve clots. **B.** This is the action of heparin. **C.** Although this may be true, it is nontherapeutic communication.
Nursing Process Phase: implementation; client need: psychosocial integrity; concern area: medical/surgical

11. Correct Answer: C. Therapeutic range is 0.5–1.5 mEq/L.

Rationales for Other Answer Choices: A. Not necessary—it's in the normal range. **B.** Holding the dose may make the range subtherapeutic. **D.** This is the antidote for $MgSO_4$.
Nursing Process Phase: implementation; client need: health promotion and maintenance; concern area: psychiatric nursing

12. Correct Answer: C. The vasodilating effect of morphine sulfate (MS) reduces the afterload and the workload of the heart, decreasing the demand for oxygen.

Rationales for Other Answer Choices: A. Its CNS suppressant effects decrease the level of consciousness. **B.** Tends to decrease the depth and rate of respirations. **D.** A

minor secondary effect due to the diaphoresis that sometimes accompanies administration.
Nursing Process Phase: planning; client need: physiological integrity; concern area: medical/surgical

13. **Correct Answer: B.**   0.4 mg : 1 mL :: 0.15 mg : x mL

$$0.4x = 0.15$$
$$x = 0.15/0.4$$
$$x = 0.375 \text{ (round to 0.38)}$$

Rationales for Other Answer Choices: A, C, and **D** are incorrect calculations.
Nursing Process Phase: planning/ client need: safe and effective care environment; concern area: pediatrics.

14. **Correct Answer: A.**   Third-generation cephalosporins such as Cefobid are highly effective against bacillilike pseudomonas, which often cause postoperative infections. They have fewer and less severe side effects.

Rationales for Other Answer Choices: B. An aminoglycoside is not usually indicated for this organism unless it becomes resistant.   **C.** This medication is not effective with this organism.   **D.** This medication is not commonly used to treat this organism.
Nursing Process Phase: planning; client need: health promotion and maintenance; concern area: maternity nursing

15. **Correct Answer: B.**   Betamethasone is a glucocorticoid that will promote the maturation of the fetus's lungs and production of surfactant.

Rationales for Other Answer Choices: A. Used for pregnancy-induced hypertension (PIH) and eclampsia.   **C.** Exosurf is a synthetic lung surfactant given to premature infants after delivery.   **D.** Used to stop preterm labor; question does not indicate that the client is in labor.
Nursing Process Phase: planning; client need: health promotion and maintenance; concern area: maternity nursing

16. **Correct Answer: B.**   Usually hyperglycemia, no effect on CNS.

Rationales for Other Answer Choices: A. Common side effects.   **C.** Common side effects.   **D.** Common side effects.
Nursing Process Phase: assessment; client need: health promotion and maintenance; concern area: medical/surgical

17. **Correct Answer: B.**   These two cancer medications are antimetabolites that alter DNA synthesis by preventing the binding of folic acid. Folic acid supplements are required to prevent massive death of the normal cells.

Rationales for Other Answer Choices: A. A female hormone that has no relation or effect on the cancer.   **C.** A male hormone that has no relationship to the administration of these agents.   **D.** Although multivitamins contain some folic acid, there is not enough to counter the effect of the chemotherapy.
Nursing Process Phase: planning; client need: safe and effective care environment; concern area: medical/surgical

18. **Correct Answer: B.**   Short-acting medications will exert their desired effect within the first 24 hours, sometimes even after the first dose.

Rationales for Other Answer Choices: A. Euphoria is experienced with overdose, restlessness with withdrawal. **C.** Therapeutic doses should not cause any unsteadiness. **D.** Not usually associated with therapeutic doses of benzodiazepines.
Nursing Process Phase: evaluation; client need: health promotion and maintenance; concern area: psychiatric nursing

19. **Correct Answer: C.** Penicillin medications have been used for many years, and often clients have allergies to them.

Rationales for Other Answer Choices: A. Important but not of highest priority. **B.** Not necessary. **D.** Generally should be given within 1 hour of mixing because of instability.
Nursing Process Phase: implementation; client need: safe and effective care environment; concern area: medical/surgical

20. **Correct Answer: D.** Dehydration may decrease the body's ability to rid itself of the chemotherapy through the kidneys; electrolyte imbalances may be worsened by the chemotherapy.

Rationales for Other Answer Choices: A. This assessment is important for psychosocial well-being but not the highest priority. **B.** Nausea and vomiting are common side effects of chemotherapy. **C.** Chemotherapy is often given through a central line, but it can also be given through peripheral IVs, depending on the medication.
Nursing Process Phase: assessment; client need: safe and effective care environment; concern area: pediatrics

21. **Correct Answer: A.** Common side effect of antibiotics.

Rationales for Other Answer Choices: B. Not symptoms of an allergic reaction. **C.** Not symptoms of a herpes infection. **D.** Not symptoms of an idiosyncratic reaction.
Nursing Process Phase: analysis; client need: physiological integrity; concern area: pediatrics

22. **Correct Answer: C.** Normal therapeutic level 10–20 μg/mL.

Rationales for Other Answer Choices: A. Seizures do not occur with therapeutic levels of this medication. **B.** Not necessary unless there are other factors present that would indicate this close monitoring. **D.** Not necessary—dose is in therapeutic range.
Nursing Process Phase: implementation; client need: safe and effective care environment; concern area: pediatrics

23. **Correct Answer: B.** Neupogen accelerates the maturation and growth of neutrophils that are often decreased by chemotherapy, increasing the WBCs.

Rationales for Other Answer Choices: A. Has no effect on immunoglobulin levels. **C.** Is not cytotoxic. **D.** Has no effect on platelet production.
Nursing Process Phase: evaluation; client need: safe and effective care environment; concern area: pediatrics

24. **Correct Answer: D.** This is a common side effect of antibiotic therapy due to alterations in the GI flora. Unless it is severe, the medication should be continued.

Rationales for Other Answer Choices: A. Gastric ulcers are not a side effect of this medication.   **B.** This is not an appropriate action.   **C.** These are not symptoms of an allergic reaction.
Nursing Process Phase: implementation; client need: health promotion and maintenance; concern area: medical/surgical

25. **Correct Answer: B.**   Daily weights would provide the most objective data of an infant's fluid status.

Rationales for Other Answer Choices: A. Assess cardiac function, not fluid status.   **C.** This assessment does not give any indication of retained fluid.   **D.** Output alone is not a good indicator of fluid balance without intake—difficult to measure accurate 24-hour urine of an infant.
Nursing Process Phase: planning; client need: health promotion and maintenance; concern area: pediatrics

26. **Correct Answer: B.**   Although some cephalosporins are effective against gram-negatives, the aminoglycosides in general are more so.

Rationales for Other Answer Choices: A. Usually are gram-positive.   **C.** Aminoglycosides have about the same effectiveness.   **D.** Most aerobic organisms are gram-positive.
Nursing Process Phase: planning; client need: safe and effective care environment; concern area: medical/surgical

27. **Correct Answer: C.**   The most serious side effect of this medication is agranulocytosis and bone marrow depression, which often lead to death.

Rationales for Other Answer Choices: A. Hypoglycemia is not a side effect of this medication.   **B.** This may cause hypotension not hypertensive crisis.   **D.** This has some mild anticholinergic side effects such as dry mouth, tachycardia, and constipation.
Nursing Process Phase: evaluation; client need: safe and effective care environment; concern area: psychiatric nursing

28. **Correct Answer: C.**   A potassium-sparing diuretic such as Aldactone is indicated when the serum potassium is low (normal 3.5–5.5 mEq/L)

Rationales for Other Answer Choices: A. A powerful loop diuretic that will lower potassium.   **B.** Blood sugar is in a normal range.   **D.** Loop diuretic that will also lower potassium.
Nursing Process Phase: planning; client need: safe and effective care environment; concern area: medical/surgical

29. **Correct Answer: A.**   These are symptoms of fluid volume deficit, often associated with DKA in diabetic clients, so the one-half strength normal saline would be the best solution for rehydration.

Rationales for Other Answer Choices: B. This is a concentrated dextrose and should not be used in diabetics.   **C.** Ringer's lactate (RL) contains potassium and should not be given to clients with elevated potassium.   **D.** The client's glucose level is not given, so it would be unsafe to use this solution.
Nursing Process Phase: implementation; client need: safe and effective care environment; concern area: medical/surgical

30. **Correct Answer: C.** After thyroid removal many clients develop hypothyroidism that must be controlled with thyroid hormone supplements.

Rationales for Other Answer Choices: A. This condition is found in children with ADHD and in clients with pheochromocytomas. **B.** Adrenergic activity is increased by thyroid hormone. **D.** Reducing metabolism will increase weight.
Nursing Process Phase: implementation; client need: health promotion and maintenance; concern area: medical/surgical

31. **Correct Answer: D.** Common symptoms of hypoglycemia.

Rationales for Other Answer Choices: A. Symptoms of diabetic ketoacidosis (DKA) or hyperglycemic hyperosmolar nonketotic coma (HHNC). **B.** Early symptoms of onset of diabetes mellitus (DM). **C.** Common findings in DKA.
Nursing Process Phase: analysis; client need: safe and effective care environment; concern area: medical/surgical

32. **Correct Answer: D.**
$$80 : 2 :: 50 : x$$
$$80x = 100$$
$$x = \frac{100}{80} = 1.25 \text{ mL}$$

Rationales for Other Answer Choices: A, B, C are incorrect.
Nursing Process Phase: planning; client need: safe and effective care environment; concern area: medical/surgical

33. **Correct Answer: D.** Renal failure can lead to death in clients receiving aminoglycoside antibiotics.

Rationales for Other Answer Choices: A. Less serious side effect. **B.** Less serious side effect. **C.** Less serious, uncommon side effect.
Nursing Process Phase: assessment; client need: safe and effective care environment; concern area: medical/surgical

34. **Correct Answer: B.** Defines the term.

Rationales for Other Answer Choices: A. An inherited bleeding disorder. **C.** A tumor of the adrenal glands—causes hypertension. **D.** Caused by a lack of intrinsic factor and low B_{12}.
Nursing Process Phase: analysis; client need: health promotion and maintenance; concern area: medical/surgical

35. **Correct Answer: C.** The hypoventilation may be secondary to CNS suppression caused by the prochlorperazine. Stimulating the client to breathe would produce increased oxygenation.

Rationales for Other Answer Choices: A. This action would be a secondary measure if **C** did not work. **B.** This action is not needed unless the client is in complete respiratory arrest. **D.** If the reading was still low after other measures were taken, this may be a choice.
Nursing Process Phase: implementation; client need: physiological integrity; concern area: medical/surgical

36. **Correct Answer: A.** This is the only medication of the group that easily crosses the blood-brain barrier.

Rationales for Other Answer Choices: B. Not effective for CNS infections.   **C.** Not effective for CNS infections.   **D.** Not effective for CNS infections.
Nursing Process Phase: analysis; client need: health promotion and maintenance; concern area: medical/surgical

37.   **Correct Answer: C.**   Additional insulin will only worsen the insulin shock and may cause death.

Rationales for Other Answer Choices: A. Will help increase the blood sugar. **B.** Will help increase the blood sugar.   **D.** Indirectly increases blood sugar and commonly used.
Nursing Process Phase: analysis; client need: safe and effective care environment; concern area: pediatrics

38.   **Correct Answer: A.**   Vitamin B_{12} does not cure the underlying pathology producing the anemia, therefore it must be taken for life.

Rationales for Other Answer Choices: B. Symptoms will return if medication is stopped.   **C.** It is unlikely that the oral form will be effective if there is no intrinsic factor.   **D.** This is the usual interval if every 3 to 4 weeks after initial treatment.
Nursing Process Phase: evaluation; client need: health promotion and maintenance; concern area: medical/surgical

39.   **Correct Answer: D.**   If the client does not know how to use the PCA and can be taught to, then the other measures are unnecessary.

Rationales for Other Answer Choices: A. This situation needs further assessment before notifying the physician.   **B.** This action is not an appropriate way to assess patency of an IV.   **C.** This action may cause the client to have an overdose of medication; also, it does not clarify the problem.
Nursing Process Phase: implementation; client need: physiological integrity; concern area: medical/surgical

40.   **Correct Answer: A.**   In general, fluid intake should be increased with all antibiotics, but particularly with UTI—it helps flush the bacteria from the urinary tract.

Rationales for Other Answer Choices: B. Renal failure is not a common side effect of this medication.   **C.** Not necessary.   **D.** Client needs to continue the medication until completed.
Nursing Process Phase: planning; client need: safe and effective care environment; concern area: medical/surgical

41.   **Correct Answer: A.**   Danazol is an antigonadotropin that suppresses the production of luteinizing hormone and FSH, reducing the engorgement caused in the ectopic endometrial tissue and the accompanying pain.

Rationales for Other Answer Choices: B. Decreases estrogen production.   **C.** Reduces LH.   **D.** Decreases the activity of the ovaries.
Nursing Process Phase: implementation; client need: health promotion and maintenance; concern area: maternity nursing

42.   **Correct Answer: C.**   This is a first-line tuberculosis (TB) medication and is used by itself for positive converters without active disease.

Rationales for Other Answer Choices: A. Antifungal medication. **B.** Not a first-line TB medication. **D.** Antiprotozoal medication, also used for gram-negative organisms.
Nursing Process Phase: planning; client need: health promotion and maintenance; concern area: medical/surgical

43. Correct Answer: B. Quick treatment is necessary to prevent liver failure. Placement of the NG tube allows for medication administration.

Rationales for Other Answer Choices: A. Important action, but lower priority at this time. **C.** The mother and child's emotional status can be treated after the medications are given. **D.** This is somewhat useful to help determine the speed of acetaminophen absorption but not a high priority.
Nursing Process Phase: planning; client need: safe and effective care environment; concern area: pediatrics

44. Correct Answer: C. This is the mode of action for this medication when used for acetaminophen toxicity.

Rationales for Other Answer Choices: A. This medication is a mucolytic, but it is not used for this effect in this situation. **B.** This medication does not have this mode of action. **D.** This medication does not have this mode of action.
Nursing Process Phase: analysis; client need: safe and effective care environment; concern area: pediatrics

45. Correct Answer: B. This medication frequently produces extrapyramidal symptoms.

Rationales for Other Answer Choices: A. Hypotension is common. **C.** Diaphoresis is uncommon—dry skin is more likely. **D.** This is a very rare side effect of this medication.
Nursing Process Phase: assessment; client need: safe and effective care environment; concern area: psychiatric nursing

46. Correct Answer: C. Beta-blockers can produce bradycardia, hypotension and heart blocks.

Rationales for Other Answer Choices: A, B, and **D** are all symptoms of Graves' disease.
Nursing Process Phase: assessment; client need: safe and effective care environment; concern area: medical/surgical

47. Correct Answer: A. Extra fluid and good hydration are necessary to purge the body of the radioactive iodine.

Rationales for Other Answer Choices: B. Should avoid contact with pregnant woman for 24 hours. **C.** It is not unusual to have some neck discomfort from the treatment. **D.** This is usually done on an outpatient basis.
Nursing Process Phase: evaluation; client need: safe and effective care environment; concern area: medical/surgical

48. Correct Answer: B. Isoniazid (INH) interferes with the absorption of pyridoxine, resulting in peripheral neuritis.

Rationales for Other Answer Choices: A. Common side effect of INH but not prevented by B$_6$.   **C.** Uncommon side effect but not prevented by B$_6$.   **D.** Not side effects of INH.
Nursing Process Phase: analysis; client need: health promotion and maintenance; concern area: medical/surgical

49. **Correct Answer: C.**   The purpose of the medications at this time is to relieve the postoperative pain. The drug-abuse problem should be dealt with at a later time when the client recovers.

Rationales for Other Answer Choices: A. Oral medications are just as addictive but work more slowly.   **B.** This measure will not help withdrawal.   **D.** This measure needs to be taken at a later time.
Nursing Process Phase: implementation; client need: safe and effective care environment; concern area: psychiatric

50. **Correct Answer: D.**   This is a common side effect of anticholinergic medications, along with dry mouth, tachycardia, and so forth.

Rationales for Other Answer Choices: A. This medication is used to treat this development in clients taking phenothiazines.   **B.** This medication causes tachycardia.   **C.** This is not a side effect of anticholinergics.
Nursing Process Phase: assessment; client need: safe and effective care environment; concern area: medical/surgical

1. In assessing a 25-year-old client with a heroin overdose, the nurse would consider which of the following the most serious complication?
   A. Flushed skin and diaphoresis
   B. Respiratory rate of 8
   C. Pupils dilated and nonresponsive
   D. Blood pressure (BP) 162/94

2. A client with preterm labor begins to display symptoms of tachycardia, hypotension, tremors, and headache. If she is receiving all of the following medications, which one is producing these symptoms?
   A. magnesium sulfate
   B. nifedipine
   C. terbutaline
   D. indomethacin

3. An 83-year-old nursing home client is admitted to the hospital with sepsis secondary to a serious urinary tract infection. He is started on metronidazole (Flagyl) 1000 mg q 8 h IVPB. What is the most likely reason that he is receiving this medication?
   A. He has a parasitic infection.
   B. He is allergic to other antimicrobial medications.
   C. He has an infection with a gram-negative organism.
   D. This medication has fewer side effects and causes less damage to the kidneys than other medications.

4. A client who is her 30th week of gestation is determined to have postfetal demise. She asks the nurse why she is being given a prostaglandin gel (PG) suppository at this time. The best response by the nurse is:
   A. "PG suppositories help relieve the pain you will experience when the baby is delivered."
   B. "PG suppositories will allow you to relax and decrease your anxiety."
   C. "PG suppositories prevent postpartum infections in cases like yours."
   D. "PG suppositories cause labor to start."

5. A 3-year-old child is taking doxycycline (Vibramycin) liquid for acute gastroenteritis. An important nursing measure in relation to this medication is to:
   A. Take the medication through a straw
   B. Monitor the child for aplastic anemia
   C. Check his hearing frequently
   D. Take with milk to prevent gastrointestinal upset

6. In planning care for a client who is in her 39th week of gestation and is to be induced with oxytocin (Pitocin), the nurse recognizes the safest way to administer the medication is:
   A. Deep IM to reduce the discomfort
   B. Mainline IV to maximize the effectiveness
   C. As a secondary solution IV piggyback
   D. Orally because of its poor absorption IM

7. A client who has been in labor for 6 hours is still having irregular and weak contractions. When oxytocin (Pitocin) is started, the client tells the nurse she is afraid of this medication because when her sister had it, her baby died. The best response by the nurse would be:
   A. "This is a very dangerous medication, but we'll keep a close watch on your condition."
   B. "Complications are rare, and we are prepared to handle any development."
   C. "You seem to be anxious. Tell me more about your fears."
   D. "I'm sure you'll be fine. Your sister's situation was a lot different from yours."

8. The nurse knows the teaching concerning sulfonamides is successful when the client states:
   A. "I must always take this medication with food to prevent a stomachache."
   B. "If I stop taking this medication before the course of treatment is finished, the bacteria will become resistant."
   C. "Taking aspirin with this medication will decrease its effectiveness."
   D. "I need to reduce my fluid intake to prevent kidney failure."

9. A client in active labor complains of severe backache with each contraction. The best time for the nurse to administer the meperidine (Demerol) IV is when:
   A. The contraction is at its peak.
   B. The contraction begins to peak.
   C. The uterus is at rest.
   D. The contraction ends.

10. A 5-month-old infant with a congenital cyanotic heart defect is to receive potassium chloride (KCL) IV. The nurse should:
    A. Give the medication immediately to prevent dysrhythmias associated with hypokalemia
    B. Give the medication over 1 hour to prevent irritation of the vein
    C. Assess the urinary output as adequate before giving the medication
    D. Evaluate the CBC results as normal prior to administration

11. The nurse suspects that a 3-month-old child who is being treated for an infection with IV ceftizoxime (Cefizox) is becoming fluid overloaded when she assesses:
    A. Swelling at the IV insertion site
    B. Vomiting after each medication administration
    C. Rectal temperature of 97.2°F
    D. Bubbling crackles in both bases

12. In planning care for an 8-year-old client with status asthmaticus who is receiving theophylline (Aminophylline) IV, the nurse would monitor the client for:
    A. Constipation
    B. Bradycardia
    C. Drowsiness
    D. Headache

13. A 10-year-old child develops Reye's syndrome secondary to aspirin use during a viral infection. In caring for this child, the nurse should:
    A. Avoid administering IM injections if possible
    B. Do hourly urine outputs with a urometer
    C. Perform neuro assessment every 4 hours
    D. Turn the child side to side every shift

14. The nurse would know that the teaching of the parents of a child who is to take sodium salicylate at home posthospitalization for rheumatic fever was successful if the parents state:
    A. "The medication may becoming toxic if my child develops blurred vision and itching."
    B. "The medication may becoming toxic if my child develops chills and fever."
    C. "The medication may becoming toxic if my child develops an acetone odor to his breath."
    D. "The medication may becoming toxic if my child develops tinnitus and nausea."

15. A client with histoplasmosis would best be treated with an:
    A. Antibiotic
    B. Antifungal
    C. Antiviral
    D. Antiprotozoan

16. The mother of a 3-year-old child who had just ingested a large number of iron tablets at home phones the ER concerning the use of syrup of ipecac for her child. The nurse instructs the mother to:
    A. Give the medication with a glass of milk
    B. Not give the medication because iron is not that toxic
    C. Have the child drink a large glass of tepid water after taking the medication
    D. Wait at least 30 minutes before giving the medication

17. The nurse instructs a client who is taking carbamazepine (Tegretol) that one of the best ways to help prevent injuries from the tonic-clonic–type seizures he experiences because of his epilepsy is to:
    A. Avoid becoming fatigued by physical activity
    B. Do not play any competitive or contact sports
    C. Take an extra dose of medication if he should develop the flu or other infections
    D. Identify factors that consistently precede a seizure

18. Which of the following side effects should the nurse include in a teaching plan for a postmenopausal woman who is to be started on estrogen therapy?
    A. Deep vein thrombosis
    B. Narrowing of visual fields
    C. Renal calculi
    D. Uterine atony

19. As a result of taking a cephalosporin medication, a patient develops hypoprothrombinemia. The primary reason for developing this condition is:
    A. Bone marrow shutdown
    B. Suppression of the platelet production
    C. Killing of the intestinal bacteria
    D. Destruction of the adrenal cortex

20. In planning care for a client who is receiving sulfamethoxazole (Gantanol), the nurse should instruct the client to:
    A. Chew the tablets completely before swallowing
    B. Not to be concerned by the blue urine
    C. Drink 2 to 3 L of fluid per day
    D. Call the physician if tinnitus occurs

21. A physician orders nystatin (Mycostatin) 50 mL PO for a hospitalized client receiving IV antibiotics. The best action for the nurse would be to:
    A. Question the order because the route of administration is incorrect.
    B. Give the medication as ordered because the client is obviously very ill.
    C. Question the order because the dose is too large.
    D. Question the order because the medication does not work when given with antibiotics.

22. Which of the following statements by a client with a cystitis who has been prescribed co-trimoxazole (Bactrim DS) would indicate that additional teaching was required by the nurse?
    A. "I should drink 2 to 3 quarts of water each day while I am taking these."
    B. "I can stop taking the pills after the pain and burning go away."
    C. "If I develop itching or a rash, I should call the physician right away."
    D. "I can break the pills in two if I am having trouble swallowing them."

23. Which of the following medications would be most likely used on the second-degree and third-degree burns on a client's arms?
    A. chlorambucil (Leukeran)
    B. tetracycline (Sumycin)
    C. silver sulfadiazine (Silvadene)
    D. sulfadiazine (Microsulfon)

24. A client with Parkinson's disease was started on levodopa (Larodopa). In planning care for this client, the nurse would monitor him for which of the following side effects of this medication?
    A. Diarrhea
    B. Drowsiness
    C. Nausea
    D. Headaches

25. A 54-year-old client with Parkinson's disease has been taking levodopa (Larodopa) for the past 3½ years. The home health-care nurse assigned to his care suspects that he is developing "on-off syndrome" because he:
    A. Takes the medication one day, then forgets to take it the next
    B. Is developing toxic symptoms and needs to be taken off it for several weeks before being put back on
    C. Fluctuates from being symptom-free to demonstrating full-blown Parkinson's symptoms
    D. Only needs to take the medication once a week to remain symptom free

26. The nurse would know that teaching of a client who was receiving levodopa (Larodopa) was successful if the client states:
    A. "When my shaking stops, I can stop taking this medication."
    B. "If my urine turns dark, I need to call the physician immediately."
    C. "I can drink my usual martini each night as long as I take it with food."
    D. "I should avoid eating pork, beef, liver, bananas, and egg yolks."

27. Before discharge, the nurse should teach the mother of a 9-year-old client taking carbamazepine (Tegretol) for a recently diagnosed seizure disorder to:
    A. Avoid washing the child's clothes in laundry soaps containing phosphates
    B. Limit the child's contact with large groups of strangers, such as at the shopping mall
    C. Keep the child covered or use sunscreen when outside during the summer
    D. Reduce the child's intake of dairy and milk products

28. Which of the following statements by a client would indicate that more teaching was required about the use of levodopa (Dopar) at home?
    A. "I should stop taking these pills when I feel better or start having side effects."
    B. "I need to avoid alcohol while I am taking this medication."
    C. "If I think I'm pregnant, I need to call the doctor right away."
    D. "I shouldn't take over-the-counter allergy medications while I'm on this medication."

29. The physician orders phenytoin (Dilantin) 750 mg IV over 1½ hour for a client who has just had a brain tumor removed. The best response of the nurse to this order is to:
    A. Give the medication as ordered
    B. Give the medication, but question the order
    C. Refuse to give the medication because the dosage is too great and will kill the patient
    D. Call the physician to verify the dose and route

30. A client asks the nurse why he is receiving lidocaine (Xylocaine) in his IV, when he is accustomed to his dentist giving him injections of the medication in his mouth before dental work. The best response by the nurse is:
    A. "The medication is much more effective IV, and you will feel no pain at all in your mouth."
    B. "When given IV, this medication reduces the irritability of the cells in your heart and helps prevent dysrhythmias."
    C. "As an IV medication, it will help you relax and rest so that your heart can heal."
    D. "This medication will help increase your urine output so that you will be less likely to develop renal failure after your accident."

31. Which of the following assessments would indicate to the nurse that the lidocaine hydrochloride (Xylocaine) therapy a client was receiving was effective?
    A. PR interval of 2.80 sec
    B. QRS complex of 0.16/sec
    C. Premature ventricular contractions now 3/min down from 12/min 15 minutes before
    D. ST segment now normal, changed from elevated 2 hours before

32. A client with an order for nitroglycerine sublingual is having chest pain. What is the first action the nurse should take at this time?
    A. Take his pulse and blood pressure.
    B. Assess if he is allergic to nitroglycerine.
    C. Administer the sublingual nitrate immediately.
    D. Evaluate the type and degree of pain.

33. The best action for the nurse to take if a client develops orthostatic hypotension after receiving diltiazem (Cardizem) is to:
    A. Start IV fluids at 150 mL/h
    B. Monitor the BP q 5 min
    C. Hold the medication and notify the physician
    D. Assist with position changes

34. What would be the best response by the nurse to a client with a recent artificial mitral valve replacement who asks the nurse, "Why must I take warfarin sodium (Coumadin) after I go home?"
    A. "The medication thins your blood so that your heart doesn't have to work so hard to pump the blood."
    B. "Clots have a tendency to form in the new valve, and this medication will prevent that."
    C. "The new valve will open and close more smoothly if the blood is anticoagulated."
    D. "All postoperative clients have a higher risk of clots in their legs or lungs, and medication prevents it."

35. In planning care for a client in hypertensive crisis who is being given nitroprusside (Nipride) IV, the nurse recognizes that nitroprusside:
    A. Increases sodium and water excretion
    B. Prevents angiotensin I from converting to angiotensin II
    C. Reduces systemic vascular resistance
    D. Decreases the contractility of the myocardial fibers

36. A 23-year-old woman is being treated for lupus erythematosus with prednisone (Deltasone) 40 mg tid. For which of the following side effects should the nurse monitor this client?
    A. Hypothermia
    B. Hyperglycemia
    C. Hypotension
    D. Hyperkalemia

37. Which of the following assessments would most concern the nurse who is caring for a client in hypertensive crisis who has been receiving IV nitroprusside (Nipride) for the past 32 hours?
   A. Dilated pupils and pink skin
   B. Deep, rapid respirations and bounding pulses
   C. Hyperactive reflexes and loud heart sounds
   D. Insomnia and mild hypertension

38. Which of the following statements made by a postoperative client who is to use a patient-controlled analgesia (PCA) pump with meperidine (Demerol) would indicate to the nurse that he correctly understood the use of the pump?
   A. "I can get pain medication every 10 minutes by pushing the button."
   B. "I can get pain medication every time I push the button."
   C. "I should notify the nurse when the pain is gone."
   D. "The pump will give me pain medication automatically when I start to hurt."

39. The nurse recognizes that polystyrene sulfonate (Kayexalate) would be appropriate for a client who had which of the following?
   A. Serum potassium of 7.1 mEq/L
   B. Resting BP of 182/104
   C. Serum sodium of 156 mEq/L
   D. Urine protein of +3

40. A 58-year-old client with chronic bronchitis is being discharged with two inhalers, one with beclomethasone (Vanceril) and the other with metaproterenol (Alupent) to use at home. Which of the following would be the most appropriate for the nurse to include in the teaching plan for this client?
   A. Use the Vanceril first, followed by the Alupent.
   B. Use the Vanceril only in the morning and the Alupent in the afternoon.
   C. Use the Alupent first, followed by the Vanceril.
   D. Use the Alupent in the morning and the Vanceril in the afternoon and evening.

41. Which of the following would the nurse observe a client for who was receiving vasopressin tannate (Pitressin)?
   A. Hyperactive deep tendon reflexes
   B. Increased heart rate
   C. Elevated blood pressure
   D. Constricted pupils

42. A client who is receiving his first dose of gentamicin (Garamycin) IV for a severe postoperative infection tells the nurse he feels "itchy." The nurse also observes a rash on the client's arms and face. Which of the following actions should the nurse take next?
   A. Take the client's vital signs.
   B. Assess the client's orientation.
   C. Stop the Garamycin infusion.
   D. Quickly call the physician.

43. Which of the following assessments made by a nurse would indicate that the infusion rate needs to be slowed for a 72-year-old client who is receiving IV nitroglycerine for chest pain after a myocardial infarction (MI)?
   A. Chest pain is now a 3 on a 1 to 10 scale, down from a 9 when the client was admitted.
   B. Serum potassium of 4.2 mEq/L has increased from a 3.2 mEq/L 2 hours ago.
   C. Pulse rate of 108 beats per minute (BPM) has increased from 91 BPM.
   D. BP of 90/71 decreased from 128/88 upon admission.

44. The nurse suspects that a 42-year-old client is having an anaphylactic allergic reaction to a dose of cephadrin (Anspor) IV he had just received. Which of the following symptoms manifested by the client would most likely lead the nurse to this conclusion?
   A. Nausea and vomiting
   B. Itchy rash and hives
   C. Hypertension and tachycardia
   D. Sudden wheezing and urticaria

45. Which of the following would be the best action for the nurse to take to prevent the development of side effects in a client who was receiving pentamidine isethionate (Pentam 300)?
   A. Take daily weights to detect fluid retention.
   B. Have the client lie down while receiving the medication to prevent hypotension.
   C. Keep the client NPO until after the dose is given, then give a calorie-restricted diet.
   D. Restrict the client's fluid intake to 1500 mL/24 h to prevent urinary calculi.

46. A client suffers from "acid indigestion" and reports taking large amounts of calcium carbonate (TUMS) for relief. During the teaching phase of the nursing process, the nurse explains that this practice may cause which result?
   A. Respiratory alkalosis with numbness and dizziness
   B. Respiratory acidosis with weakness and tachycardia
   C. Metabolic acidosis with muscle twitching and tremors
   D. Metabolic alkalosis with nausea, vomiting, and convulsions

47. Which of the following statements by a client would indicate to the nurse that the teaching about methenamine hippurate (Hiprex) was not understood?
   A. "I will avoid over-the-counter antacids containing sodium bicarbonate."
   B. "I must weigh myself daily and write it down."
   C. "I have to take this medication with food to prevent my stomach from hurting."
   D. "Taking the medication with cranberry juice or ascorbic acid will help clear the infection."

48. Prior to discharge, a client with a renal transplant is given instructions concerning the corticosteroids he will be taking at home. Which of the following statements by the client would indicate to the nurse that he understood these instructions?
- **A.** "I can't eat any salt."
- **B.** "I should stop taking the medication if I develop swelling or if my blood pressure goes up."
- **C.** "I must take the medication every day and not skip doses."
- **D.** "I will use these urine dipsticks you gave me to test for urine protein every day."

49. In planning care for a 4-year-old child with nephrosis, which outcome would the nurse expect after the administration of a course of prednisone?
- **A.** Increased diuresis
- **B.** Reduced serum sodium levels
- **C.** Reduced urinary protein levels
- **D.** Increased white blood cell count

50. Which of the following statements made by the parents of a 4-year-old child who just received a kidney transplant would indicate to the nurse that they understood how to administer the child's daily dose of cyclosporine (Sandimmune) oral solution?
- **A.** "We should mix the medication in chocolate milk just before the child drinks it."
- **B.** "The medication should be kept cold to reduce the sour taste that it has."
- **C.** "We should give the liquid 1 hour before or 2 hours after meals to maximize the effectiveness."
- **D.** "We should use a plastic cup when mixing the medication with water before administering."

ANSWERS/RATIONALES

1. **Correct Answer: B.** Respiratory depression is the most serious effect of narcotic medications and may lead to death.

Rationales for Other Answer Choices: A. Common but noncritical effect of narcotics. **C.** Expected reaction after a narcotic overdose. **D.** Expect hypotension with narcotic overdose.
Nursing Process Phase: assessment; client need: safe and effective care environment; concern area: psychiatric nursing

2. **Correct Answer: C.** These are common side effects of tocolytic medications like terbutaline—note the tremors.

Rationales for Other Answer Choices: A. Hypotension is a side effect of magnesium sulfate ($MgSO_4$), but the other symptoms are rare. **B.** Calcium channel blockers do not cause tremors or tachycardia. **D.** Prostaglandin inhibitors may produce headaches and hypertension.
Nursing Process Phase: analysis; client need: health promotion and maintenance; concern area: maternity nursing

3. **Correct Answer: C.** This antiprotozoal medication is highly effective against gram-negative organisms frequently found in urinary tract infections (UTIs).

Rationales for Other Answer Choices: A. Rarely are UTIs caused by parasites. **B.** Not enough information in the question to select this answer. **D.** Do not know what other medications are indicated.
Nursing Process Phase: planning; client need: safe and effective care environment; concern area: medical/surgical

4. **Correct Answer: D.** Prostaglandin E_2 vaginal suppositories or gel are used to induce labor in cases in which there is second- or third-trimester fetal demise. They stimulate smooth muscle and cause the uterus to contract.

Rationales for Other Answer Choices: A. Have no analgesic effects. **B.** Have no antianxiety effects. **C.** Have no antibiotic effects.
Nursing Process Phase: implementation; client need: health promotion and maintenance; concern area: maternity nursing

5. **Correct Answer: A.** This medication is generally not given to children under 8 years of age because it stains the teeth. If it is used, it should be taken through a straw to avoid teeth staining.

Rationales for Other Answer Choices: B. This condition is not a side effect of this medication. **C.** Ototoxicity is not a side effect. **D.** Milk inactivates the medication.
Nursing Process Phase: planning; client need: health promotion and maintenance; concern area: medical/surgical

6. **Correct Answer: C.** After the main IV is started, the oxytocin is piggybacked into it so it can be stopped quickly if complications develop, but an IV access is still maintained.

Rationales for Other Answer Choices: A. Is given IM after delivery. **B.** Should never be used as the primary or main IV. **D.** Not used because of poor oral absorption.
Nursing Process Phase: planning; client need: health promotion and maintenance; concern area: maternity nursing

7. **Correct Answer: C.** Most therapeutic of the responses; it acknowledges the client's fears, and the open-ended statement allows her to ventilate her feelings.

Rationales for Other Answer Choices: A. Statement would only reinforce her fear. **B.** Not completely true—less therapeutic than **C.** **D.** Blank reassurance does not acknowledge her anxiety.
Nursing Process Phase: implementation; client need: psychosocial integrity; concern area: maternity nursing

8. **Correct Answer: B.** This is true of all antibiotics.

Rationales for Other Answer Choices: A. This works best on an empty stomach. **C.** This has no effect on the medication. **D.** Should increase the fluid intake.
Nursing Process Phase: evaluation; client need: health promotion and maintenance; concern area: medical/surgical

9. **Correct Answer: B.** During the onset of a contraction, the blood flow to the uterus and fetus is decreased, so the IV medication will be less likely to cause weakening of contractions or fetal respiratory depression.

Rationales for Other Answer Choices: A. There is insufficient time for the medication to reach the mother before it reaches the fetus. **C.** The mother and fetus share the same circulation. **D.** There is full placental circulation at the end of a contraction.
Nursing Process Phase: implementation; client need: health promotion and maintenance; concern area: maternity nursing

10. **Correct Answer: C.** Unless there is normal renal function, the child can become rapidly hyperkalemic, which is more difficult to treat.

Rationales for Other Answer Choices: A. Avoid giving the medication until normal renal function has been determined. **B.** Time to be determined by the concentration. **D.** No significance to complete blood count (CBC); it is better to evaluate chemistries.
Nursing Process Phase: analysis; client need: safe and effective care environment; concern area: pediatrics

11. **Correct Answer: D.** Fluid excess often produces left-sided congestive heart failure manifested by wet lung sounds.

Rationales for Other Answer Choices: A. May indicate an infiltrated IV. **B.** May indicate an adverse reaction to the medication. **C.** Symptom not associated with over-hydration.
Nursing Process Phase: assessment; client need: safe and effective care environment; concern area: pediatrics

12. **Correct Answer: D.**   Headache, nervousness, and insomnia are common side effects of the medication.

Rationales for Other Answer Choices: A. Causes vomiting and diarrhea.   **B.** Causes tachycardia.   **C.** Causes insomnia.
Nursing Process Phase: planning; client need: safe and effective care environment; concern area: pediatrics

13. **Correct Answer: A.**   Because of the liver involvement of this condition, the bleeding times are prolonged. IM injections should be avoided, but if necessary, pressure should be applied to the site for 3 to 5 minutes.

Rationales for Other Answer Choices: B. Not required for this condition; renal involvement is rare.   **C.** During the acute stage, should be done every hour.   **D.** Should be turned every 2 hours to prevent skin breakdown.
Nursing Process Phase: implementation; client need: safe and effective care environment; concern area: pediatrics

14. **Correct Answer: D.**   These are common toxic symptoms of salicylate medications (Aspirin).

Rationales for Other Answer Choices: A. May indicate an allergic reaction.   **B.** Symptoms of infection.   **C.** Symptom of diabetic ketoacidosis (DKA).
Nursing Process Phase: evaluation; client need: safe and effective care environment; concern area: pediatrics

15. **Correct Answer: B.**   Histoplasmosis is a serious fungal infection.

Rationales for Other Answer Choices: A. Not effective for fungal infections.   **C.** Not effective for fungal infections.   **D.** Generally not used for fungal infections.
Nursing Process Phase: analysis; client need: safe and effective care environment; concern area: medical/surgical

16. **Correct Answer: C.**   Syrup of ipecac will best induce vomiting when taken with 100 to 200 mL of tepid water or other clear liquids.

Rationales for Other Answer Choices: A. Milk may counteract the effect of the medication and delay or prevent vomiting.   **B.** Iron is highly toxic to children (and adults), and excessive oral iron needs to be removed quickly.   **D.** Needs to be given as soon as possible.
Nursing Process Phase: implementation; client need: safe and effective care environment; concern area: pediatrics

17. **Correct Answer: D.**   Many clients have an "aura" 30 to 90 seconds prior to their seizures. If the clients can identify and recognize them, they can assume a safe position prior to the onset of the seizures.

Rationales for Other Answer Choices: A. Although in some individuals fatigue can precipitate a seizure, avoiding fatigue does not help prevent injury.   **B.** If the seizures are under control, sports are not contraindicated.   **C.** Client should take the medication as prescribed—extra doses can lead to toxicity.
Nursing Process Phase: implementation; client need: physiological integrity; concern area: medical/surgical

18. **Correct Answer: A.** Estrogen therapy increases the clotting tendencies. If the woman should experience any leg pain, redness, or swelling, she needs to call the physician.

Rationales for Other Answer Choices: B. Glaucoma is not associated with estrogen therapy. **C.** These are not caused by estrogen therapy. **D.** This is not caused by estrogen therapy.
Nursing Process Phase: planning; client need: health promotion and maintenance; concern area: medical/surgical

19. **Correct Answer: C.** Condition is secondary to treatment with antibiotics that kill off the intestinal flora, preventing synthesis and absorption of vitamin K.

Rationales for Other Answer Choices: A. Causes aplastic anemia. **B.** Causes thrombocytopenia. **D.** Causes Addison's disease.
Nursing Process Phase: planning; client need: health promotion and maintenance; concern area: medical/surgical

20. **Correct Answer: C.** It is always a good idea to drink extra fluid when on any type of antibiotic. Sulfa medications may cause urinary crystal formation if client is dehydrated.

Rationales for Other Answer Choices: A. Should not be chewed, although if large they may be crushed and taken with food. **B.** Do not produce blue urine. **D.** Not a side effect.
Nursing Process Phase: planning; client need: health promotion and maintenance; concern area: medical/surgical

21. **Correct Answer: C.** Normal dose is 5–10 mL (500,000 U).

Rationales for Other Answer Choices: A. Right route. **B.** Would be even sicker if he took this much. **D.** Often given with antibiotics because of superinfections.
Nursing Process Phase: planning; client need: safe and effective care environment; concern area: medical/surgical

22. **Correct Answer: B.** The entire prescription should be completed, even though the symptoms subside before it is completed. Resistant organisms may develop if it is not finished.

Rationales for Other Answer Choices: A. True statement—extra fluid should always be taken when client is on antibiotics. **C.** These may be signs of an allergic reaction. **D.** These are large pills that may be difficult to swallow. Can be broken if scored, but they should not be crushed.
Nursing Process Phase: evaluation; client need: health promotion and maintenance; concern area: medical/surgical

23. **Correct Answer: C.** This is a commonly used topical antimicrobial when there is burn injury.

Rationales for Other Answer Choices: A. Anticancer medication. **B.** Broad spectrum antibiotic; PO or IV. **D.** Broad spectrum antibiotic; PO or IV.
Nursing Process Phase: planning; client need: health promotion and maintenance; concern area: medical/surgical

24. **Correct Answer: C.** This is a common side effect of this medication; hypotension, dry mouth, weakness, ulcers, and anemia are other side effects.

Rationales for Other Answer Choices: A. Tends to cause constipation. **B.** Increases alertness. **D.** Not a common side effect.
Nursing Process Phase: planning; client need: safe and effective care environment; concern area: medical/surgical

25. **Correct Answer: C.** When symptom-free, the client is "on"; when symptoms develop, he is "off." These may last from a few minutes to several days. This relatively common syndrome develops after 2 years of levodopa therapy and is probably due to a tolerance to the medication.

Rationales for Other Answer Choices: A. This is noncompliance due to forgetfulness. **B.** Toxicity is not associated with the syndrome. **D.** Typically, clients need larger or more frequent doses of this medication.
Nursing Process Phase: analysis; client need: health promotion and maintenance; concern area: medical/surgical

26. **Correct Answer: D.** These foods contain high levels of protein and pyridoxine (vitamin B_6), which are metabolized into amino acids and compete with the brain receptor sites for dopamine.

Rationales for Other Answer Choices: A. Client must continue to take the medication until the physician changes or stops it. **B.** This is a common side effect but has no significance. **C.** All alcohol should be avoided when taking this medication.
Nursing Process Phase: evaluation; client need: safe and effective care environment; concern area: medical/surgical

27. **Correct Answer: C.** Photosensitivity is a common side effect of this medication.

Rationales for Other Answer Choices: A. Although this may be good for the environment, there is no interaction with the medication. **B.** The medication does not affect the immune system. **D.** These are no interactions with dairy products.
Nursing Process Phase: planning; client need: safe and effective care environment; concern area: pediatrics

28. **Correct Answer: A.** This medication needs to be continued and never stopped suddenly.

Rationales for Other Answer Choices: B. Alcohol should be avoided. **C.** This medication is contraindicated in pregnancy. **D.** Client should avoid all over-the-counter (OTC) central nervous system (CNS) drugs, such as antihistamines.
Nursing Process Phase: evaluation; client need: safe and effective care environment; concern area: medical/surgical

29. **Correct Answer: A.** This is an appropriate loading dose for this medication for clients who are at high risk for seizures.

Rationales for Other Answer Choices: B. If there is a question, do not give this medication. **C.** Untrue. **D.** Not necessary; both dose and route are "right."
Nursing Process Phase: evaluation; client need: safe and effective care environment; concern area: medical/surgical

30. **Correct Answer: B.** Lidocaine IV is used to treat ventricular dysrhythmias (premature ventricular contractions [PVCs], ventricular tachycardia [VT], ventricular fibrillation [VF]), particularly in clients who have suffered an MI.

Rationales for Other Answer Choices: A. Causes no anesthetic effect unless the client receives an overdose. **C.** May cause some drowsiness as a side effect, but it is not used for this purpose. **D.** Has no effect on renal output.
Nursing Process Phase: implementation; client need: safe and effective care environment; concern area: medical/surgical

31. **Correct Answer: C.** Lidocaine is used to treat ventricular dysrhythmias, such as PVCs, and its effectiveness would be indicated by a decrease in the number of ectopic beats.

Rationales for Other Answer Choices: A. This is abnormal—indicates a first-degree atrioventricular (A-V) block. **B.** This is abnormal—indicates a ventricular conduction defect or ectopic beat. **D.** Not an effect of lidocaine.
Nursing Process Phase: evaluation; client need: safe and effective care environment; concern area: medical/surgical

32. **Correct Answer: D.** There are many causes for chest pain, and nitroglycerine (NTG) should not be used unless the pain is cardiac in origin.

Rationales for Other Answer Choices: A. Important but can be done later. **B.** Important but can be done if client is going to be given NTG. **C.** Must assess the pain first.
Nursing Process Phase: assessment; client need: health promotion and maintenance; concern area: medical/surgical

33. **Correct Answer: D.** This is a fairly common side effect of this medication and can be managed with slow position changes.

Rationales for Other Answer Choices: A. Not necessary. **B.** Generally not required with simple postural hypotension. **C.** Only if the hypotension is severe or if other symptoms, such as bradycardia, are present.
Nursing Process Phase: implementation; client need: physiological integrity; concern area: medical/surgical

34. **Correct Answer: B.** All artificial structures placed in the body tend to produce clots.

Rationales for Other Answer Choices: A. Untrue statement—anticoagulants do *not* thin the blood. **C.** Not true. **D.** Although this is true, the incidence is very low for all postoperative clients, and most are not started on anticoagulants.
Nursing Process Phase: implementation; client need: health promotion and maintenance; concern area: medical/surgical

35. **Correct Answer: C.** Nitroprusside is a member of the nitrate family of medications; it causes vasodilation and reduction of afterload.

Rationales for Other Answer Choices: A. Mode of action (MOA) of diuretics. **B.** MOA of angiotensin-converting enzyme (ACE) inhibitors. **D.** MOA of beta-blockers and calcium channel blockers.
Nursing Process Phase: planning; client need: safe and effective care environment; concern area: medical/surgical

36. Correct Answer: B. One of the side effects of glucocorticoids is to increase the blood sugar, producing hyperglycemia.

Rationales for Other Answer Choices: A. This is not a side effect of this medication. **C.** Glucocorticoids increase fluid retention and raise the blood pressure. **D.** Glucocorticoids increase urinary output and may lower the potassium.
Nursing Process Phase: assessment; client need: safe and effective care environment; concern area: medical/surgical

37. Correct Answer: A. These are signs of nitroprusside toxicity; other signs include shallow respirations, weak pulses, suppressed reflexes, distant heart sounds, somnolence, coma, and severe hypotension.

Rationales for Other Answer Choices: B, C, and **D** are not symptoms of nitroprusside toxicity.
Nursing Process Phase: assessment; client need: safe and effective care environment; concern area: medical/surgical

38. Correct Answer: A. Depending on the time lockout, pain medication can be delivered by pushing the button every 10 to 60 minutes.

Rationales for Other Answer Choices: B. The machine has a time lockout on the administration of medication to prevent overdose. **C.** This is not necessary, although the nurse should assess the effectiveness of the medication periodically. **D.** Although the PCA pump can be set to deliver continuous IV analgesic medications, it cannot know when the client hurts.
Nursing Process Phase: evaluation; client need: safe and effective care environment; concern area: medical/surgical

39. Correct Answer: A. Kayexalate is an ion-exchange resin that exchanges sodium ions for potassium ions in the large intestine. It is given as an enema or can be given orally to lower high serum-potassium levels (normal 3.5–5.5 mEq/L).

Rationales for Other Answer Choices: B. Not used for hypertension. **C.** May actually increase serum-sodium levels (normal 135–148 mEq/L). **D.** Not used for elevated urine proteins.
Nursing Process Phase: analysis; client need: safe and effective care environment; concern area: medical/surgical

40. Correct Answer: C. Metaproterenol (Alupent) is a bronchodilator that opens the air passages so that the steroid medication (beclomethasone) can penetrate deeper into the lungs and reduce the inflammation of the bronchioles and alveoli better.

Rationales for Other Answer Choices: A. This sequence would reduce the effectiveness of the steroid medication. **B.** Both inhalers should be used together according to the physician's prescription, usually 3 to 4 times a day. **D.** Both inhalers should be used together according to the physician's prescription, usually 3 to 4 times a day.
Nursing Process Phase: planning; client need: health promotion and maintenance; concern area: medical/surgical

41. Correct Answer: C. This medication is used for the treatment of diabetes insipidus and causes fluid retention, which can lead to hypertension.

Rationales for Other Answer Choices: A, B, and **D** are not side effects of this medication.
Nursing Process Phase: assessment; client need: safe and effective care environment; concern area: medical/surgical

42. Correct Answer: C. These are signs of an allergic reaction. Stopping the medication immediately will prevent anaphylaxis.

Rationales for Other Answer Choices: A. Important but lower priority. **B.** Not high priority at this time. **D.** Can be done later when the client is stable.
Nursing Process Phase: implementation; client need: safe and effective care environment; concern area: medical/surgical

43. Correct Answer: D. This is a significant drop in BP caused by the vasodilating effects of the medication. Further reduction in BP may produce hypotension.

Rationales for Other Answer Choices: A. The goal is to make the client pain-free; the medication has not achieved this goal yet. **B.** Potassium is not affected by this medication. **C.** As the blood pressure drops, the pulse rate often increases. Usual parameter is 110 BPM.
Nursing Process Phase: evaluation; client need: safe and effective care environment; concern area: medical/surgical

44. Correct Answer: D. Anaphylactic reactions cause bronchial spasms/constriction and rashes.

Rationales for Other Answer Choices: A. Nausea and vomiting are side effects, and hypertension is not associated with anaphylactic shock. **B.** This answer is included in **D**. **C.** Hypotension is associated with anaphylactic reactions.
Nursing Process Phase: assessment; client need: safe and effective care environment; concern area: medical/surgical

45. Correct Answer: B. The two major side effects of this medication are hypotension and hypoglycemia. Having the client lie down will prevent falls from postural hypotension.

Rationales for Other Answer Choices: A. This does not cause fluid retention. **C.** Client should eat before the administration because of possible hypoglycemia. **D.** Client should increase the fluid intake to 2 to 3 liters per day.
Nursing Process Phase: implementation; client need: safe and effective care environment; concern area: medical/surgical

46. Correct Answer: D. One cause for metabolic alkalosis is ingesting base-containing medications, which increase the bicarbonate levels. These are symptoms of metabolic alkalosis.

Rationales for Other Answer Choices: A. Respiratory alkalosis is caused by hyperventilation. **B.** Respiratory alkalosis is caused by hypoventilation and retention of car-

bon dioxide. **C.** Metabolic acidosis is caused by many diseases, including renal failure and insulin-dependent diabetes mellitus (IDDM).
Nursing Process Phase: planning; client need: safe and effective care environment; concern area: pediatrics

47. **Correct Answer: B.** Hiprex is a urinary tract antiseptic used to treat UTI. It does not affect the weight nor increase fluid retention.

Rationales for Other Answer Choices: A. Best results occur when the urine pH is acid (below 5); antacids make the pH alkaline. **C.** Hiprex is irritating to the stomach and needs to be taken with food. **D.** The substances also acidify the urine.
Nursing Process Phase: client need: safe and effective care environment; concern area: medical/surgical

48. **Correct Answer: C.** Corticosteroids are a vital part of the antirejection regimen posttransplant. Although the dosage may be gradually tapered, the client should not skip doses.

Rationales for Other Answer Choices: A. A low-sodium diet is recommended because of the sodium retention that occurs with steroids, but salt should not be avoided altogether. **B.** These are rather common side effects; the physician should be notified, but the medication should not be stopped. **D.** Proteinuria is a possible side effect, but it does not need to be checked daily.
Nursing Process Phase: evaluation; client need: safe and effective care environment; concern area: medical/surgical

49. **Correct Answer: C.** Steroids are used in children with nephrosis to reduce glomerular inflammation and increase the reabsorption of proteins into the vascular system.

Rationales for Other Answer Choices: A. Diuresis should be reduced after treatment. **B.** No direct effect on sodium levels. **D.** WBCs may be decreased because of the immune suppression effect of steroids.
Nursing Process Phase: planning; client need: health promotion and maintenance; concern area: pediatrics

50. **Correct Answer: A.** Cyclosporine oral solution is a mixture of alcohol and vegetable oil, best given with chocolate milk or orange juice at room temperature just after mixing.

Rationales for Other Answer Choices: B. Should be given at room temperature. **C.** Needs to be given with food or meals. **D.** Best to use glass to reduce the adherence of the oil to the side of the container.
Nursing Process Phase: evaluation; client need: safe and effective care environment; concern area: pediatrics

1. Before discharging a client who is taking carbamazepine (Tegretol), the nurse should teach him that:
   A. Blood dyscrasias are possible side effects, and hematologic monitoring is essential.
   B. Diplopia is a possible side effect, and bifocal eyeglasses are essential.
   C. Hyperpyrexia is a side effect, and cooling baths are essential.
   D. Respiratory depression is a side effect, and oxygen therapy is essential.

2. A 62-year-old chronic schizophrenic woman who has been a 15-year inpatient in a state hospital is noted to manifest bizarre repetitive movements of her mouth, tongue, hands, and feet. Her mouth involuntarily grimaces, and her tongue intermittently protrudes. Her fingers repetitively flex, and she often rocks back and forth. She has been treated for 12 years with moderate doses of phenothiazines. The most common clinical phenomenon that the nurse is observing is:
   A. Conversion reaction
   B. Tardive dyskinesia
   C. Decerebrate posturing
   D. Huntington's chorea

3. A client is to be discharged on (haloperidol) Haldol 5 mg PO tid. The nurse who completes the discharge medication teaching should instruct the client about medication compliance and:
   A. Hypertensive crisis
   B. Agranulocytosis, seizures
   C. Photosensitivity, agranulocytosis
   D. Dermatitis

4. Extrapyramidal reactions (acute dystonia, akathesia, Parkinsonism) can be managed by support from the nurse and a stat dose of which medication?
   A. dopamine (Intropin)
   B. levodopa (Dopar)
   C. benztropine (Cogentin)
   D. captopril (Capoten)

5. After several hours on the psychiatric unit, a client becomes severely agitated, displays looseness of association, and attacks the housekeeping staff with a lamp. Neurological examination is completed after the client is placed in full leather restraints (FLR). The examination is normal. Thus the treatment team decides to rapidly tranquilize the client with haloperidol (Haldol). The nurse knows that the rapid tranquilization schedule will be:
   A. 2 mg q h (IM)
   B. 5 mg q h (IM)
   C. 10 mg q h (IM)
   D. 20 mg q h (IM)

6. The nurse is teaching a client recently diagnosed with a seizure disorder about carbamazepine (Tegretol) prior to discharge. Which statement by the client would indicate to the nurse that the teaching was effective?
   A. "If I drink alcohol while taking this medication, I should do so only before bedtime to help me sleep."
   B. "If I go out in the bright sun, I should be covered or use lots of sunscreen."
   C. "If I get drowsy or start having stomach pains, I should stop taking the medication for several days."
   D. "For the medication to be most effective, I need to take it 1 hour before meals with very little water."

7. After taking a medication, a pediatric client begins to have difficulty breathing and breaks out in a red, itchy rash. Which type of reaction is he most likely having?
   A. Idiosyncratic
   B. Unpredictable
   C. Anaphylactic
   D. Adverse

8. A 37-year-old male client is admitted for obsessive-compulsive disorder and panic attacks. He has been increasingly bothered by a series of rituals to control his fears of substances in the air. The client reports that he spends 10 to 12 hours each day meticulously cleaning his house and its air. The client is started on alprazolam (Xanax) and an antidepressant (doxepin). In planning care for this client, the nurse should anticipate that alprazolam:
   A. Has serious adverse reactions
   B. Has a slow onset of action
   C. Is administered subcutaneously
   D. In high doses can suppress panic attacks

9. A 44-year-old female client has been incapacitated with unipolar depression for 4 years. She has had a slight improvement with amitriptyline (Elavil), but the physician decides to prescribe a monoamine oxidase inhibitor (MAOI). When medication teaching is complete, the nurse informs the client that:
   A. Anticholinergic symptoms do not occur with the MAOIs
   B. Hypertensive crises may occur if one consumes foods high in tyramine content
   C. MAOIs have few interactions with other drugs
   D. The onset of therapeutic effects is 5 days

10. The nurse would recognize that an antidepressant a client was taking was causing anticholinergic side effects if the nurse observed:
    A. Bradycardia
    B. Delirium
    C. Sedation
    D. Diarrhea

11. The greatest risk for a client being discharged on antidepressants is:
    A. Hypotension
    B. Seizures
    C. Suicide/overdose
    D. Narrow-angle glaucoma

12. The nurse understands that antidepressants are used in the treatment of the following syndromes (in addition to depression):
    A. Hysterical personality disorder
    B. Chronic pain syndrome
    C. Phobias
    D. Dementia

13. A 72-year-old woman is brought to the hospital for psychiatric evaluation. Her daughter states that her mother has "changed from being an outgoing, happy person to someone who keeps to herself and shows no interest in life." Over the past 4 months the client has lost weight, has been irritable, has been slow to understand concepts, and cries often. A medical diagnosis of affective disorders is made (major depression, unipolar). The client is started on amoxapine. In planning care for this client, the nurse recognizes that this medication has:
    A. Low-sedative effects, low-anticholinergic effects
    B. High-sedative effects, high-anticholinergic effects
    C. High-sedative effects, low-anticholinergic effects
    D. Low-sedative effects, high-anticholinergic effects

14. Prior to administering lithium carbonate to a client for the first time, the nurse would assess him carefully for:
    A. Agitation
    B. Dehydration
    C. Agedness
    D. Hypothermia

15. The nurse suspects that a client who is being treated with lithium carbonate is developing toxicity when he develops which of the following symptoms?
    A. Diarrhea, vomiting, muscular weakness
    B. Higher temperature, thirst, constipation
    C. Anuria, spiked t-waves, hypersalivation
    D. Tachycardia, dry mouth, urinary retention

16. In planning care for the client taking lithium, the nurse would carefully monitor the therapeutic range, which is:
    A. 0.1 to 0.4 mEq/L
    B. 0.5 to 1.5 mEq/L
    C. 1.6 to 1.8 mEq/L
    D. 2.5 to 5 mEq/L

17. The nurse understands that a medication with an agonist effect:
    A. Binds with a receptor site to produce an effect
    B. Inhibits or counteracts effects of hormones and other medications
    C. Works only on one specific receptor site
    D. Is a precursor to another neurotransmitter

18. A 40-year-old male client is admitted to the emergency room with rapid speech, grandiose delusions, insomnia, and hypersexual behavior. His history reveals similar past episodes interspersed with periods of psychomotor retardation, hypersomnia, and weight gain. As the nurse completes the health history, he or she would ask the client if he has a history of taking:
    A. diazepam (Valium)
    B. chlorpramazine (Thorazine)
    C. lithium carbonate (Eskalith)
    D. imipramine (Tofranil)

19. A 5-year-old child is being discharged with a prescription for cyclophosphamide (Cytoxan). The nurse should teach the parents the importance of:
    A. Increasing the child's fluid intake
    B. Monitoring the child's bowel movements
    C. Decreasing the child's contact with children
    D. Preventing the child from becoming self-conscious about hair loss.

20. A 10-year-old female client is receiving chemotherapy for the treatment of leukemia. During this clinic visit, she stated that her handwriting has really gotten bad, and she has not had a bowel movement in 5 days. Considering that the child is on all of the following drugs, which one would most likely cause the symptoms she is having?
    A. cyclophosphamide (Cytoxan)
    B. prednisone (Deltasone)
    C. vincristine (Oncovin)
    D. methotrexate (Mexate)

21. A 4-year-old boy is receiving chemotherapy for a brain tumor. Which of the following nursing actions are most important during the nadir (period of greatest immunosuppression) occurring as a result of chemotherapy?
    A. Maintain normal growth and development by allowing him to play with other children on the unit.
    B. Withhold blood transfusions to decrease the risk associated with invasive procedures.
    C. Closely monitor the administration of chemotherapeutic agents.
    D. Assess the child for subtle signs of infection.

22. The nurse would know that the discharge teaching to the parents of a 7-year-old boy who will be taking cyclophosphamide (Cytoxan) at home was successful if the parents state:
    A. "We need to give the Cytoxan at noon."
    B. "We need to give the Cytoxan in the morning."
    C. "We need to give the Cytoxan at bedtime."
    D. "We need to give the Cytoxan with any meal."

23. A 17-year-old male client with a brain tumor is receiving intravenous fluorouracil (Adrucil). His IV is at a keep-open rate for medications. After his second dose of fluorouracil (Adrucil), the client becomes nauseated, starts vomiting, and refuses to eat or drink. Besides giving him the prn antiemetic that has been ordered, the nurse should request from the physician an order to:
   A. Withhold the next dose of Adrucil
   B. Increase the IV rate to 100 mL/h
   C. Place him on NPO status
   D. Force fluids orally

24. After a 6-month-old infant has had two febrile seizures, she is started on phenobarbital. In planning care for this child, the nurse should be aware that phenobarbital:
   A. Helps control seizure activity
   B. Cures the seizure condition
   C. Decreases anxiety associated with seizures
   D. Helps prevent elevated temperatures which cause the seizures

25. While teaching a pregnant client about care during pregnancy, the nurse explains that teratogens are:
   A. Safe to use because they promote normal development of the fetus
   B. Not related to pregnancy but useful in the control of seizure disorders
   C. Medications, toxins, radiation, and viruses that may cause birth defects in the fetus.
   D. Dangerous to the fetus only during the third trimester of pregnancy.

26. The physician orders mebendazole (Vermox) for the treatment of enterobiasis in a 14-year-old female client. Before administering this medication, it is important to determine if the child:
   A. Is pregnant
   B. Is allergic to eggs
   C. Is allergic to penicillin
   D. Has eaten within the past 2 hours

27. A 6-year-old child has been started on mebendazole (Vermox) for the treatment of enterobiasis. In planning care for this client, it is important for the nurse to realize that:
   A. It is recommended that the entire family be treated
   B. Active immunity results from past medication administration
   C. Medication should be given until there are no worms evident in the stool
   D. Child should be isolated from siblings and peers until course of medication is completed

28. Which of the following statements by a client would indicate to the nurse that the teaching concerning home use of digoxin (Lanoxin) had been successful?
   A. "I should avoid taking laxatives and antacids when I'm taking the Lanoxin."
   B. "I must check my pulse before I take the medication, and I should not take it if it's over 100 beats per minute (BPM)."
   C. "I cannot eat fresh fruits or vegetables while I'm taking Lanoxin because they will upset my stomach."
   D. "When I feel better and the swelling goes down in my legs, I can stop taking the medication."

29. A 28-year-old client is started on IV ritodrine to help stop her preterm labor. An increase in blood plasma volume is sometimes associated with this medication. What laboratory test(s) results would the nurse use to confirm development of this side effect?
    A. Elevated serum electrolytes
    B. Decreased serum glucose
    C. Decreased hemoglobin and hematocrit
    D. Elevated serum BUN and creatinine

30. A client is admitted in labor to a perinatal unit at 27 weeks gestation with twin fetuses. Which of the following would not be a contraindication to starting IV ritodrine at this time?
    A. Spontaneously ruptured membranes
    B. Temperature greater than 100.6°F.
    C. Cervical dilation of 4 cm or greater
    D. Bloody show

31. A gravida 1 para 0 client has been receiving magnesium sulfate ($MgSO_4$) for 12 hours for her pregnancy-induced hypertension (PIH). For which of the following assessments would the nurse turn off the magnesium sulfate?
    A. Respiratory rate under 12/min
    B. Urine output of 35 mL/h
    C. Deep tendon reflexes (DTRs) of 2+ no clonus
    D. Blood pressure (BP) 128/84 after prolonged BP of 188/104

32. A client with severe preeclampsia has been receiving IV magnesium sulfate for 12 hours. Which of the following is not a sign of overdose?
    A. Absence of DTRs
    B. Respiration rate slower than 12/min
    C. Urinary output less than 30 mL/h
    D. Decrease in blood pressure

33. While the labor and delivery nurse is running IV oxytocin (Pitocin) to augment labor, she notices that the fetal monitor is showing late decelerations and loss of beat-to-beat variability. What is the first thing the nurse should do?
    A. Administer oxygen by mask to the mother.
    B. Turn off Pitocin.
    C. Turn the mother to her left side.
    D. Increase the rate of the primary IV.

34. Ritodrine hydrochloride has been infusing IV for several hours to stop a client's preterm labor. Since there are no contraindications for inhibiting labor and the client is 30 weeks' gestation, what other standard tocolytic therapy might the nurse anticipate to be used in place of ritodrine?
    A. indomethacin
    B. meperidine (Demerol) and hydroxyzine (Vistaril) IM
    C. magnesium sulfate
    D. morphine sulfate

35. A client who is gravida 2 para 1 at 40 weeks has been 4 cm for 3 hours. Her physician wants the nurse to augment her with oxytocin (Pitocin). What concentration would the nurse mix in order to start the augmentation?
   A. 20 U Pitocin in 1000 mL
   B. 10 U Pitocin in 500 mL
   C. 10 U Pitocin in 1000 mL
   D. 10 U Pitocin in 250 mL

36. While assessing a client who has been taking large doses of diuretics for congestive heart failure, the nurse notes symptoms of tetany. The nurse understands that these symptoms are most likely associated with:
   A. Hyponatremia
   B. Hypokalemia
   C. Hypermagnesemia
   D. Hypocalcemia

37. A client is receiving verapamil (Calan) and metoprolol tartrate (Lopressor) for coronary artery disease and myocardial infarction. The nurse should monitor the client for which of the following drug interactions?
   A. Increased pulmonary depressant effects
   B. Decreased pulmonary depressant effects
   C. Decreased cardiodepressant effects
   D. Increased cardiodepressant effects

38. A client is receiving tocainide (Tonocard) PO for ventricular ectopy. The nurse knows that the primary action of this antiarrhythmic is to suppress ventricular automaticity in the:
   A. Sinoatrial (S-A) node
   B. Atrioventricular (A-V) node
   C. His-Purkinje fibers
   D. Bundle of His

39. A client is admitted with a low potassium level and is prescribed parenteral potassium chloride 40 mEq/L stat. Which of the following would be an appropriate method to administer the drug?
   A. IV push
   B. Concentrated IV infusion
   C. Diluted IV infusion
   D. IM

40. Which of the following symptoms would the nurse observe in an adult client who was developing salicylism?
   A. Respiratory depression and acidosis
   B. Rash and bronchial wheezing
   C. Bleeding from the gums and blood in the urine
   D. Respiratory alkalosis and tachypnea

41. Which of the following statements by a client who started on allopurinol (Zyloprim) 300 mg daily for treatment of gout would indicate the need for additional teaching?
   A. "Ultraviolet light exposure to the eyes may cause cataracts."
   B. "I should maintain adequate fluid intake to reduce the frequency of attacks."
   C. "I need to immediately report the development of a rash or itching."
   D. "Medical supervision may be discontinued after the maintenance dose is prescribed."

42. A client with a gastric ulcer is being discharged with prescriptions for ranitidine (Zantac) and the antacid Maalox TC (chewable tablets). What medication teaching should the nurse include prior to discharge?
    A. Take the Maalox and ranitidine (Zantac) at the same time to maximize the effectiveness.
    B. Take the ranitidine (Zantac) with food at mealtimes and the Maalox one hour after meals.
    C. Take the Maalox at meal times with food and the ranitidine (Zantac) 2 hours after meals.
    D. If you develop diarrhea while taking these two medications, stop taking the ranitidine (Zantac) for 24 hours.

43. A 22-year-old male client with second- and third-degree burns of his legs and lower abdomen returns to his room after whirlpool and debridement therapy. He is scheduled to receive silver sulfadiazine (Silvadene) cream on all burned areas. Which of the following methods should the nurse use?
    A. Sterile technique after debridement.
    B. Sterile technique just before the next debridement session
    C. Aseptic technique after debridement
    D. Aseptic technique before next debridement

44. A client with hemorrhagic gastritis is to receive cimetidine (Tagamet) 300 mg IVPB q 6 hours. The medication comes from the pharmacy mixed in 50 mL of normal saline. At what rate would the nurse set the volumetric IV pump to run to infuse the medication in 15 minutes?
    A. 25 mL/h
    B. 75 mL/h
    C. 100 mL/h
    D. 200 mL/h

45. In teaching a client who is receiving amitriptyline hydrochloride (Elavil) to control her chronic depression, the nurse should include the fact that the therapeutic effects of this drug are generally seen in:
    A. 3 to 4 weeks
    B. 3 to 4 months
    C. 3 to 4 days
    D. 3 to 4 hours

46. A 70-year-old female client who is admitted to the adult psychiatric unit for severe depression is to be started on amitriptyline hydrochloride (Elavil) PO. Which of the following nursing actions would be indicated with the initiation of drug therapy?
    A. Decrease the patient's fluid intake at night.
    B. Elevate the patient's side-rails at night.
    C. Administer drug prior to meals.
    D. Maintain the patient on bed rest for 2 days.

47. A 26-year-old female client who is admitted for chemotherapy to treat Hodgkin's disease is receiving vincristine sulfate (Oncovin) 0.01 mg/kg per week. The nurse should counsel the client on which of the following common adverse effects?
    A. Alopecia
    B. Hirsutism
    C. Irritability
    D. Gingivitis

48. A 48-year-old female client who has idiopathic parkinsonism with tremors and rigidity is started on benztropine mesylates (Cognetin) 1 mg PO daily. The nurse should instruct the client that suppression of tremors and rigidity will occur at which of the following?
   A. After 1 week of drug therapy
   B. After 1 month of drug therapy
   C. After first dose
   D. After 2 to 3 days of drug therapy

49. A 25-year-old female client is admitted to the emergency room with acetaminophen overdose. The nurse should plan to administer which of the following drugs as the antidote?
   A. albumin
   B. acetylcysteine (Mucomyst)
   C. acyclovir (Zovirax)
   D. naloxone (Narcan)

50. An elderly client at the outpatient clinic tells the nurse that he has problems with constipation and asks the nurse which laxative is best for him to take, bisacodyl (Dulcolax) or psyllium (Metamucil). The best response by the nurse is:
   A. "Take the biscodyl (Dulcolax) because it is more effective and works quickly."
   B. "It would be best to use the psyllium (Metamucil) because it is easier on the GI tract."
   C. "Tell me more about your constipation and what you take for it now."
   D. "You could take either of the medications and have good results."

ANSWERS/RATIONALES

1. **Correct Answer: A.** Carbamazepine has severe hematologic toxicities. Blood dyscrasias such as anemia, leukopenia, and thrombocytopenia occur once in every 20,000 patients. Red cells, white cells, platelets, and reticulocytes are monitored monthly on an outpatient basis.

Rationales for Other Answer Choices: B. Does not affect vision. **C.** Temperature regulation not affected. **D.** Respiratory centers affected only by large overdoses.
Nursing Process Phase: planning; client need: health promotion and maintenance; concern area: medical/surgical

2. **Correct Answer: B.** The client is suffering from tardive dyskinesia. This syndrome was first described in the early 1960s but was first recognized as pathological in the later 1960s. It is most common in clients who are female, aged, and have been treated chronically with an antipsychotic. It can occur as soon as 1 to 2 months after institution of antipsychotic drug treatment. Tardive dyskinesia is thought to be due to basal ganglia dopenergic hypersensitivity. The condition may be permanent.

Rationales for Other Answer Choices: A. Conversion reaction is a type of anxiety disorder that produces physical symptoms, such as pain. **C.** Abnormal posturing is a result of increased intracranial pressure. **D.** Huntington's chorea is a genetic disorder.
Nursing Process Phase: analysis; client need: safe and effective care environment; concern area: psychiatric nursing

3. **Correct Answer: B.** The client who receives Haldol should be taught that drug compliance is important and that the side effects of Haldol include agranulocytosis, seizures, impotence, sedation, orthostatic hypotension, extrapyramidal side effects, and neuroleptic malignant syndrome.

Rationales for Other Answer Choices: A. Hypertensive crises is a side effect of monoamine oxidase inhibitors. **C.** Photosensitivity is a side effect of phenothiazines. **D.** Dermatitis is a side effect for nurses and clients handling phenothiazine in the oral liquid form.
Nursing Process Phase: planning; client need: psychosocial integrity; concern area: psychiatric nursing

4. **Correct Answer: C.** The term *extrapyramidal side effects* refers to a group of movement disorders that result from the ability of antipsychotic agents to disrupt function of the extrapyramidal motor system (the same neuronal network that is responsible for the movement disorders of Parkinson's disease).

Rationales for Other Answer Choices: A. Dopamine is used to increase cardiac output and maintain blood pressure. **B.** Levodopa is used to treat the dopamine depletion that occurs in Parkinson's disease. **D.** Captopril is an antihypertensive.

Nursing Process Phase: implementation; client need: safe and effective care environment; concern area: psychiatric nursing

5. **Correct Answer: B.** If Haldol is used as a rapid tranquility agent, 5 mg IM q h will be given until the client is sedated or improved. Rapid tranquilization is used not only in psychiatry but also in the care of violent medical clients.

Rationales for Other Answer Choices: A, C, and **D** are improper dosages and times.
Nursing Process Phase: implementation; client need: psychosocial integrity; concern area: psychiatric nursing

6. **Correct Answer: B.** One of the important side effects of this medication is photosensitivity, and clients need to protect themselves from sunburns.

Rationales for Other Answer Choices: A. Client should avoid drinking all alcohol while taking this medication. **C.** Client should never stop taking this medication suddenly because of rebound effect and increased seizure activity. **D.** Medication should be taken with a full glass of water and can be taken with food.
Nursing Process Phase: evaluation; client need: safe and effective care environment; concern area: medical/surgical

7. **Correct Answer: C.** These are symptoms of a severe allergic reaction, especially the difficulty in breathing, which may indicate bronchospasms.

Rationales for Other Answer Choices: A. These are reactions that would be the opposite of what the desired action is (e.g., giving a person a sleeping pill makes him agitated and anxious). **B.** Unpredictable reactions are reactions that have never happened before and are not documented; anaphylactic reactions are predictable in persons allergic to the medication. **D.** Adverse reactions are not as severe as anaphylactic reactions.
Nursing Process Phase: assessment; client need: safe and effective care environment; concern area: pediatrics

8. **Correct Answer: D.** This medication is given in high doses for the suppression of panic attacks often seen in clients with this disorder.

Rationales for Other Answer Choices: A. Alprazolam is relatively safe, with few adverse side effects. **B.** Alprazolam has an intermediate onset of action. **C.** The drug is given by mouth.
Nursing Process Phase: planning; client need: psychosocial integrity; concern area: psychiatric nursing

9. **Correct Answer: B.** Hypertensive crisis may follow ingestion of foods that contain tyramine (aged cheese, broad beans, chianti wine, chocolate, pickled herring). The reaction involves a sharp headache, nuchal rigidity, and subarachnoid hemorrhage.

Rationales for Other Answer Choices: A. Anticholinergic side effects do occur with monoamine oxidase inhibitors. **C.** MAOIs interact with diet pills, over-the-counter (OTC) cold medication, and nasal decongestants. **D.** The onset of therapeutic effect is 2 to 4 weeks, not 5 days.
Nursing Process Phase: implementation; client need: safe and effective care environment; concern area: psychiatric nursing

10. **Correct Answer: B.** Anticholinergic side effects commonly interfere with treatment compliance. Symptoms that the nurse should be aware of include dry mouth, blurred vision, constipation, tachycardia, agitation, seizures, urinary retention, and delirium.

Rationales for Other Answer Choices: A, C, and **D** are not anticholinergic symptoms.
Nursing Process Phase: assessment; client need: safe and effective care environment; concern area: psychiatric nursing

11. **Correct Answer: C.** Most antidepressants have a narrow therapeutic index and can be lethal in overdose. Thus, a careful evaluation of the client's risk of suicide must be undertaken upon discharge. Generally, no more than a week's supply of any antidepressant should be prescribed for clients upon discharge.

Rationales for Other Answer Choices: A. Hypotension is usually transient and not severe. **B.** Seizures are a rare complication of use of these medications. **D.** Narrow angle glaucoma is not caused by these medications.
Nursing Process Phase: analysis; client need: safe and effective care environment; concern area: psychiatric nursing

12. **Correct Answer: B.** Antidepressants are generally prescribed in major depressive disorders, bulimia, chronic pain disorders, pathological crying or laughing, and panic disorders.

Rationales for Other Answer Choices: A. Antidepressants are not effective for the treatment of hysteria. **C.** Antidepressants are not used to treat phobias unless there is a secondary diagnosis of depression. **D.** Antidepressants are not used to treat dementia.
Nursing Process Phase: analysis; client need: health promotion and maintenance; concern area: psychiatric nursing

13. **Correct Answer: A.** There are pharmacodynamic (receptor) effects (which are not well understood) that predispose the aged to pronounced anticholinergic effects. In addition, the aged are more prone to postural hypotension and falling. Thus, low-sedative, low-anticholinergic drugs should be used with this age group.

Rationales for Other Answer Choices: B, C, and **D** are untrue about amoxapine, a tricyclic antidepressant.
Nursing Process Phase: planning; client need: psychosocial integrity; concern area: psychiatric nursing

14. **Correct Answer: B.** Lithium therapy may be associated with diminution of renal concentrating ability and occasionally causes symptoms of polyuria and polydipsia. Dehydration of a client taking lithium may result in lithium retention and toxicity.

Rationales for Other Answer Choices: A. This medication is given for manic behavior. **C.** Age is relatively unimportant when administering this medication. **D.** Hypothermia is not an important factor.
Nursing Process Phase: assessment; client need: safe and effective care environment; concern area: psychiatric nursing

15. **Correct Answer: A.** Although side effects from lithium may be multiple, the range of symptoms generally progresses as follows: diarrhea, vomiting, drowsiness, and muscular weakness occur as early side effects with serum lithium levels below 2.0 mEq/L. At higher levels, ataxia, tinnitus, blurred vision, and large dilute output of urine may be seen. Serum lithium levels above 3.0 mEq/L may produce a complex clinical picture of multiple organ involvement.

Rationales for Other Answer Choices: B. Side effects of phenothiazines. **C.** Not side effects of lithium. **D.** Side effects of anticholinergics.
Nursing Process Phase: assessment; client need: safe and effective care environment; concern area: psychiatric nursing

16. **Correct Answer: B.** Therapeutic lithium levels range from 0.5 –1.5 mEq/L. During the acute phase of mania, serum lithium concentrations fluctuate because of several variables, such as gastrointestinal absorption, renal output, age, diet, salt intake, and perspiration.

Rationales for Other Answer Choices: A. This range is too low. **C** and **D.** These ranges are too high.
Nursing Process Phase: analysis; client need: safe and effective care environment; concern area: psychiatric nursing

17. **Correct Answer: A.** Statement defines the term.

Rationales for Other Answer Choices: B. Statement defines antagonist effect. **C.** Statement defines specific binding effect. **D.** Statement does not answer the question.
Nursing Process Phase: planning; client need: safe and effective care environment; concern area: medical/surgical

18. **Correct Answer: C.** The client portrays a classic picture of manic-depressive illness. The client's age, sex, and behavioral symptoms would suggest that the nurse assess this client's history with lithium carbonate, the drug of choice for manic-depressive illness.

Rationales for Other Answer Choices: A. Symptoms not typical of anxiety disorders. **B.** Symptoms not typical of psychotic disorders. **D.** Symptoms not typical of depressive disorders.
Nursing Process Phase: assessment; client need: psychosocial integrity; concern area: psychiatric nursing

19. **Correct Answer: A.** Cytoxan, an antineoplastic medication, can cause renal irritation and hemorrhagic cystitis. It is important to increase fluid intake to help prevent these complications. Encouraging parents to increase fluid intake as well as encouraging frequent emptying of the bladder throughout the day is important.

Rationales for Other Answer Choices: B. Monitoring of bowel movements is important with Vincristine but not with Cytoxan. **C.** Although the child will have increased susceptibility to infection, she should still be encouraged to have contact with healthy

children rather than decreasing contact with them.   **D.** Teaching parents ways to help manage self-consciousness about hair loss is important, but it is unrealistic to teach them that they can prevent it from occurring.
Nursing Process Phase: planning; client need: safe and effective care environment; concern area: pediatrics

20.   **Correct Answer: C.**   Vincristine is the drug that is most likely to cause neurological and neuromuscular side effects. Severe constipation, paralytic ileus (especially in children), and peripheral neuropathy are all of concern with vincristine. If these side effects cannot be managed, the child may have to be taken off the medication.

Rationales for Other Answer Choices: A. Not common side effects of Cytoxan. **B.** Not common side effects of prednisone.   **D.** Not common side effects of Mexate.
Nursing Process Phase: analysis; client need: safe and effective care environment; concern area: pediatrics

21.   **Correct Answer: D.**   The most important intervention during the period of greatest immunosuppression is to watch for subtle signs of infection, the number one cause of mortality in the immunosuppressed child.

Rationales for Other Answer Choices: A. Continuation of normalization is important, but if bone marrow suppression is great enough, the child may have to be put into reverse isolation.   **B.** Special precautions are taken with any invasive procedure to help prevent infection, but if the child needs to have blood components, they are administered.   **C.** Monitoring the administration of chemotherapy is an ongoing process and is not specific to the period of greatest immunosuppression.
Nursing Process Phase: implementation; client need: safe and effective care environment; concern area: medical/surgical

22.   **Correct Answer: B.**   It is preferred that Cytoxan be given in the morning. This will allow a full day to force fluids and increase the number of times the child voids, which will help prevent hemorrhagic cystitis.

Rationales for Other Answer Choices: A. Noon is too late in the day.   **C.** Bedtime is the worst time to give this medication.   **D.** Cytoxan should be given only with breakfast; lunch and supper are too late.
Nursing Process Phase: evaluation; client need: safe and effective care environment; concern area: medical/surgical

23.   **Correct Answer: B.**   Chemotherapy medications can cause renal irritation and hemorrhagic cystitis. It is important to increase fluid intake to help prevent these complications. Because the client has decreased PO intake, increasing IV rate will help get the required amount of fluid.

Rationales for Other Answer Choices: A. This is a common side effect of medication and is not a reason to withhold the medication.   **C.** The client should be allowed to gauge his own oral intake rather than forcing NPO status on him.   **D.** Forcing fluids with a child who has nausea and vomiting is not appropriate.

Nursing Process Phase: implementation; client need: safe and effective care environment; concern area: pediatrics

24. Correct Answer: A. Phenobarbital is used for its anticonvulsant effect in children with a history of febrile seizures. It helps to decrease the number and severity of the seizures.

Rationales for Other Answer Choices: B. Phenobarbital does not cure febrile seizures. Children usually outgrow this problem around 6 years of age. **C.** Although phenobarbital can be used to decrease anxiety, it is not used for this purpose with febrile seizures or with 6-month-old infants. **D.** Families do need to be taught to use antipyretics for elevated temperatures in children with a history of febrile convulsions; however, phenobarbital is not an antipyretic.
Nursing Process Phase: planning; client need: health promotion and maintenance; concern area: pediatrics

25. Correct Answer: C. Statement defines teratogen.

Rationales for Other Answer Choices: A. Teratogens by definition produce birth defects and are unsafe to use. **B.** Untrue statement—teratogens have no use for seizure disorders. **D.** Cause the most damage during the first trimester but may also affect the fetus in the second and third as well.
Nursing Process Phase: implementation; client need: health promotion and maintenance; concern area: obstetrics

26. Correct Answer: A. Safety of mebendazole (Vermox) in pregnancy has not been established, and therefore it is important to determine if the girl is pregnant or not before this medication is administered.

Rationales for Other Answer Choices: B. There is no known relationship between allergies to eggs and adverse reactions to mebendazole (Vermox). **C.** There is no known relationship between allergies to penicillin and adverse reactions to mebendazole (Vermox). **D.** Vermox can be given without regard to food. Food in GI tract reportedly does not affect drug action.
Nursing Process Phase: planning; client need: safe and effective care environment; concern area: medical/surgical

27. Correct Answer: A. It is recommended that the entire family be treated. Enterobiasis infestations are highly contagious, and reinfestation is common.

Rationales for Other Answer Choices: B. There is no known immunization to prevent the condition or immunity, which results from having contracted it. **C.** The dosage is 100 mg as a single dose, with a second course 3 weeks later if the pinworm infestation has not been eliminated. **D.** Good hand washing is recommended in the home. In the hospital setting, children are placed on enteric precautions. However, isolation from the other children is not necessary.
Nursing Process Phase: planning; client need: safe and effective care environment; concern area: medical/surgical

28. Correct Answer: A. Antacids and laxatives may alter the effectiveness of digoxin because of changes in electrolytes.

Rationales for Other Answer Choices: B. Hold rate is 60 BPM.   **C.** Client should increase intake of these to keep potassium at a normal level.   **D.** Client should never stop taking this medication without the physician's approval.
Nursing Process Phase: evaluation; client need: safe and effective care environment; concern area: medical/surgical

29. **Correct Answer: C.**   If the blood plasma volume increases, dilution of the RBCs will cause a decrease in hemoglobin and hematocrit.

Rationales for Other Answer Choices: A. Electrolyte levels (K⁻ and Na⁺) change with ritodrine use, which helps in the assessment of cardiac irritability and muscle contraction.   **B.** Serum glucose increases with ritodrine use but will not tell about plasma volumes.   **D.** Serum blood urea nitrogen (BUN) and creatinine are indicative of kidney function, not blood plasma levels.
Nursing Process Phase: assessment; client need: health promotion and maintenance; concern area: maternity nursing

30. **Correct Answer: D.**   Loss of the mucus plug does not indicate advanced labor.

Rationales for Other Answer Choices: A. If preterm labor is advanced (cervical dilation of 4 cm or greater), ritodrine will not be effective.   **B.** If a client has a temperature of 100.6°F, she needs to be further assessed for chorioamnionitis, pyelonephritis, or upper respiratory infection before using ritodrine because cardiovascular, respiratory, and kidney functions are affected by the drug. If chorioamnionitis is present, the fetuses have a greater chance of survival in the neonatal intensive care unit (ICU).   **C.** If preterm labor is advanced (amniotic membranes are ruptured), ritodrine will not be effective.
Nursing Process Phase: analysis; client need: health promotion and maintenance; concern area: maternity nursing

31. **Correct Answer: A.**   A respiratory rate below 12 is life-threatening, because the magnesium has affected the respiratory musculature and respiratory center in the brain.

Rationales for Other Answer Choices: B. Normal minimal urine output is 30 mL/h.   **C.** DTRs are expected to become normal or decreased.   **D.** A normal blood pressure would be a welcome sign.
Nursing Process Phase: assessment; client need: health promotion and maintenance; concern area: medical/surgical

32. **Correct Answer: D.**   This is an expected outcome.

Rationales for Other Answer Choices: A. Early indicators of magnesium toxicity also include sedation, confusion, profound thirst, muscle weakness, and diminished DTRs.   **B.** Respiratory rates under 12 are dangerous.   **C.** Because magnesium is excreted by the kidneys, toxicity can develop rapidly if renal function is impaired.
Nursing Process Phase: assessment; client need: health promotion and maintenance; concern area: maternity nursing

33. **Correct Answer: B.**   In order to take the added stress of contractions away, the Pitocin should be stopped first. By stopping Pitocin, if contractions are causing the uteroplacental insufficiency, the heart rate pattern should improve in about 5 minutes.

Rationales for Other Answer Choices: A. The client should be given oxygen by face mask at 7 to 10 L/min and the physician notified if all other measures fail. **C.** The second action, to correct any hypotension, is to turn the client to her left side. **D.** The third action is to increase the primary IV rate.

Nursing Process Phase: implementation; client need: health promotion and maintenance; concern area: maternity nursing

34. **Correct Answer: C.** In most parts of the United States either ritodrine or magnesium sulfate is the first-line drug of choice for preterm labor. If one does not work, the other may be tried.

Rationales for Other Answer Choices: A. Indomethacin is experimental at this time because it can cause persistent fetal circulation problems in the newborn. **B.** Demerol and Vistaril actually can potentiate contraction patterns, not stop them. **D.** Morphine sulfate may also potentiate preterm labor and cause respiratory depression in an already compromised newborn.

Nursing Process Phase: planning; client need: health promotion and maintenance; concern area: maternity nursing

35. **Correct Answer: C.** IV Pitocin is usually diluted 10 U Pitocin in 1000 mL. 1.0 U/min equals 6 mL/h so that it is easy to regulate dosage in small increments. It is increased every 30 minutes until contractions are 2 to 3 minutes apart and lasting 40 to 60 seconds.

Rationales for Other Answer Choices: A, B, and **D** are not standard mixtures.

Nursing Process Phase: implementation; client need: health promotion and maintenance; concern area: maternity nursing

36. **Correct Answer: D.** Calcium is lost along with sodium and potassium through the renal system. Tetany is one of the primary symptoms of low calcium levels.

Rationales for Other Answer Choices: A. Low sodium levels may produce disorientation, weakness, syncope. **B.** Low potassium levels lead to cardiac dysrhythmias. **C.** Low magnesium levels produce few symptoms.

Nursing Process Phase: assessment; client need: safe and effective care environment; concern area: medical/surgical

37. **Correct Answer: D.** Calan (Verapamil) inhibits the influx of calcium into the myocardium, resulting in decreased myocardial excitation and contraction and a small decrease in heart rate. Metoprolol tartrate (Lopressor) blocks beta-adrenergic receptors, which in turn depress myocardial automaticity and heart rate. Therefore, use of beta-blockers with calcium channel blockers enhances the cardiodepressant (negative inotropic and chronotropic) effects.

Rationales for Other Answer Choices: A, B, and **C** are not expected effects.

Nursing Process Phase: planning; client need: safe and effective care environment; concern area: medical/surgical

38. **Correct Answer: C.** Tocainide suppresses ventricular ectopy by decreasing automaticity and excitability in the His-Purkinje fibers, which are located within the ventricles.

Rationales for Other Answer Choices: A. S-A node not affected by this medication. **B.** A-V node not affected by this medication. **D.** Bundle of His included in answer **C.**
Nursing Process Phase: planning; client need: safe and effective care environment; concern area: medical/surgical

39. **Correct Answer: C.** Potassium chloride should be diluted with appropriate intravenous solution (usually dextrose) and administered via slow IV infusion. In order to prevent life-threatening hypokalemia and risk of vascular irritation, never give an intravenous infusion greater than 40 mEq/L in 100 mL.

Rationales for Other Answer Choices: A. Never give potassium chloride IV push. **B.** Never give potassium chloride in concentrated amounts by any other route. **D.** Never give potassium chloride IM.
Nursing Process Phase: planning; client need: safe and effective care environment; concern area: medical/surgical

40. **Correct Answer: D.** The respiratory centers in the CNS are directly stimulated by elevated salicylate (aspirin) levels, increasing the respiratory rate.

Rationales for Other Answer Choices: A. These symptoms are not commonly associated with high salicylate levels. **B.** These are symptoms of allergic reaction to salicylates. **C.** These are side effects of salicylates.
Nursing Process Phase: assessment; client need: safe and effective care environment; concern area: medical/surgical

41. **Correct Answer: D.** Allopurinol is used for long-term management of gout, and the client should continue medical supervision to monitor for side effects and effectiveness of the medication.

Rationales for Other Answer Choices: A. True statement, although not necessarily related to the medication. **B.** Adequate fluid intake helps rid the body of uric acid and prevents gout attacks. **C.** This is good practice for any client on a medication.
Nursing Process Phase: evaluation; client need: safe and effective care environment; concern area: medical/surgical

42. **Correct Answer: B.** Antacids decrease absorption of ranitidine when taken at the same time—should be taken at least 1 hour apart.

Rationales for Other Answer Choices: A. Antacids decrease the effectiveness. **C.** Antacids generally are not taken with meals. **D.** It is more likely that the antacid will cause diarrhea; never stop taking medications without physician's approval.
Nursing Process Phase: implementation; client need: safe and effective care environment; concern area: medical/surgical

43. **Correct Answer: A.** Silver sulfadiazine (Silvadene) should be applied, using sterile technique, to burn areas after debridement to prevent infection. It should be reapplied to areas where it has been wiped off. Burned areas are generally kept covered with medication at all times.

Rationales for Other Answer Choices: B. This would allow the burn wounds to be exposed for too long a time, increasing the risk of infection. **C.** Sterile technique must be used to prevent infection. **D.** Sterile technique must be used.

Nursing Process Phase: implementation; client need: safe and effective care environment; concern area: medical/surgical

44. **Correct Answer: D.** $\dfrac{\text{amount to infuse (mL)}}{\text{time to infuse (h)}} = \dfrac{50}{0.25} = 200 \text{ mL/h}$

Rationales for Other Answer Choices: A. Incorrect calculation. **B.** Incorrect calculation. **C.** Incorrect calculation.
Nursing Process Phase: planning; client need: safe and effective care environment; concern area: medical/surgical

45. **Correct Answer: A.** As with many antidepressants, it takes 3 to 4 weeks to achieve a therapeutic blood level.

Rationales for Other Answer Choices: B. Blood levels should be achieved before this time. **C.** There are no therapeutic effects in this short a time. **D.** Time is much too short.
Nursing Process Phase: planning; client need: psychosocial integrity; concern area: psychiatric nursing

46. **Correct Answer: B.** Amitriptyline hydrochloride (Elavil) has sedative and anticholinergic properties (blurred vision, dry mouth, constipation, confusion, and orthostatic hypotension). Nursing interventions to prevent falling or injury are important, especially with initial drug therapy, until the client adapts to the side effects.

Rationales for Other Answer Choices: A. This nursing action is not necessary if the client is instructed to put on the call light when she needs to void. **C.** This nursing action is not necessary. **D.** Client safety needs to be monitored, but she does not need bed rest.
Nursing Process Phase: implementation; client need: safe and effective care environment; concern area: psychiatric nursing

47. **Correct Answer: A.** Alopecia (loss of hair) generally occurs in about 70% of the clients who receive vincristine sulfate (Oncovin). It is a reversible adverse effect, and regrowth of hair may begin prior to the end of treatment.

Rationales for Other Answer Choices: B. Hirsutism is a side effect of corticosteroids. **C.** Irritability is not associated with this medication. **D.** Gingivitis is not associated with this medication.
Nursing Process Phase: analysis; client need: safe and effective care environment; concern area: medical/surgical

48. **Correct Answer: D.** Improvements in symptoms may not occur until 2 to 3 days after oral administration of drug is begun, and the effects of the drug may continue after it is stopped (6–10 hours).

Rationales for Other Answer Choices: A. Suppression of tremors starts sooner than this. **B.** Suppression of tremors starts sooner than this. **C.** It is too early to see any effects.
Nursing Process Phase: planning; client need: safe and effective care environment; concern area: psychiatric nursing

49. Correct Answer: B. Acetylcysteine (Mucomyst) is the antidote for acetaminophen poisoning. It neutralizes the hepatotoxic metabolism of acetaminophen.

Rationales for Other Answer Choices: A. Albumin is used to expand vascular volume in shock. **C.** Acyclovir is an antiviral drug used in herpes infections. **D.** Narcan is used for narcotic overdose.
Nursing Process Phase: planning; client need: safe and effective care environment; concern area: medical/surgical

50. Correct Answer: C. Need more information concerning the severity of the constipation and alternative methods to treat it.

Rationales for Other Answer Choices: A. Produces stimulation of sensory nerve endings in the linings of the intestinal mucosa and is used for severe constipation. **B.** Increases the fluid content and bulk of the stool and is used for minor constipation. **D.** Need to determine which would be most appropriate based on client condition.
Nursing Process Phase: implementation; client need: safe and effective care environment; concern area: medical/surgical

1. Upon admission, the nurse notes that the client is allergic to diazepam (Valium). The physician has ordered clonazepam (Klonopin) 1.5 mg PO tid for this client. The best action by the nurse is:
   A. Give the medication as ordered.
   B. Hold the medication, and notify the physician.
   C. Give the medication, but monitor the client closely for allergic reactions for 4 hours.
   D. Give a trial dose of 0.75 mg, and monitor for effect.

2. Which of the following facts should the nurse include in the discharge teaching about the mode of action of surfactant laxatives?
   A. These medications increase the bulk of the stool and promote bowel movements.
   B. This type of laxative draws water into the stool to soften it.
   C. You should avoid taking this medication if you have a bowel obstruction.
   D. These laxatives reduce the surface tension of the stool, allowing water to enter and soften it.

3. A client has been started on a sustained-release amphetamine. In planning care for this client, the nurse recognizes that the best time to administer sustained-release amphetamines is:
   A. In the evening only
   B. In the midafternoon
   C. With meals
   D. At least 10 hours before bedtime

4. In planning care for a client with schizophrenia, the nurse recognizes that all antipsychotic drugs are derivatives of phenothiazine. Most importantly, they differ from each other in:
   A. Degree of sedation manifested
   B. Potential to cause tardive dyskinesia
   C. Potency and side effect
   D. Method of administration

5. Before administering a phenothiazine to a client, the nurse notes that the choice of drug for treatment is based upon:
   A. Client response to psychotherapy
   B. Capacity to decrease psychotic symptoms with a minimum of side effects
   C. Capacity to decrease target symptoms regardless of side effects
   D. Degree of side effects caused by treatment

287

6. Which of the following factors is the most important for the nurse to include in the discharge instructions for a client who has been prescribed a bulk-forming laxative?
A. Increase your fluid intake to 2 to 3 liters per day.
B. Take supplemental fat-soluble vitamins to maintain nutritional status.
C. You can expect diarrhea after 24 hours.
D. Avoid eating dairy products while taking this medication.

7. Sometimes when clients begin to feel better as they leave a treatment institution, they stop taking their neuroleptic medication. Severe symptoms develop, and the client must reenter the hospital. The name of this syndrome is:
A. The therapeutic-window syndrome
B. The closed-door syndrome
C. The merry-go-round syndrome
D. The on-off syndrome

8. A female client is to take chlorpromazine (Thorazine) at home for her psychotic condition. In planning her discharge, the nurse should explain to the client and her significant other that the medication may turn the:
A. Stools black
B. Stools white
C. Urine reddish-brown
D. Urine greenish

9. If a client were receiving phenytoin (Dilantin) for seizures and the doctor ordered chlorpromazine (Thorazine) as a neuroleptic drug, you would expect the doctor to:
A. Monitor serum levels of phenytoin
B. Decrease the dosage of phenytoin
C. Monitor serum levels of Thorazine
D. Taper the client off phenytoin

10. A client who is being started on chlorpromazine asks the nurse, "Why do I need to take this medication?" The best explanation by the nurse is:
A. "This medication is to help you organize your thoughts."
B. "This medication is to keep you from having nightmares."
C. "This medication will help you to sleep."
D. "This medication will help you to stop shaking."

11. Butyrophenones, phenothiazines, dihydroidolones, and thioxanthenes belong to the group of drugs called:
A. Anxiolytics
B. Antidepressants
C. Anticholinergics
D. Antipsychotics

12. In planning care for a client who is taking chlorpromazine (Thorazine), the nurse recognizes that it is important to notify the doctor and document signs and symptoms of tardive dyskinesia because:
A. Tardive dyskinesia is always reversible
B. Tardive dyskinesia is potentially irreversible
C. The doctor may increase the neuroleptic
D. The doctor will order an antidepressant

13. A 55-year-old female client who had been taking haloperidol (Haldol Decanoate) 100 mg for 3 years discontinues the medication on her own. During the admission interview, the nurse notes that the client is blinking her eyes continuously, periodically her tongue protrudes, and she drools. The nurse recognizes this syndrome as:
    A. Neuroleptic-induced catatonia
    B. Tardive dyskinesia
    C. Dystonia
    D. Akathisia

14. To control and/or prevent extrapyramidal signs and symptoms while a client is taking fluphenazine (Prolixin) 0.5 mg qid, it would be important for the nurse to administer:
    A. levodopa (Dopar) 0.5 mg qid
    B. diazepam (Valium) 5 mg qid
    C. methocarbamol (Robaxin) 1 g qid
    D. benztropine (Cogentin) 2 mg qid

15. Which of the following medications exerts its antiemetic effect by stimulating the motility of the upper gastrointestinal (GI) tract?
    A. dimenhydrinate (Dramamine)
    B. metoclopramide (Reglan)
    C. prochlorperazine (Compazine)
    D. trimethobenzamine (Tigan)

16. While assessing a 31-year-old male client who is taking haloperidol (Haldol) for hallucinations, the nurse observes that he suddenly becomes diaphoretic, extremely rigid, and is unable to speak. His blood pressure was 100/60 one half hour ago, but now it is 150/70; temperature, 101.2°F; pulse, 126; respiration, 32. All of the following medications are ordered prn:

    acetaminophen (Tylenol) tab ii for temperature greater than 101°F.
    bromocriptine (Parlodel 7.5) mg PO
    methocarbamol (Robaxin) 2 mg IM
    Notify the physician

    What would be the best nursing action at this time?
    A. Give Tylenol tab ii and encourage fluids.
    B. Give Robaxin 2 mg IM and notify the physician.
    C. Give Tylenol tab ii, Robaxin 2 mg, and notify the physician.
    D. Hold the Haldol, give Parlodel 7.5 mg, and notify the physician.

17. A pediatric client who receives gentamicin (Garamycin) 50 mg IVPB q 6 hours at 10 A.M., 4 P.M., 10 P.M., and 4 A.M. is to have a peak and trough drawn. At what time should the nurse instruct the laboratory to draw the trough level?
    A. 10:45 A.M.
    B. 12 noon
    C. 9:30 A.M.
    D. 5:00 A.M.

18. A client who has been taking haloperidol (Haldol) for a week has begun to tremble. The nurse would know that this is a sign of:
    A. Dystonia
    B. Dyskinesia
    C. Parkinsonism
    D. Akathisia

19. A major disadvantage of antipsychotic or neuroleptic drugs is the incidence of side effects. One of the categories of side effects is that of extrapyramidal reactions. Included as extrapyramidal reactions are:
    A. Dystonia and dystrophic muscular weakness
    B. Parkinsonism and akinesia
    C. Dystonia and tardive dyskinesia
    D. Parkinsonism and tardive dyskinesia

20. A client asks the nurse, "Why am I getting haloperidol decanoate or depot injections instead of my oral medication?" The best answer by the nurse is:
    A. "You are getting these injections because they have a longer half-life."
    B. "You are getting these injections because they are more slowly absorbed."
    C. "You are getting these injections because they are less irritating to the tissues."
    D. "You are getting these injections because they increase compliance with the medication regimen."

21. The best method for a home health nurse to administer a monthly dose of haloperidol decanoate 150 mg IM to a home-care psychotic client is to use a:
    A. 1-in., 20-gauge needle and administer deep IM in the gluteal
    B. 1-in., 25-gauge needle and administer IM in the deltoid
    C. 2-in., 21-gauge needle and administer deep IM in the gluteal
    D. 1-in., 21-gauge needle and administer IM in the deltoid

22. After 2 weeks of treatment with haloperidol (Haldol) 5 mg PO bid, a hospitalized 41-year-old male client continues to scratch himself and insists that he hears voices. The physician increases the Haldol to 5 mg tid either PO or IM. The nurse's rationale for giving this client his Haldol IM instead of PO would be:
    A. He will not swallow pills.
    B. He will not take any PO medications.
    C. The medication works faster if given IM.
    D. He continues to hallucinate.

23. A client who hears voices that tell him to hurt himself refuses to swallow his haloperidol (Haldol) 5 mg pills. The physician then orders the Haldol concentrate, which the nurse will give:
    A. By deep IM injection into a large muscle
    B. Orally undiluted
    C. Diluted in coffee or tea
    D. Diluted in apple or orange juice

24. In preparing a care plan for a client with schizophrenia who is to be started on fluphenazine decanote (Prolixin), the nurse recognizes that the medication's mode of action is to:
    A. Increase the release of norepinephrine and serotonin available for binding sites
    B. Block dopamine receptors in the brain and alter dopamine release and turnover
    C. Prevent the reuptake of norepinephrine and serotonin by presynaptic neurons
    D. Stimulate dopamine receptors

25. A nine-year-old girl is being treated with trimethoprim-sulfamethoxazole (Bactrim) for urinary tract infection. While the child is on this medication, the nurse should monitor her:
    A. Intake and output
    B. Serum creatinine
    C. Hearing ability
    D. Liver enzymes

26. In which of the following situations would the use of terbutaline be contraindicated?
    A. Transfer of a high-risk labor client to a tertiary facility
    B. Temporary cessation of contractions during fetal distress
    C. Use as tocolytic therapy in preterm labor
    D. Prevention of postpartum hemorrhage caused by subinvolution

27. A pregnant client who is gravida 3, para 2 is admitted with severe pregnancy-induced hypertension. Her physician wants to start IV magnesium sulfate at 2 g/h. What are the initial side effects the nurse should explain to the client?
    A. Hypotension, decreased respirations
    B. Hypoflexia and flaccid paralysis
    C. Flushing, sweating, irritability
    D. Vomiting and diarrhea

28. A client with intestinal cancer is started on total parenteral nutrition (TPN) at 25 mL/h for the first 12 hours. The nurse understands that this rate was selected because it:
    A. Helps prevent catheter site infections
    B. Reverses the negative nitrogen balance the client has because of his cancer
    C. Allows the client's body to adjust to the increased glucose levels
    D. Reverses fluid volume deficit caused by low oral intake of fluids

29. In order to keep a client at 27 weeks' gestation with ruptured membranes from having contractions while betamethasone (Celestone) is being administered, the physician orders IV ritodrine. The nurse should monitor the client for which of the following side effects during administration?
    A. Maternal bradycardia
    B. Drowsiness
    C. Increased urinary output
    D. Cardiac arrhythmias

30. A client who is at 27 weeks gestation with spontaneously ruptured membranes and no contractions is admitted to the preterm labor unit. Which of the following medications will the nurse most likely administer to promote fetal lung maturation?
    A. betamethasone
    B. prostaglandin E_2
    C. magnesium sulfate
    D. ritodrine

31. A postpartum client who has 40 U of oxytocin (Pitocin) in her IV bag after the placenta is delivered continues to hemorrhage even after uterine massage. Her vital signs are pulse, 120; BP, 90/50; respirations, 26. The nurse anticipates the physician will order which of the following to stop the atony and hemorrhage?
    A. ibuprofen
    B. prostaglandin $F_{2\alpha}$
    C. ephedrine
    D. Methergine

32. A client who has delivered after a 14-hour labor has oxytocin (Pitocin) added to the IV bottle to help:
    A. Prevent uterine atony and hemorrhage
    B. Decrease milk let-down
    C. Prolong uterine involution
    D. Relieve pain

33. A pregnant client's contractions are firm, lasting 90 seconds, and are 1 to 2 minutes apart. While the IV oxytocin (Pitocin) is infusing at 10 μg/min, the fetal heart rate begins to lose beat-to-beat variability. What would be the most appropriate action by the nurse?
    A. Leave the Pitocin at 10 μg/min, and turn the client on her left side.
    B. Discontinue the Pitocin.
    C. Decrease the Pitocin to 5 μg/min.
    D. Increase the Pitocin to 15 μg/min in order to shorten the labor and decrease the time of fetal distress.

34. In planning care for a 32-year-old gravida 1, para 0 client who is at 42 weeks gestation and is admitted for induction of labor, the nurse should include what important information about oxytocin (Pitocin) prior to its administration IV?
    A. IV Pitocin will lower blood pressure.
    B. IV Pitocin is diluted and given as a piggyback.
    C. IV Pitocin has a long half-life.
    D. IV Pitocin is a natural diuretic.

35. Which of the following side effects should the nurse warn a client about in the home use of timolol maleate (Timoptic)?
    A. Tachycardia, tachypnea
    B. Electrolyte imbalances, dysrhythmia
    C. Abdominal discomfort, bradycardia
    D. CNS stimulation, insomnia

36. Which of the following would be most important to teach a pregnant client who has recently been diagnosed with gestational diabetes about the side effects of insulin?
    A. Hypoglycemic reactions have a gradual onset.
    B. Symptoms of hyperglycemic reactions include tremors and cool, moist skin.
    C. Hypoglycemic reactions are caused by too much insulin.
    D. Hyperglycemic symptoms appear suddenly.

37. When a client fails to begin labor after 34 weeks pregnancy, the physician plans to induce labor. The nurse prepares:
    A. A SC dose of methylergonovine (Methergine)
    B. IM ergovine (Ergotrate)
    C. An IV infusion of ritodrine (Yutopar)
    D. An IV infusion of oxytocin (Pitocin)

38. Which of the following statements by a client with a gastric ulcer would indicate to the nurse that additional information on antacid preparations to be taken at home is required?
    A. "Antacid tablets should be thoroughly chewed."
    B. "Liquid antacids are generally less effective than tablets."
    C. "Antacids do not alter gastric acid secretion."
    D. "Do not take antacids with other drugs unless specifically instructed to do so."

39. A client who is approximately 160 pounds overweight is started on amphetamine (Dexedrine) for weight loss. The nurse should instruct the client:
    A. "Take the medication just before bedtime for best results."
    B. "The use of this medication for obesity is recommended for 2 weeks."
    C. "There will be very few side effects from short-term use."
    D. "Take 50 mg twice a day."

40. When reviewing the product information available on a medication, the nurse finds that it is *teratogenic.* The nurse would know that this medication should not be administered to a(n):
    A. Asthmatic client
    B. Pregnant client
    C. Child
    D. Client with renal failure

41. A client is being monitored in the cardiac care unit following a myocardial infarction (MI) when he suddenly develops ventricular fibrillation (VF). In this emergency situation, the nurse should prepare to administer which antiarrhythmic drug?
    A. osmolal (Brevibloc)
    B. procainamide (Pronestyl)
    C. lidocaine (Xylocaine)
    D. verapamil (Calan)

42. Which of the following would best indicate to the nurse that the dose of lithium ordered for a newly diagnosed 22-year-old male client with bipolar disorder is appropriate?
    A. Appropriate behavior response
    B. Absence of side effects
    C. Development of slight weight gain
    D. Serum blood levels

43. When caring for a hospitalized client receiving lithium therapy, the nurse would be most concerned about lithium toxicity if the client developed:
    A. Renal failure
    B. Thrombophlebitis
    C. Liver dysfunction
    D. Anemia

44. The husband of a client who has been taking the tricyclic antidepressant drug imipramine (Trofanil) for 3 days asks the nurse why his wife shows no signs of improvement. The best response by the nurse is:
    A. "The dose is probably too low and will be increased gradually until the desired response is seen."
    B. "Since your wife has not responded after 3 days, she will most likely not get significant relief symptoms from this drug, and another drug will probably be tried."
    C. "It usually takes 2 to 4 weeks to notice any improvement in behavior."
    D. "It's difficult to assess the level of depression; only your wife knows for sure if the medication is working at this early stage of therapy."

45. A client in a psychiatric clinic who is taking antipsychotic medications complains of dry mouth and constipation. The nurse knows that these side effects are referred to as:
    A. Cholinergic side effects
    B. Anticholinergic side effects
    C. Extrapyramidal side effects
    D. Hepatobiliary dysfunction

46. Upon admission, the nurse notes that the client's physician has just ordered chlorpromazine (Thorazine). The nurse would know that the major use of chlorpromazine is to:
    A. Decrease gastric acid secretion
    B. Manage primary hypertension
    C. Reduce tissue inflammation
    D. Manage psychiatric disorders

47. A 12-year-old boy is admitted to a surgical unit with possible appendicitis. When taking the child's medication history, the nurse notes that he has been taking phenobarbital (Luminal) 40 mg tid. The nurse would suspect that this child most likely has:
    A. An eating disorder
    B. A seizure disorder
    C. Cystic fibrosis
    D. Attention deficit disorder (ADD)

48. An unconscious client with a head injury is to receive phenytoin (Dilantin) IV for seizure activity. While administering the loading dose of medication, the nurse would monitor the client for:
    A. Hypotension
    B. Apnea
    C. Tachycardia
    D. Anuria

49. The nurse is caring for a client who develops a rapid heart rate. The medication the physician will most likely use to slow the heart rate will be:
    A. phentolamine (Regitine)
    B. propranolol (Inderal)
    C. cimetidine (Tagamet)
    D. dopamine (Intropin)

50. Which of the following would the nurse expect to observe in a client who had just received a treatment with acetylcysteine (Mucomyst)?
    A. Increased cough effort
    B. Suppressed cough reflex
    C. Thick, tenacious sputum
    D. Decreased viscosity of sputum

ANSWERS/RATIONALES

1. **Correct Answer: B.** Klonopin should not be taken if the client is allergic to other benzodiazepines such as Valium.

Rationales for Other Answer Choices: A. May cause an allergic reaction—there are often cross-allergies among benzodiazepines. **C.** Should not be given. **D.** It is illegal to give trial doses without an order.
Nursing Process Phase: implementation; client need: safe and effective care environment; concern area: psychiatric nursing

2. **Correct Answer: D.** Surfactant is a substance that reduces surface tension, allowing water to penetrate.

Rationales for Other Answer Choices: A. Mode of action (MOA) of bulk laxatives, like psyllium. **B.** MOA of disaccarhide laxatives, like lactulose. **C.** True statement but does not answer the question.
Nursing Process Phase: planning; client need: physiological integrity; concern area: medical/surgical

3. **Correct Answer: D.** An amphetamine is a stimulant and may interfere with sleep, so it should be given early in the day.

Rationales for Other Answer Choices: A. Given late in the day will interfere with sleep. **B.** May be too late. **C.** Only with breakfast or lunch, not supper.
Nursing Process Phase: planning; client need: safe and effective care environment; concern area: psychiatric nursing

4. **Correct Answer: C.** Phenothiazines are similar to chlorpromazine, the prototype, but differ from it in potency and degree of side effects.

Rationales for Other Answer Choices: A. Sedation is related to some degree to potency. **B.** All tend to produce this side effect over time. **D.** Most can be given PO or IM, and sometimes IV.
Nursing Process Phase: planning; client need: psychosocial integrity; concern area: psychiatric nursing

5. **Correct Answer: B.** Since all phenothiazines are similar, choice is based on client response to drugs that decrease psychotic (or target) symptoms with the fewest side effects.

Rationales for Other Answer Choices: A. Psychotherapy is dependent on client response to medication. **C.** Side effects always need to be considered. **D.** Need to consider the effect on the symptoms.
Nursing Process Phase: analysis; client need: psychosocial integrity; concern area: psychiatric nursing

6. **Correct Answer: A.** The client should take the medicine with a full glass of liquid and increase daily liquid intake to prevent bowel obstruction.

Rationales for Other Answer Choices: B. Nutritional status not affected by these medications. **C.** They are slow acting (24–72 hours) and mild, so they should not produce diarrhea if taken as directed. **D.** Dairy products have no effect on these medications.
Nursing Process Phase: planning; client need: physiological integrity; concern area: medical/surgical

   7. **Correct Answer: C.** Most psychotic illnesses recur, unless clients continue to take their medicines over a long period of time.

Rationales for Other Answer Choices: A. No such syndrome. **B.** No such syndrome. **D.** Occurs in Parkinson's syndrome clients taking dopamine-enhancing medications.
Nursing Process Phase: assessment; client need: psychosocial integrity; concern area: psychiatric nursing

   8. **Correct Answer: C.** Although it may turn the urine pink to reddish-brown, this is not harmful.

Rationales for Other Answer Choices: A, B, and **D** are not side effects of this medication.
Nursing Process Phase: planning; client need: health promotion and maintenance; concern area: psychiatric nursing

   9. **Correct Answer: A.** Thorazine inhibits phenytoin metabolism, so it could cause phenytoin toxicity. Also, phenothiazine medications lower the seizure potential in clients.

Rationales for Other Answer Choices: B. May need to increase the dosage to prevent seizures. **C.** Not affected by phenytoin. **D.** This action would increase the number and severity of seizures.
Nursing Process Phase: planning; client need: safe and effective care environment; concern area: medical/surgical

10. **Correct Answer: A.** Antipsychotics are used in the treatment of acute and chronic psychoses, particularly when accompanied by increased psychomotor activity.

Rationales for Other Answer Choices: B. Are not used to decrease nightmares. **C.** May indirectly help with sleep, but not the primary use. **D.** May actually increase shaking with long-term use.
Nursing Process Phase: implementation; client need: safe and effective care environment; concern area: psychiatric nursing

11. **Correct Answer: D.** All of these are neuroleptic drugs used to treat psychotic conditions.

Rationales for Other Answer Choices: A. Antianxiety medications reduce anxiety. **B.** Used to treat depression. **C.** Used for a variety of reasons, such as control of Parkinson's symptoms, bradycardia, neurotoxin poisoning, and so forth.
Nursing Process Phase: analysis; client need: safe and effective care environment; concern area: psychiatric nursing

12. **Correct Answer: B.** Early intervention to eliminate the drug at the first signs of tardive dyskinesia may cause the symptoms to remit if the medication is discontinued.

Rationales for Other Answer Choices: **A.** Is not reversible.   **C.** Will make the condition worse.   **D.** Does not affect the condition.
Nursing Process Phase: planning; client need: psychosocial integrity; concern area: psychiatric nursing

13. **Correct Answer: B.**   Tardive dyskinesia is characterized by involuntary movements. If tardive dyskinesia is suspected, notify the doctor at once. Movements may interfere with swallowing, breathing, gait, and may result in falls.

Rationales for Other Answer Choices: **A.** Involves a type of paralysis.   **C.** Dystonia is marked by severe muscle spasms of the face, jaw, tongue, or back. Needs immediate intervention.   **D.** Akathisia is a type of motor restlessness in which the client cannot sit or stand still.
Nursing Process Phase: analysis; client need: safe and effective care environment; concern area: psychiatric nursing

14. **Correct Answer: D.**   Cogentin is an anti-Parkinsonism drug used to help prevent extrapyramidal signs and symptoms.

Rationales for Other Answer Choices: **A.** Levodopa (which restores dopamine levels) is not used for pseudoparkinsonism. It is used in idiopathic Parkinsonism.   **B.** Valium is an anxiolytic used for anxiety.   **C.** Robaxin is a muscle relaxant.
Nursing Process Phase: implementation; client need: safe and effective care environment; concern area: psychiatric nursing

15. **Correct Answer: B.**   Reglan increases the motility of the upper gastrointestinal (GI) system and blocks dopamine in the chemoreceptor trigger zone (CTZ).

Rationales for Other Answer Choices: **A.** This medication is an antihistamine antiemetic.   **C.** This medication is a phenothiazine antiemetic.   **D.** Antihistamine antiemetic.
Nursing Process Phase: planning; client need: safe and effective care environment; concern area: medical/surgical

16. **Correct Answer: D.**   The signs and symptoms are of neuroleptic malignant syndrome. It can be reversed if there is early intervention, but it is potentially fatal. Supportive treatment is necessary, but emergency treatment is a dopamine antagonist and a muscle relaxant.

Rationales for Other Answer Choices: **A.** The fever is of secondary importance at this time.   **B.** Robaxin is not a drug of choice; the neuroleptic must be stopped immediately.   **C.** Combines **A** and **B**.
Nursing Process Phase: implementation; client need: safe and effective care environment; concern area: psychiatric nursing

17. **Correct Answer: C.**   The trough level is the minimum level and usually occurs just prior to the next dose of medication.

Rationales for Other Answer Choices: **A.** This would be a good time to draw the peak.   **B.** Would not be a good time for either—it is in the middle of the time span.   **D.** Would not be a good time for either—it is in the middle of the time again.
Nursing Process Phase: planning; client need: safe and effective care environment; concern area: pediatrics

18. **Correct Answer: C.** Pseudo-Parkinsonism usually develops after about 5 days of treatment.

Rationales for Other Answer Choices: A. Takes several weeks for this to develop. **B.** Not the symptoms associated with this disorder. **D.** Not the symptoms associated with this condition.
Nursing Process Phase: analysis; client need: safe and effective care environment; concern area: psychiatric nursing

19. **Correct Answer: B.** Extrapyramidal reactions include Parkinsonism, dystonia, dyskinesia, and akathisia.

Rationales for Other Answer Choices: A. Dystrophic muscular weakness is not a symptom. **C.** Tardive dyskinesia is not a symptom. **D.** Tardive dyskinesia is not a symptom.
Nursing Process Phase: assessment; client need: safe and effective care environment; concern area: psychiatric nursing

20. **Correct Answer: D.** "Depot" means deposit or storage, so a depot drug is one that is injected for slow absorption. Although decanoate or deposit medications have longer half-lives and are more slowly absorbed than their short-acting counterpart IM medications, the rationale for giving them is to increase compliance in the taking of medications.

Rationales for Other Answer Choices: A. True, but not the rationale. **B.** True, but not the rationale. **C.** Untrue statement.
Nursing Process Phase: implementation; client need: psychosocial integrity; concern area: psychiatric nursing

21. **Correct Answer: C.** Haldol is very irritating and must be given deep IM, which is best accomplished with a 2-inch, 21-gauge needle and given into a muscle larger than the deltoid.

Rationales for Other Answer Choices: A. Needle is too short. **B.** Needle too short; deltoid not appropriate. **D.** Needle too short; deltoid not appropriate.
Nursing Process Phase: implementation; client need: health promotion and maintenance; concern area: psychiatric nursing

22. **Correct Answer: B.** Haldol IM is reserved for clients who are uncooperative with PO medication regimen, need long-acting decanoate, or are severely agitated.

Rationales for Other Answer Choices: A. Haldol may be taken as a liquid concentrate if pills cannot be swallowed. **C.** Although IM administration is quicker, there is no reason in this case to hurry. **D.** Hallucination is a target symptom and does not necessitate immediate response by giving IM injection.
Nursing Process Phase: planning; client need: safe and effective care environment; concern area: psychiatric nursing

23. **Correct Answer: D.** *Concentrate* refers to oral liquid preparation. It has a very unpleasant taste and is irritating to the gastric mucosa, so it is best diluted in orange juice or apple juice and followed by a glass of water.

Rationales for Other Answer Choices: A. IM injection is for Haldol Decanoate. **B.** Taste is too unpleasant to be taken this way. **C.** Haldol liquid forms a precipitant when mixed with coffee or tea.
Nursing Process Phase: implementation; client need: safe and effective care environment; concern area: psychiatric nursing

24. **Correct Answer: B.** Antipsychotic medications block receptor sites for the neurotransmitter dopamine in the brain and have a peripheral anticholinergic and alpha-adrenergic blockade effect.

Rationales for Other Answer Choices: A. Serotonin-enhancing antidepressants act by increasing the release of norephinephrine and serotonin. **C.** Tricyclic antidepressants act by preventing the reuptake of norepinephrine and serotonin. **D.** Dopamine stimulates dopamine receptors in the renal beds and mesentery.
Nursing Process Phase: planning; client need: safe and effective care environment; concern area: psychiatric nursing

25. **Correct Answer: A.** Because of the possibility of renal calculi formation and the need for increased fluid intake, children on this drug should have intake and output (I & O) monitored.

Rationales for Other Answer Choices: B. Renal compromise is more of a problem with the elderly than with children on this drug. **C.** Altered hearing is not a problem with children on this drug; it is a problem with children on aminoglycosides. **D.** Liver compromise is more often a problem with the elderly than with children on this drug.
Nursing Process Phase: assessment; client need: safe and effective care environment; concern area: pediatrics

26. **Correct Answer: D.** To stop postpartum bleeding, a medication that increases the contractions of the uterus is needed.

Rationales for Other Answer Choices: A, B, and **C.** Terbutaline is ideal for short-term tocolysis in all three situations. Knowledge of the drug of choice in critical situations is paramount for the nurse and eliminates wasted time in a situation in which time is crucial.
Nursing Process Phase: planning; client need: health promotion and maintenance; concern area: maternity nursing

27. **Correct Answer: C.** It is common for clients to experience flushes, sweating, and irritability initially with the bolus.

Rationales for Other Answer Choices: A. Hypotension and decreased respirations are symptoms of magnesium sulfate overdose. **B.** Hypoflexia and flaccid paralysis are symptoms of magnesium sulfate overdose. **D.** Diarrhea and vomiting are associated with oral use.
Nursing Process Phase: planning; client need: health promotion and maintenance; concern area: maternity nursing

28. **Correct Answer: C.** The high glucose content of total parenteral nutrition (TPN) can cause hyperglycemia if started at too great a rate initially.

Rationales for Other Answer Choices: A. Catheter-site infections are best prevented by good aseptic technique. **B.** The negative nitrogen balance is reversed with higher rates of TPN. **D.** The rate will need to be higher to affect fluid volume deficit.

Nursing Process Phase: planning; client need: safe and effective care environment; concern area: medical/surgical

29. **Correct Answer: D.** Ritodrine causes many side effects, including tremors, cardiac arrhythmias, nervousness, tachycardia, pulmonary edema, and chest pain.

Rationales for Other Answer Choices: A. Causes tachycardia. **B.** Because of the increased restlessness, patients are unable to sleep or doze. **C.** Hourly I & O is required because of decreased urine output and glycosuria.
Nursing Process Phase: assessment; client need: health promotion and maintenance; concern area: maternity nursing

30. **Correct Answer: A.** Betamethasone is used in two doses to help fetal lung maturity for 26- to 32-weeks'-gestation fetuses. These doses are given 24 hours apart, so labor must be delayed for this medication to work.

Rationales for Other Answer Choices: B. Prostaglandin E_2 is used to induce labor in second and third trimesters. **C.** Magnesium sulfate is used to stop labor. **D.** Ritodrine is used to stop labor.
Nursing Process Phase: planning; client need: health promotion and maintenance; concern area: maternity nursing

31. **Correct Answer: D.** Methergine is an ergot derivative. Given IV, it will elevate blood pressure and work to contract uterine musculature.

Rationales for Other Answer Choices: A. Ibuprofen is an analgesic and is not used in the delivery room. **B.** Prostaglandin F_2 alpha is used as an abortifacient. **C.** Ephedrine will evaluate blood pressure but will not help with hemorrhage.
Nursing Process Phase: planning; client need: health promotion and maintenance; concern area: maternity nursing

32. **Correct Answer: A.** Pitocin postdelivery increases uterine contractions to prevent hemorrhage and atony.

Rationales for Other Answer Choices: B. Pitocin augments milk let-down. **C.** Pitocin aids in uterine involution. **D.** The contractions produced by Pitocin are uncomfortable.
Nursing Process Phase: analysis; client need: health promotion and maintenance; concern area: maternity nursing

33. **Correct Answer: C.** The contractions are too close for the length of duration. By weaning the Pitocin down, the fetus will get a chance to recover during the relaxation phase, and the heart rate variability will recover.

Rationales for Other Answer Choices: A. Will only worsen the condition. **B.** If the Pitocin is turned off completely, contractions may stop. Stopping is only necessary with late or severe variable decelerations. **D.** Never increase Pitocin when contractions are lasting 90 seconds.
Nursing Process Phase: implementation; client need: health promotion and maintenance; concern area: maternity nursing

34. **Correct Answer: B.** Pitocin must always be diluted when given IV because it is caustic to the veins. It is given piggyback in order to stop the medication if necessary and still hydrate the client.

Rationales for Other Answer Choices: A. Side effects include elevated blood pressure and water intoxication. **C.** IV Pitocin's half-life is very short. **D.** Pitocin causes fluid retention.
Nursing Process Phase: planning; client need: health promotion and maintenance; concern area: maternity nursing

35. **Correct Answer: C.** This medication is a beta-blocker, and bradycardia, abdominal discomfort, diaphoresis, and confusion are possible side effects, even with eyedrops.

Rationales for Other Answer Choices: A. Not side effects of this medication. **B.** More commonly seen with diuretics such as Diamox. **D.** Not side effects of beta-blockers.
Nursing Process Phase: intervention; client need: safe and effective care environment; concern area: medical/surgical

36. **Correct Answer: C.** Administering too much insulin, as well as unplanned exercise or lack of food intake, can produce a hypoglycemic reaction.

Rationales for Other Answer Choices: A. Hypoglycemic reactions happen quickly. **B.** These are symptoms of hypoglycemia, hyperglycemia includes dry, warm skin, frequent urination, acetone odor to breath. **D.** Hyperglycemic reactions may take several hours to appear.
Nursing Process Phase: intervention; client need: safe and effective care environment; concern area: obstetrics

37. **Correct Answer: D.** Oxytocin is the only drug used to stimulate or induce labor.

Rationales for Other Answer Choices: A. Methylergonovine is a uterine stimulant that is used only following delivery. **B.** Ergovine is a uterine stimulant that is used only following delivery. **C.** Ritodrine is used to suppress uterine contractions.
Nursing Process Phase: planning; client need: health promotion and maintenance; concern area: maternity nursing

38. **Correct Answer: B.** In general, tablets have a relatively low acid-neutralizing capacity compared with liquid antacid preparations.

Rationales for Other Answer Choices: A. Tablets must be thoroughly chewed to provide the greatest possible surface area for neutralizing acids. **C.** H_2 inhibitors alter gastric acid. **D.** Antacids alter the absorption of many drugs, and clients should be warned against taking other medications at the same time as antacids.
Nursing Process Phase: evaluation; client need: safe and effective care environment; concern area: medical/surgical

39. **Correct Answer: B.** This powerful medication should be used only short-term for weight loss.

Rationales for Other Answer Choices: A. Insomnia is a common side effect; last dose for day should be taken in late afternoon. **C.** Has many side effects, including insom-

nia, nervousness, hypertension, tachycardia, and addiction. **D.** Normal dose is 5 to 20 mg bid.
Nursing Process Phase: planning; client need: safe and effective care environment; concern area: medical/surgical

40. Correct Answer: B. The term *teratogenic* means that the medication may cause abnormal development of the fetus if used during pregnancy. Many medications have not been adequately studied; however, no medication that is known to be teratogenic should be administered to a pregnant client unless the benefits clearly outweigh the risks.

Rationales for Other Answer Choices: A. No contraindication for asthma. **C.** No contraindication for children. **D.** No contraindication for renal failure.
Nursing Process Phase: planning; client need: safe and effective care environment; concern area: maternity nursing

41. Correct Answer: C. Lidocaine is the preferred drug for treatment of ventricular tachycardia or fibrillation.

Rationales for Other Answer Choices: A. Osmolal is a beta-blocker used to slow the heart rate. **B.** Procainamide is used to treat atrial fibrillation as well as ventricular arrhythmias, but not ventricular fibrillation. **D.** Verapamil, a calcium channel blocker, is used in the treatment of supraventricular arrhythmias.
Nursing Process Phase: implementation; client need: safe and effective care environment; concern area: medical/surgical

42. Correct Answer: D. Lithium has a very low margin of safety, which necessitates monitoring blood levels frequently when starting therapy and periodically during therapy. High-risk clients may require daily blood tests. The other choices are not sensitive indicators of therapeutic levels.

Rationales for Other Answer Choices: A. Clinical effectiveness may not appear for several weeks. **B.** Side effects frequently appear early in therapy despite therapeutic blood levels and often disappear after about 6 weeks of therapy. **C.** Weight gain is a common early side effect.
Nursing Process Phase: assessment; client need: safe and effective care environment; concern area: psychiatric nursing

43. Correct Answer: A. Lithium, which is administered orally, is excreted almost exclusively (95%) by the kidneys, with no metabolism. Lithium's plasma half-life is prolonged in a patient with reduced renal function. If doses are not reduced in the presence of decreased renal function, the drug will accumulate, leading to toxicity.

Rationales for Other Answer Choices: B. Does not significantly alter lithium excretion. **C.** Does not significantly alter lithium excretion. **D.** Does not significantly alter lithium excretion.
Nursing Process Phase: analysis; client need: safe and effective care environment; concern area: psychiatric nursing

44. **Correct Answer: C.**   Tricyclic antidepressant medications inhibit reuptake of several neurotransmitters (norepinephrine, serotonin, and dopamine) in the brain, which may account for their primary action.

Rationales for Other Answer Choices: A. While this effect takes place rapidly, it usually takes several weeks for the antidepressive effects of the tricyclic drugs to become apparent. **B.** Failure to obtain an immediate antidepressive effect does not mean the drug is ineffective, inasmuch as adequate time must be allowed for a full response to the drug. **D.** The level of depression and response to therapy can be assessed through behavioral symptoms.
Nursing Process Phase: implementation; client need: psychosocial integrity; concern area: psychiatric nursing

45. **Correct Answer: B.**   All antipsychotic drugs can produce the same side effects as atropine. These effects are due to the same mechanism: blocking the action of acetylcholine receptors. Some anticholinergic effects are rather mild, and others may be dangerous. Anticholinergic side effects include dry mouth, visual disturbance, increased intraocular pressure, tachycardia, urinary retention or frequency, and constipation.

Rationales for Other Answer Choices: A. Cholinergic side effects are those produced by medications like epinephrine (tachycardia, central nervous system [CNS] stimulation, increased blood pressure, diaphoresis). **C.** Extrapyramidal side effects are similar to symptoms of Parkinsonism (shuffling gait, drooling, tremors, muscular rigidity). **D.** Long-term use may affect the liver, leading to jaundice, edema, and increased liver enzymes.
Nursing Process Phase: analysis; client need: safe and effective care environment; concern area: psychiatric nursing

46. **Correct Answer: D.**   Chlorpromazine is an antipsychotic drug often considered the prototype with which other antipsychotic drugs are compared. Chlorpromazine is also used to treat nausea and vomiting.

Rationales for Other Answer Choices: A. No direct effect on gastric acid. **B.** May lower BP as a side effect, but not a primary medication. **C.** Has no anti-inflammatory effects.
Nursing Process Phase: analysis; client need: safe and effective care environment; concern area: psychiatric nursing

47. **Correct Answer: B.**   Phenobarbital is a barbiturate used for sedation, hypnosis, and management of seizure disorders. The major use in children is for chronic seizure disorders. In addition, since it is administered three times a day rather than at bedtime, it is unlikely to be intended as a sedative/hypnotic.

Rationales for Other Answer Choices: A, C, and **D** are not treated with sedative/hypnotic drugs.
Nursing Process Phase: analysis; client need: safe and effective care environment; concern area: pediatrics

48. **Correct Answer: A.** A common result of IV administration of phenytoin is sudden drop in blood pressure.

Rationales for Other Answer Choices: B. Not associated with this medication. **C.** May cause bradycardia. **D.** Not associated with this medication.
Nursing Process Phase: evaluation; client need: safe and effective care environment; concern area: medical/surgical

49. **Correct Answer: B.** Propranolol is a beta-blocking medication that reduces sympathetic (beta) stimulation of the heart, slowing the heart rate.

Rationales for Other Answer Choices: A. Phentolamine is an alpha-blocker that reduces the client's blood pressure but not the heart rate. **C.** Cimetidine is used to decrease gastric acid production and has no effect on the heart rate. **D.** Dopamine is a sympathomimetic drug that would most likely increase the heart rate.
Nursing Process Phase: planning; client need: safe and effective care environment; concern area: medical/surgical

50. **Correct Answer: D.** Acetylcysteine breaks the molecular bonds of the mucus, allowing the client to cough it out more easily.

Rationales for Other Answer Choices: A. Should reduce the amount of effort to cough out the secretions. **B.** Has no effect on the cough center directly. **C.** Should be just the opposite.
Nursing Process Phase: assessment; client need: physiological integrity; concern area: medical/surgical

1. Which of the following would indicate to the nurse that the IV amino-caproic acid (Amicar) a client was receiving was effective?
   A. Urine output increases to 45 mL/h from 22 mL/h.
   B. BP increases to 110/66 from 88/42.
   C. Gastric drainage from a nasogastric (NG) tube turns a greenish yellow from bright red.
   D. Serum ammonia level increases from 42 μg/dL to 55 μg/dL.

2. A 5-year-old child is admitted to the pediatric unit with nausea, vomiting, and a temperature of 101.5°F. Which of the following would the nurse expect if the child is to be given an IV medication?
   A. Prolonged action of the medication because of systemic dehydration
   B. Reflex tachycardia because of the large volume of fluid being given IV
   C. Reduced duration of the therapeutic effect
   D. Reduction in vomiting and increased level of consciousness

3. An HIV-positive, 23-year-old male client is beginning a course of treatment with zidovudine (AZT). Which of the following statements by the client would indicate to the nurse that he understood the nurse's instructions about the medication?
   A. "If I am asleep, I can put off taking the medication until I wake up because I need rest to keep up my resistance."
   B. "This medication will cure my HIV in 6 months to a year."
   C. "After I have been on this medication for several weeks I can resume going to bars and dances."
   D. "If I get a sore throat or fever, I should call the physician."

4. Which information should the nurse include in the teaching plan for a client who is taking bulk-forming laxatives?
   A. The volume of the stool is increased as water is absorbed into the fecal contents.
   B. They produce a liquid stool that cleanses the bowel.
   C. They can interfere with vitamin A absorption.
   D. They work within 1 to 2 hours.

5. A client develops joint pain and swelling in the great toe of his right foot after his eighth treatment with chlorambucil (Leukeran) for Hodgkin's disease. Which of the following nursing actions would be most effective in preventing this side effect?
   A. Ambulate the client the length of the hall tid to promote joint mobility.
   B. Encourage the client to drink 2 to 3 liters of fluid per day.
   C. Administer an ordered prn dose of acetaminophen (Tylenol) 650 mg PO.
   D. Keep the foot of the bed elevated during administration of the medication.

6. A client is given methylergonovine maleate (Methergine) 0.2 mg by mouth. Which of the following responses would indicate to the nurse that the medication was achieving its desired effect?
   A. Respiratory rate of 16 breaths per minute (BPM)
   B. Blood pressure (BP) of 124/78
   C. Apical pulse of 72 beats per minute (BPM)
   D. Uterine fundus firm and in the midline

7. Which of the following statements made by the parents of a 4-year-old girl who is being treated with permethrin (Nix) for pediculosis would indicate to the nurse that they understood instructions about the medication?
   A. "She must take the pills twice a day with at least a full glass of water."
   B. "After washing her hair with her usual shampoo, we leave the medication on for 10 minutes."
   C. "We have to shampoo her hair every day for a week with this medication."
   D. "We need to check her stools each day to see if there are any live worms remaining."

8. For which of the following clients would the nurse question an order for a carbonic anhydrase inhibitor? A client with:
   A. Tonic-clonic seizures
   B. Open-angle glaucoma
   C. Drug-induced edema
   D. A pulmonary obstruction

9. For which of the following clients would Ensure be most appropriate? A client who:
   A. Requires primarily protein replacement
   B. Has a lactose intolerance
   C. Is unable to take any oral fluids
   D. Requires 2200 calories per day

10. A 44-year-old client who has smoked two and one-half packs of cigarettes per day since age 13 is admitted with acute respiratory failure. While receiving an IV theophylline drip (Aminophylline) at 15 mg/h, he develops tachycardia, restlessness, nausea, and vomiting. Which would be the most appropriate initial action by the nurse?
    A. Administer the client's ordered prn antiemetic.
    B. Bring the emergency anaphylaxis medication kit to the bedside.
    C. Call the physician.
    D. Stop the theophylline infusion.

11. A 56-year-old male client with severe chronic obstructive pulmonary disease (COPD) who is intubated and connected to a positive pressure volume cycled ventilator is to be started on Sustical feedings via percutaneous endoscopic gastrostomy (PEG) tube. In planning care for this client, the nurse should anticipate that:
    A. Full-strength feedings will be started at 100 mL/h, then increased to 150 mL/h after 8 hours.
    B. The feeding will not provide enough calories to sustain a severely ill client for an extended period of time.
    C. The client can begin to eat soft food after 7 days on the tube feeding.
    D. Half-strength feeding will be started at 50 mL/h, then titrated for rate and concentration according to the client's tolerance.

12. A 69-year-old client with a long history of recurrent congestive heart failure (CHF) is admitted to the intensive care unit and has a pulmonary artery catheter placed for monitoring. The most important assessment the nurse makes prior to beginning the administration of dopamine (Intropine) IV is the client's:
    A. Neurological status
    B. White blood cell count
    C. Serum sodium level
    D. Hydration status

13. In planning care for a client with a serum uric acid level of 10.4 mg/dL, the nurse would anticipate teaching the client about the side effects of which of the following medications?
    A. zidovudine (AZT)
    B. probenecid (Benemid)
    C. furosemide (Lasix)
    D. vincristine (Oncovin)

14. A 78-year-old female who weighs 94 pounds is to receive Sustical 240 mL between meals as a nutritional supplement. The most important factor for the nurse to consider prior to administering this product is:
    A. The client must have an intact digestive system.
    B. The product provides 20 cal/mL.
    C. When given by itself, it is nutritionally incomplete.
    D. It has a low-carbohydrate, but high-protein content.

15. In teaching a female client about the metabolic effects of conjugated estrogen (Premarin), the nurse includes the fact that this medication:
    A. Reduces blood cholesterol and protein synthesis
    B. Decreases sodium and water retention
    C. Decreases the production of oils from the sebaceous glands
    D. Increases milk production postpartum

16. A client with tonic-clonic seizures is to be started on primidone (Mysoline) by mouth. The nurse would hold the primidone if the client has a known allergy to:
    A. phenytoin (Dilantin)
    B. prochlorperazine (Compazine)
    C. phenobarbital (Luminal)
    D. propranolol (Inderal)

17. A client is being discharged to home with a prescription for amiodarone (Cordarone) for the control of:
  A. Hypertension
  B. CHF
  C. Atrial fibrillation
  D. Premature ventricular contractions

18. A client asks the nurse why he is being switched from chlorpromazine (Thorazine) to clozapine (Clozaril). The best answer by the nurse to this question is:
  A. "You are building up a resistance to the Thorazine, so the Clozaril will be more effective."
  B. "Clozaril produces fewer extrapyramidal reactions than the Thorazine."
  C. "Your schizophrenia has improved to the point where you no longer need the more potent Thorazine."
  D. "You had better ask your physician, because nurses are not allowed to give this information to clients."

19. While evaluating a client's list of medications, the nurse notes which of the following medications as increasing the risk for developing cataracts?
  A. Acetaminophen
  B. Nifedipine
  C. Ibuprofen
  D. Aspirin

20. Which of the following would best indicate to the nurse that the doxepin (Sinequan) a client was taking was achieving a positive therapeutic effect?
  A. The client is better able to cope with day-to-day stressors from the environment.
  B. The client reports fewer auditory hallucinations and better thought organization.
  C. The client's BP is now 134/88, down from 162/98 a week ago.
  D. The client displays less paranoid ideation in discussing his illness.

21. A nurse working in a psychiatric unit notes that a client who has been taking a phenothiazine has developed akathisia as manifested by the client's:
  A. Expressionless face
  B. Forgetting what he had for breakfast
  C. Need to be in continual motion
  D. Frequent focal seizures

22. While obtaining the admission assessment and history of a 55-year-old male client, the nurse notes that he takes colchicine 0.6 mg PO each morning. Based on this information, the nurse would anticipate that the client would:
  A. Have fluid restrictions of 1000 mL/d
  B. Be required to ambulate tid the length of the hall
  C. Receive a purine-restricted diet
  D. Be uncooperative and disoriented after dark

23. Which of the following laboratory values from a client who was taking didanosine (ddI, Videx) would most concern the nurse?
  A. Serum amylase 306 U/L
  B. Serum glutamic-oxaloacetic transaminase (SGOT) of 32 U/L
  C. White blood cell (WBC) count of 13,000
  D. Serum potassium 5.2 mEq/L

24. The physician orders imipenem/cilastatin (Primaxin) IVPB 1 g q 6 hours for a 22-year-old male client with osteomyelitis. The most appropriate action by the nurse in response to this order is to:
   A. Hold the medication, and notify the physician that the dose is too large
   B. Skin test the client for an allergic reaction before giving the first dose
   C. Give the medication as ordered
   D. Give half the dose of medication, observe for side effects, then give the second half 30 minutes later

25. For which of the following clients would an ER nurse question an order for an antiemetic? A client:
   A. With metastatic cancer
   B. Who is pregnant
   C. With wide-angle glaucoma
   D. Who has a bleeding gastric ulcer

26. A 43-year-old male client who experiences an acute attack of gout after eating "Surf and Turf" at a local steak house is given colchicine 1.2 mg PO initially, then 0.6 mg q 1 hour. At this rate of administration, the nurse realizes that the maximum cumulative dose of this medication will be reached in:
   A. 4 hours
   B. 6 hours
   C. 9 hours
   D. 10 hours

27. Which of the following would the nurse anticipate for a client who was started on levothyroxine (Synthroid) for treatment of hypothyroidism?
   A. Reduction in protein synthesis
   B. Well-regulated growth in an adult
   C. Increase in cholesterol levels
   D. Increased rate and force of cardiac contraction

28. A client is to be started on clozapine (Clozaril) for treatment of chronic schizophrenia. The nurse would give the medication as ordered if the dosage regimen was:
   A. 300 mg bid for 2 days, then increase to 400 mg bid for maintenance dose
   B. Loading dose of 300 mg times three over a 24-hour period, then a maintenance dose of 300 mg qid
   C. 25 mg bid, increasing by 25 mg/d for 2 weeks up to a target dose of 350 mg/d
   D. 50 mg/d until symptoms decrease, then 25 mg/d

29. Which of the following statements made by a client would indicate to the nurse that the discharge teaching concerning the use of amiodarone (Cordarone) had been understood?
   A. "When the physician says I can stop taking this medication, I can go to the beach and get a good suntan."
   B. "The side effects of this medication may not begin to show up for several weeks or even months after I start taking it."
   C. "If my pulse drops below 100 beats per minute, I should call the physician right away."
   D. "If I miss a dose of medication, I should take it as soon as I remember that I missed it."

30. After administering the first dose of primidone (Mysoline) PO to a 21-year-old female client diagnosed with seizure disorder, the nurse should caution the client to:
    A. Avoid food for at least 1 hour to decrease nausea
    B. Keep the head of her bed elevated to lessen dizziness
    C. Avoid sudden changes in position to decrease orthostatic hypotension
    D. Drink 2 to 3 liters of fluid to help flush the medication from the system

31. Which of the following statements by a client would indicate that the nurse's teaching concerning digoxin (Lanoxin) was successful?
    A. "I can expect some swelling in my feet and ankles while I'm taking this medication."
    B. "If I miss a dose, I should eliminate it and not take two the next day."
    C. "I can stop taking this medication in 2 months when my heart heals after the heart attack."
    D. "If I should develop nausea or vomiting, I need to stop taking the medication."

32. A 20-year-old female client is brought into the ER by her boyfriend, complaining of shortness of breath, dizziness, and a fluttering feeling in her chest. When connected to the monitor, her electrocardiogram (ECG) pattern shows a rapid heart rate (220 BPM) with QRS complexes measuring 0.1 second but no visible P waves. If all of the following medications are available for the nurse to give IV, which should she administer to treat this dysrhythmia?
    A. amiodarone (Cordarone)
    B. lidocaine HCL (Xylocaine)
    C. adenosine (Adenocard)
    D. atropine sulfate

33. Which of the following side effects would be most important for the nurse to assess a client for after receiving meperidine (Demerol) 50 mg IV?
    A. Hyperthermia
    B. Bradypnea
    C. Bradycardia
    D. Hyperpraxia

34. Which of the following statements by the nurse would be the best response to a client about why the nurse is giving promethazine hydrochloride (Phenergan) suppository prior to his weekly dose of chemotherapy?
    A. "Phenergan will help you relax so that the chemotherapy will work better."
    B. "Phenergan reduces the pain at the IV site where the chemotherapy is being administered."
    C. "Phenergan helps control the nausea and vomiting often associated with chemotherapy administration."
    D. "Phenergan reduces the fever that most clients who are getting chemotherapy experience after administration."

35. Which of the following statements made by the father of a 4-month-old girl with transposition of the great vessels who is to be given digoxin (Lanoxin) liquid at home would indicate to the nurse that he understood the instructions about the side effects of the medication?
    A. "If the baby becomes sleepy, I should skip the next dose of Lanoxin."
    B. "I should wait 6 hours before feeding the baby if she has loose stools."
    C. "I need to call the physician if the baby develops hiccoughs that last more than 1 hour."
    D. "I will bring the baby into the clinic if she vomits several times."

36. The nurse would withhold an emergency dose of protamine sulfate for an overdose of heparin if the client were allergic to:
    A. Sulfonamides
    B. Strawberries
    C. Fish
    D. Aspirin

37. When explaining the medication glyburide (Micronase) to a newly diagnosed type 2 diabetic client, the nurse should include the statement:
    A. "Micronase works by increasing the insulin secretions of the pancreas."
    B. "Micronase works by blocking insulin absorption in the cells."
    C. "Micronase works by reducing the breakdown of the insulin in the blood."
    D. "Micronase works by replacing the insulin your body does not make."

38. Which of the following should the nurse include in the care plan of a 24-year-old male client who is being started on lithium carbonate (Eskalith)?
    A. Monitor for the development of Chvostek's sign.
    B. Observe for vomiting and diarrhea.
    C. Maintain 1 g sodium diet.
    D. Instruct client in self-testicular examination (STE).

39. Which of the following data obtained by the nurse while assessing a 12-year-old female client who is being treated with phenytoin (Dilantin) for an idiopathic seizure disorder should be reported to the physician?
    A. She began her first menstrual cycle 2 days ago.
    B. She avoids eating citrus fruits.
    C. She has had nausea and vomiting for the past 12 hours.
    D. She is on the track team at school and runs several miles each day.

40. Which of the following would be the most appropriate statement for the nurse to include in the discharge instructions to a client with a prescription for naproxen (Naprosyn)?
    A. "Make sure you take the medication with food or meals."
    B. "Limit your intake of foods containing potassium, such as citrus fruits, bananas, and meats."
    C. "You must drink 2 to 3 liters of fluid each day while taking this medication."
    D. "Eat no more than 2 g of sodium each day to prevent edema."

41. Which of the following assessments would be important for a client admitted to the hospital who had been on long-term ibuprofen (Motrin) therapy for an injured back?
   A. Bleeding time
   B. Serum potassium
   C. Levels of T_3 and T_4
   D. Blood pressure

42. Which of the following statements made by a client who was being discharged with a prescription for rifampin (Rifadin) would indicate to the nurse that additional teaching was required?
   A. "After taking the medication for several weeks, I will no longer be contagious."
   B. "If my stools appear white, I need to call the physician."
   C. "I should take the medication at the same time each day."
   D. "When I begin to gain weight and stop coughing, I can stop taking the medication."

43. A 22-year-old college student is admitted to the intensive care unit after having ingested 50 tablets of acetaminophen (Tylenol) in an attempt to commit suicide because of a poor grade on a test. The nurse would anticipate which of the following changes in laboratory values?
   A. Decrease in serum potassium
   B. Decrease in blood urea nitrogen (BUN)
   C. Increase in serum bilirubin
   D. Increase in WBCs

44. If a nursing student does all of the following while administering heparin sodium 3500 units subcutaneously to a post–myocardial infarction (MI) client, which would indicate that she requires further instruction?
   A. Aspirating to make sure the needle is not in a vein
   B. Selecting a ½-inch, 24-gauge needle for administration
   C. Injecting the medication into a different site than was used for the last injection
   D. Using an area approximately 2 inches to the left of the umbilicus for the injection site

45. The nurse will closely monitor the client receiving streptokinase (Streptase) during and after administration for development of:
   A. Urinary retention
   B. Hypertension
   C. Urticaria
   D. Peripheral edema

46. Which of the following activities reported by a 46-year-old female client who is taking conjugated estrogen (Premarin) for postmenopausal syndrome would be of most concern to the clinic nurse?
   A. Joining a gourmet cooking club
   B. Starting to jog 2 miles per day
   C. Beginning smoking cigarettes after a 4-year abstinence
   D. Drinking a glass of wine with supper each day

47. In planning care for a malnourished client who has an inflammatory bowel disease, the nurse realizes that which of the following nutritional supplements is most appropriate?
    A. Ensure
    B. Ensure Plus
    C. Vivonex
    D. Sustical

48. While obtaining a history from the parents of a 4-year-old child, the nurse discovers that the child has been recently treated with permethrin (Nix). Which would be an appropriate action by the nurse in response to this information?
    A. Obtain a stool sample for ova and parasite.
    B. Assess the child for appropriate mental ability and motor development.
    C. Carefully examine the hair and scalp.
    D. Put on a mask and sterile gown to keep the child from getting a respiratory infection.

49. Which of the following assessments would indicate to the nurse that a client was developing a side effect directly related to his treatment with chlorambucil (Leukeran)?
    A. Joint pain and swelling in the great toe of his right foot
    B. BP increased to 158/100
    C. Oral temperature of 96.8°F
    D. Constipation and abdominal distention

50. A client who is receiving diltiazem (Cardizem) by IV infusion in his left hand complains that the hand hurts. In assessing the IV site, the nurse notes the hand is swollen, but there is a good blood return in the IV tubing. What would be the most appropriate action by the nurse at this time?
    A. Elevate the right hand on a pillow to reduce the swelling.
    B. Apply a cool compress to the infusion site for 30 minutes to reduce the sensation of pain.
    C. Slow the rate of the medication infusion, and assess again after 1 hour.
    D. Discontinue the IV infusion.

ANSWERS/RATIONALES

1. **Correct Answer: C.** Amicar is a hemostatic medication that prevents fibrinolysis and stabilizes clot formation. It is an antidote for streptokinase and heparin and can be used with any severe bleeding disorder, such as gastric ulcers.

Rationales for Other Answer Choices: A. Has no direct effect on urine output. **B.** Does not directly effect BP. **D.** Normal serum ammonia levels are 15 to 45 μg/dL—this medication has no effect on them.
Nursing Process Phase: evaluation; client need: safe and effective care environment; concern area: medical/surgical

2. **Correct Answer: C.** Metabolism in children increases dramatically with an increased body temperature, reducing the half-life of medications.

Rationales for Other Answer Choices: A. The child will be quickly rehydrated with IV fluids. **B.** The heart rate should return to normal when rehydrated. **D.** Unable to make this conclusion without knowing what medications are being given.
Nursing Process Phase: planning; client need: physiological integrity; concern area: pediatrics

3. **Correct Answer: D.** These are early signs of infection that may develop into more severe infections in the immune-suppressed HIV client.

Rationales for Other Answer Choices: A. Should take doses of AZT as scheduled, even if it means interrupting sleep. **B.** Does not cure HIV—client remains contagious. **C.** Should avoid crowds and exposure to infections.
Nursing Process Phase: evaluation; client need: safe and effective care environment; concern area: medical/surgical

4. **Correct Answer: A.** These add bulk to the stool by absorbing water from the body, stimulating peristalsis of the large intestine.

Rationales for Other Answer Choices: B. Stool will be formed but will be soft. **C.** No known problem with vitamin absorption. **D.** Slow acting—12 to 24 hours.
Nursing Process Phase: planning; client need: physiological integrity; concern area: medical/surgical

5. **Correct Answer: B.** Increasing the fluid intake will help prevent uric acid build-up and eliminate the uric acid from the body.

Rationales for Other Answer Choices: A. May not be possible to ambulate a client with Hodgkin's—does not prevent the gout. **C.** Provides only temporary relief of symptoms—anti-inflammatory medications are more effective. **D.** Does not help prevent the development of gout.
Nursing Process Phase: implementation; client need: safe and effective care environment; concern area: medical/surgical

6. **Correct Answer: D.** Methergine, an oxytocic class medication, is used postpartum to prevent postpartum hemorrhage caused by subinvolution.

Rationales for Other Answer Choices: A. Has no direct effect on the respiratory system. **B.** May cause an increase in BP because of vasoconstriction. **C.** May increase the heart rate but is not its primary use.
Nursing Process Phase: evaluation; client need: health promotion and maintenance; concern area: maternity nursing

7. **Correct Answer: B.** Nix is a rinse that coats the entire head of hair after the child has shampooed with the usual shampoo and must be left on for 10 minutes before rinsing.

Rationales for Other Answer Choices: A. No oral form of this medication. **C.** It is not a shampoo—too frequent use can lead to neurotoxicity. Once a week is frequent enough. **D.** Is not used for gastrointestinal (GI) parasites.
Nursing Process Phase: evaluation; client need: safe and effective care environment; concern area: pediatrics

8. **Correct Answer: D.** The metabolic acidosis produced by a carbonic anhydrase inhibitor could not be easily compensated for by the respiratory system in a client with an obstruction or other respiratory condition.

Rationales for Other Answer Choices: A. No contraindication for seizure disorders. **B.** One of the primary uses for this medication. **C.** Has a powerful diuretic effect.
Nursing Process Phase: implementation; client need: safe and effective care environment; concern area: medical/surgical

9. **Correct Answer: B.** Ensure is lactose-free and can be used with clients who have lactose intolerance.

Rationales for Other Answer Choices: A. Ensure has a relatively high percentage of carbohydrates and a lower percentage of protein. **C.** All nutritional supplements can be given by feeding or gastrostomy tube. **D.** Ensure delivers approximately 1 cal/mL; Ensure Plus provides approximately 1.5 cal/mL.
Nursing Process Phase: analysis; client need: safe and effective care environment; concern area: medical/surgical

10. **Correct Answer: D.** These are symptoms of theophylline toxicity, and the medication needs to be stopped to prevent worsening of the condition.

Rationales for Other Answer Choices: A. This could be done after the aminophylline is stopped. **B.** Not required—these are not symptoms of an anaphylactic reaction. **C.** This is the second action to be taken.
Nursing Process Phase: implementation; client need: safe and effective care environment; concern area: medical/surgical

11. **Correct Answer: D.** This is a typical initial rate and concentration for Sustical.

Rationales for Other Answer Choices: A. Starting with a large volume of full-strength feeding can cause diarrhea and GI cramping. **B.** An adult client will need ap-

proximately 2000 mL of Sustical per day to maintain nutritional status.   **C.** If the client were able to eat, the PEG tube would not have been inserted.
Nursing Process Phase: planning; client need: safe and effective care environment; concern area: medical/surgical

12. **Correct Answer: D.**   Positive inotropic medications like dopamine cause vaso-constriction and raise BP. It should not be given to clients who are dehydrated.

Rationales for Other Answer Choices: A. Lower priority—generally not affected by this medication.   **B.** Not affected.   **C.** May be lowered with increased urination secondary to dopamine.
Nursing Process Phase: assessment; client need: safe and effective care environment; concern area: medical/surgical

13. **Correct Answer: B.**   Normal uric acid level is 3.5 to 8.0 mg/dL. It is increased in gout, and Benemid is a commonly used uricosuric agent that lowers uric acid levels.

Rationales for Other Answer Choices: A. Antiviral medication used with HIV.   **C.** Diuretic used for CHF, edema, and so forth.   **D.** Anticancer medication.
Nursing Process Phase: planning; client need: safe and effective care environment; concern area: medical/surgical

14. **Correct Answer: A.**   These milk-based products require an intact digestive system for breakdown and absorption.

Rationales for Other Answer Choices: B. Provides 1 cal/mL.   **C.** These are nutritionally complete products.   **D.** All are high in carbohydrates and fats, lower in protein.
Nursing Process Phase: planning; client need: physiological integrity; concern area: medical/surgical

15. **Correct Answer: A.**   These are two of the common metabolic effects of this medication.

Rationales for Other Answer Choices: B. It increases sodium and water retention, resulting in edema.   **C.** It increases secretions of oil, leading to acne.   **D.** It decreases milk production.
Nursing Process Phase: planning; client need: safe and effective care environment; concern area: medical/surgical

16. **Correct Answer: C.**   Primidone is converted into a metabolite form of phenobarbital in the liver—cross allergies are common.

Rationales for Other Answer Choices: A, B, and **D** do not have common cross-allergies with primidone.
Nursing Process Phase: implementation; client need: safe and effective care environment; concern area: medical/surgical

17. **Correct Answer: D.**   Often touted as an "oral lidocaine," amiodarone is used to prevent life-threatening ventricular dysrhythmia unresponsive to less toxic agents.   ·

Rationales for Other Answer Choices: A. Has no direct effect on BP. **B.** Does not increase the force of contraction. **C.** Not effective for this dysrhythmia.
Nursing Process Phase: analysis; client need: safe and effective care environment; concern area: medical/surgical

18. **Correct Answer: B.** Clozaril has fewer extrapyramidal side effects and less incidence of tardive dyskinesia but carries a higher risk of hematologic abnormalities.

Rationales for Other Answer Choices: A. Most clients do not become sufficiently resistant to Thorazine to require a switch in medication. **C.** Both medications have equal potency. **D.** Untrue statement—nurses can and should provide this information to clients.
Nursing Process Phase: implementation; client need: psychosocial integrity; concern area: psychiatric nursing

19. **Correct Answer: B.** A known side effect of nifedipine and steroid medications.

Rationales for Other Answer Choices: A, C, D. These analgesic medications may actually prevent the formation of cataracts.
Nursing Process Phase: assessment; client need: safe and effective care environment; concern area: medical/surgical

20. **Correct Answer: A.** Doxepin is a tricyclic antidepressant that is also used as an antianxiety agent. The goal of therapy is to have the client overcome depression/anxiety and be able to resume normal activities of daily living.

Rationales for Other Answer Choices: B. This medication is not appropriate for psychotic disorders and may actually cause hallucinations during early therapy. **C.** Has no direct effect on blood pressure. **D.** Not appropriate for treatment of paranoia.
Nursing Process Phase: evaluation; client need: psychosocial integrity; concern area: psychiatric nursing

21. **Correct Answer: C.** Akathisia is often manifested by continual pacing and non-purposeful movements of the extremities.

Rationales for Other Answer Choices: A. Masklike face is a common side effect. **B.** Not associated with these medications. **D.** Phenothiazines may lower the seizure threshold.
Nursing Process Phase: evaluation; client need: safe and effective care environment; concern area: psychiatric nursing

22. **Correct Answer: C.** Colchicine is an anti-inflammatory medication used to treat gout. Purines are protein substances found in many meats, fish, meat extracts, and so forth that promote uric acid production and make gout worse.

Rationales for Other Answer Choices: A. Fluid intake of 2 to 3 liters per day should be encouraged. **B.** Ambulation may or may not be appropriate. **D.** Colchicine is not used for disorientation or hostile behavior.
Nursing Process Phase: planning; client need: safe and effective care environment; concern area: medical/surgical

23. **Correct Answer: A.** Pancreatitis is a serious side effect of this medication, indicated by a serum amylase one and a half to two times normal (normal = 30–170 U/L [SI units]).

Rationales for Other Answer Choices: B. ddI may increase liver enzymes, but this value is in the normal range (8–33 U/L at 98.6°F SI units). **C.** Although an elevated WBC (normal 5000–10,000) may indicate an infection, low WBC count in the population that takes ddI would be of more concern. **D.** The diarrhea caused by this medication will lower the potassium (normal 3.5–5.5 mEq/L), not increase it.
Nursing Process Phase: analysis; client need: safe and effective care environment; concern area: medical/surgical

24. **Correct Answer: C.** For severe infections, such as bone infections, a normal adult dose is 0.5 to 1 g q 6–8 h IVPB.

Rationales for Other Answer Choices: A. Dose is appropriate for this client. **B.** Not necessary for this medication—it has a very low incidence of allergic reaction. **D.** Not an acceptable nursing measure.
Nursing Process Phase: implementation; client need: safe and effective care environment; concern area: medical/surgical

25. **Correct Answer: B.** Most antiemetics have teratogenic effects and are high risk for causing fetal defects during pregnancy.

Rationales for Other Answer Choices: A. Often used because of side effects of chemotherapy. **C.** No contraindication for this condition. **D.** Can be used to control vomiting of blood.
Nursing Process Phase: intervention; client need: safe and effective care environment; concern area: obstetrics

26. **Correct Answer: C.** A total cumulative dose of 6 mg is considered maximum for this medication ($8 \times 0.6 = 4.8 + 1.2 = 6$).

Rationales for Other Answer Choices: A. Will have only 3 mg total. **B.** Will have only 4.2 mg total. **D.** Will have 6.6 mg, exceeding the recommended total.
Nursing Process Phase: planning; client need: safe and effective care environment; concern area: medical/surgical

27. **Correct Answer: D.** Thyroid hormones have positive inotropic and chronotropic effects on the heart, producing a general increase in cardiac output.

Rationales for Other Answer Choices: A. Thyroid is an anabolic hormone and increases protein synthesis and muscle mass. **B.** Not a significant factor. **C.** May actually lower cholesterol because of increased metabolism.
Nursing Process Phase: planning; client need: physiological integrity; concern area: medical/surgical

28. **Correct Answer: C.** This is a normal dosage regimen for this medication. It is increased gradually so that the client can adjust to the side effects.

Rationales for Other Answer Choices: A. Total dose should be only between 300 and 450 mg/d after several weeks of adjustment period. **B.** This is an excessive amount of this medication, which is sure to produce severe side effects.   **D.** Dosage is too low to be effective.

Nursing Process Phase: planning; client need: psychosocial integrity; concern area: psychiatric nursing

29. **Correct Answer: B.**   It is not unusual for the side effects of this medication to take several weeks to as much as a year to manifest themselves.

Rationales for Other Answer Choices: A. Side effects persist for up to 4 months after the medication is stopped; photosensitivity is one of the side effects.   **C.** Pulse should be monitored, but if it is above 100 for a sustained period of time, the physician should be called.   **D.** If a dose is missed, the client should call the physician before taking any more of the medication.

Nursing Process Phase: evaluation; client need: safe and effective care environment; concern area: medical/surgical

30. **Correct Answer: C.**   Orthostatic hypotension is a common side effect of this medication, and sudden position changes can lead to syncope and falls.

Rationales for Other Answer Choices: A. May be taken with food if nausea occurs. **B.** Lowering the head of the bed would be more effective in preventing dizziness. **D.** Drinking this much fluid is a good practice for any client, but it is not necessary with this medication.

Nursing Process Phase: implementation; client need: safe and effective care environment; concern area: medical/surgical

31. **Correct Answer: B.**   Trying to "catch up" on once-a-day doses of digoxin by taking two pills the following day can lead to toxicity.

Rationales for Other Answer Choices: A. Edema may indicate that the medication is not effective.   **C.** Client should be re-evaluated by the physician before stopping medication. **D.** Nausea and vomiting are early signs of toxicity, but digoxin level should be evaluated.

Nursing Process Phase: evaluation; client need: safe and effective care environment; concern area: medical/surgical

32. **Correct Answer: C.**   Adenosine is an antidysrhythmic that is used to treat paroxysmal supraventricular tachycardia (PSVT), which is identified by a rapid heart rate with normal QRS complexes (0.6–1.1 sec) and no visible P waves. Also, the symptoms displayed by this client are classical for PSVT, as well as her age range and sex.

Rationales for Other Answer Choices: A. Used to treat ventricular dysrhythmias marked by wide QRS complexes. **B.** Also used to treat ventricular dysrhythmias. **D.** Used to treat slow heart rates and A-V blocks.

Nursing Process Phase: implementation; client need: safe and effective care environment; concern area: medical/surgical

33. **Correct Answer: B.**   Narcotic medications like meperidine often slow the respiratory rate.

Rationales for Other Answer Choices: A. Elevated temperature not a side effect of this medication.   **C.** Although narcotics may slow the heart rate some, they usually do not decrease it below normal (60 BPM).   **D.** Narcotics do not cause excessive activity or restlessness often seen in anxiety disorders.

Nursing Process Phase: assessment; client need: safe and effective care environment; concern area: medical/surgical

34.   Correct Answer: C.   Phenergan is used primarily as an antiemetic, particularly in clients who are receiving chemotherapy.

Rationales for Other Answer Choices: A. Although it does have a sedative effect as a side effect, this is not its primary use.   **B.** Has no analgesic effect by itself, although it will potentiate narcotic pain medications.   **D.** Although hypothermia is a side effect of all phenothiazines, this is not a primary use.

Nursing Process Phase: implementation; client need: safe and effective care environment; concern area: medical/surgical

35.   Correct Answer: D.   GI upset and vomiting are early signs of digoxin toxicity. The digoxin level needs to be evaluated.

Rationales for Other Answer Choices: A. Should wake the child and give the medication—skipping doses may be dangerous.   **B.** No need to wait this long—the child will become very hungry.   **C.** Hiccoughs not a side effect of digoxin.

Nursing Process Phase: evaluation; client need: safe and effective care environment; concern area: pediatrics

36.   Correct Answer: C.   The sperm of salmon and other fish is the primary source for protamine sulfate and is likely to produce severe anaphylactic reactions in persons allergic to fish.

Rationales for Other Answer Choices: A, B, D have no cross-allergies with protamine sulfate.

Nursing Process Phase: planning; client need: safe and effective care environment; concern area: medical/surgical

37.   Correct Answer: A.   This is a second-generation antidiabetic medication that lowers the blood sugar by stimulating the pancreas to increase its levels of insulin production.

Rationales for Other Answer Choices: B. Blocking insulin absorption would increase the blood sugar levels.   **C.** Glyburide does not have this mode of action.   **D.** This is the mode of action of insulin injections.

Nursing Process Phase: planning; client need: safe and effective care environment; concern area: medical/surgical

38.   Correct Answer: B.   These are early signs of toxicity—the lithium level will need to be evaluated. Also, prolonged vomiting and diarrhea may lead to electrolyte imbalances that can make the toxicity worse.

Rationales for Other Answer Choices: A. Chvostek's sign (spasms of the facial muscles following a tap on the side of the face) is usually associated with tetany caused by calcium imbalances.   **C.** Client will need an adequate sodium intake (3–4 g/d) to prevent toxicity.   **D.** STE, while important, is not specific to this medication.

Nursing Process Phase: planning; client need: safe and effective care environment; concern area: psychiatric nursing

39. Correct Answer: C. Prolonged nausea and vomiting may be signs of early Dilantin toxicity.

Rationales for Other Answer Choices: A. No relationship to Dilantin therapy. **B.** May indicate mouth discomfort but can be treated independently by the nurse. **D.** Exercise is not a contraindication for Dilantin therapy.
Nursing Process Phase: assessment; client need: safe and effective care environment; concern area: medical/surgical

40. Correct Answer: A. Naproxen, like many of the nonsteroidal anti-inflammatory drugs (NSAIDs), is irritating to the gastric mucosa and can cause gastritis or ulcers if taken on an empty stomach.

Rationales for Other Answer Choices: B. Naproxen has no effect on potassium in the body. **C.** Increasing fluid intake is a good health practice but not specific to naproxen. **D.** No relationship between naproxen and fluid retention.
Nursing Process Phase: implementation; client need: safe and effective care environment; concern area: medical/surgical

41. Correct Answer: A. NSAIDs such as ibuprofen impair platelet aggregation and prolong the bleeding times.

Rationales for Other Answer Choices: B, C, D. This medication has no effect on these.
Nursing Process Phase: assessment; client need: safe and effective care environment; concern area: medical/surgical

42. Correct Answer: D. This is an antituberculosis medication that needs to be taken for at least 6 months to as much as a year to adequately treat the disease.

Rationales for Other Answer Choices: A. Clients are usually not contagious after 2 to 3 weeks of therapy. **B.** White or clay-colored stools may indicate that the rifampin is causing liver damage. **C.** Taking the medication at the same time each day promotes compliance and maintains even blood levels.
Nursing Process Phase: evaluation; client need: safe and effective care environment; concern area: medical/surgical

43. Correct Answer: C. The most serious consequence of acetaminophen overdose (OD) is liver failure, which would be indicated by an increase in bilirubin.

Rationales for Other Answer Choices: A. Potassium is not directly affected by Tylenol, although vomiting secondary to treatment for overdose may lower the potassium. **B.** Renal toxicity is another potential consequence of Tylenol OD—indicated by increased BUN. **D.** WBCs are not affected by Tylenol.
Nursing Process Phase: planning; client need: safe and effective care environment; concern area: medical/surgical

44. Correct Answer: A. When heparin is given SC, it should never be aspirated or rubbed after administration.

Rationales for Other Answer Choices: B. This is an appropriate needle for this medication. **C.** A different injection site should be selected each time. **D.** This is an appropriate location for the injection of this medication.

Nursing Process Phase: evaluation; client need: safe and effective care environment; concern area: medical/surgical

45. **Correct Answer: C.**   Allergic reactions such as urticaria, warm, flushed skin, and fever are fairly common with this medication because it is made from a protein produced by the streptococcus organism.

Rationales for Other Answer Choices: A. Not a side effect of this medication. **B.** May produce hypotension when the blood vessels open.   **D.** Not a side effect of this medication.
Nursing Process Phase: assessment; client need: safe and effective care environment; concern area: medical/surgical

46. **Correct Answer: C.**   Smoking and estrogen together increase the risk for vascular disease and clot formation.

Rationales for Other Answer Choices: A. No increase in risk with this activity. **B.** This activity decreases the risk of vascular disease.   **D.** Recent studies indicate that wine may protect the vascular system when taken in moderate amounts.
Nursing Process Phase: planning; client need: safe and effective care environment; concern area: obstetrics

47. **Correct Answer: C.**   Vivonex is an elemental formulation that contains dipeptides, tripeptides, and crystalline amino acids that require little digestion and leave no GI residue. Most appropriate for clients who have GI abnormalities, including partial bowel obstruction, inflammatory bowel disease, radiation enteritis, fistulas, or short bowel syndrome.

Rationales for Other Answer Choices: A. Ensure is polymeric formulation that is best for clients with a fully functioning GI system.   **B.** Ensure Plus is a high-calorie polymeric formulation that is best for clients with a fully functioning GI system.   **D.** Sustical is polymeric formulation that is best for clients with a fully functioning GI system.
Nursing Process Phase: planning; client need: safe and effective care environment; concern area: medical/surgical

48. **Correct Answer: C.**   Nix is a rinse that is used to treat head lice and scabies in children and adults.

Rationales for Other Answer Choices: A. Medication has no effect on intestinal parasites. **B.** An appropriate action—but is not related to the medication.   **D.** Not necessary to place the child in protective isolation for using this medication.
Nursing Process Phase: implementation; client need: safe and effective care environment; concern area: pediatrics

49. **Correct Answer: A.**   Leukeran is an alkylating antineoplastic medication used for a number of different types of cancer. One of its side effects is to raise the uric acid level and produce the symptoms of gout.

Rationales for Other Answer Choices: B. Produces hypotension as a side effect. **C.** Produces elevated temperature as side effect.   **D.** Produces diarrhea as a side effect.
Nursing Process Phase: assessment; client need: safe and effective care environment; concern area: medical/surgical

50. Correct Answer: D. A blood return is not always indicative of patency of an IV. The pain and swelling are good indicators that the IV has infiltrated.

Rationales for Other Answer Choices: A. Should be done after the IV is discontinued. **B.** Can be done after the IV is discontinued. **C.** Not an appropriate nursing action in this situation.
Nursing Process Phase: implementation; client need: safe and effective care environment; concern area: medical/surgical

Appendices

APPENDIX A

COMMONLY USED ABBREVIATIONS IN PHARMACOLOGY

a	before	IM	intramuscular
ABGs	arterial blood gases	in, in.	inches
ac	before meals	inhal., inhaln	inhalation
ACE	angiotensin-converting en-zyme	IPPB	intermittent positive pressure breathing
AD	right ear	IU	international unit
ADHD	attention deficit hyperactivity disorder	IV	intravenous
		K	potassium
agit	shake	kg	kilogram
ad lib	as desired	L, l, lit	liter
ANS	autonomic nervous system	LA	long acting
AS	left ear	liq	liquid; solution
AU	both ears	m	meter
AV	atrioventricular	µg, mcg	microgram (1/1,000,000 of a gram)
bid	two times a day		
bin	twice a night	mg	milligram (1/1000 of a gram)
BPM	beats per minute (heart rate)	min(s)	minute(s)
c	with	mL, ml	milliliter (1/1000 of a liter)
cap	capsule	mm	millimeter
CAL	chronic airway limitations (new term)	mo	month
		MS	musculoskeletal; morphine sulfate
cc	cubic centimeter (mililiter)		
CNS	central nervous system	Na	sodium
COPD	chronic obstructive pulmonary disease	neuro	neurological
		ng	nanograms
CR	controlled release	NGT	nasogastric tube
CSF	cerebral spinal fluid	noct	at night
CV	cardiovascular	OD	right eye
CVP	central venous pressure	o d	once a day; each day
d	day	oint	ointment
D/C	discontinue; stop	ophth	ophthalmic
dL, dl	deciliter (100 liters)	OS	left eye
dr, d	dram(s)	os	mouth
endo	endocrine	OTC	over-the-counter
ER	extended release	OU	both eyes
elix	elixir	oz	ounce(s)
ext	extract	p	after
g, gm, GM	gram(s)	pc	after meals
GI	gastrointestinal	PCA	patient controlled analgesia
gr	grain(s)	PO	by mouth; oral
gt(t)	drop(s)	prn	as needed
GU	genitourinary	q, Q	every
hemat	hematologic	qd	every day
h, hr	hour(s)	qh	every hour
HS, hs	hour of sleep	qid	four times a day
id	the same	qod	every other day

qwk	every week	SR	sustained release
q 15 min	every 15 minutes	ss	one half
q 1 h	every hour	stat	immediately
q 2 h	every 2 hours	supp	suppository
q 4 h	every 4 hours	syr	syrup
q 6 h	every 6 hours	tab	tablet(s)
q 8 h	every 8 hours	tb(s), T	table spoon(s)
q 12 h	every 12 hours	tid	three times a day
rect., R, or rect	rectal	top, top.	topical
resp	respiratory	tsp, t	teaspoon
RTU	ready to use	U	unit(s)
Rx	prescription	UK	unknown
s	without	ung	ointment
SC	subcutaneous	vag	vaginal
sec(s)	second(s)	wk	week
SL	sublingual	yr	year
sol or sol.	solution		

APPENDIX B

COMMONLY USED MEASUREMENT CONVERSIONS

METRIC SYSTEM EQUIVALENTS

1 gram	= 1000 milligrams
1000 grams	= 1 kilogram
0.000001 gram	= 1 microgram
1000 micrograms	= 1 milligram
1 liter	= 1000 milliliters
1 milliliter	= 1 cubic centimeter
1 meter	= 100 centimeters
1 meter	= 1000 millimeters
1 centimeter	= 10 millimeters

METRIC UNITS TO APPROXIMATE APOTHECARY EQUIVALENTS

Liquid

1 liter	= 1 quart		
500 milliliters	= 1 pint		
250 milliliters	= 1 cup (8 ounces)		
30 milliliters	= 1 ounce	= 8 fluidrams	= 450 minims
15 milliliters	= 1 tbs	= 4 fluidrams	= 225 minims
4–5 milliliters	= 1 teaspoon	= 1 fluidrams	= 60 minims
1 milliliter	= 15 minims		

Weight

1 grain	= 60 milligrams = 0.06 gram
15 grains	= 1 gram
30 grams	= 1 ounce
16 ounces	= 1 pound
1 kilogram	= 2.2 pounds
5 grains	= 300 (325) milligrams
10 grains	= 600 (650) milligrams

APPENDIX C

COMMONLY USED OR PROTOTYPICAL MEDICATIONS

acetaminophen (Tylenol)
acetazolamide Na (Diamox)
acetylcysteine (Mucomyst)
adenosine (Adenocard)
allopurinol (Zyloprim)
alprazolam (Xanax)
aluminum hydroxide (Amphogel)
aminocaproic acid (Amicar)
amiodarone (Cordarone)
amitriptyline (Elavil)
amoxicillin (Amoxil)
amphetamine (Dexedrine)
ampicillin (Omnipen, et al.)
aspirin
atropine
benztropine (Cogentin)
bisacodyl (Dulcolax)
calcium carbonate (Tums)
captopril (Capoten)
carbamazepine (Tegretol)
cefaclor (Ceclor)
cefoxitin (Mefoxin)
ceftazidime (Fortaz)
cephadrine (Anspor, Velosef)
cephalexin (Keflex)
chloral hydrate (Noctec)
chlorambucil (Leukeran)
chloramphenicol (Chloromycetin)
chlordizepoxide (Librium)
chlorothiazide (Diuril)
chlorpromazine (Thorazine)
chlorpropamide (Diabinese)
cimetidine (Tagamet)
clozapine (Clozaril)
codeine phosphate
colchicine (Novocolchine)
cyclophosphamide (Cytoxan)
dexamethasone (Decadron)
dextromethorphan (DM)
diazepam (Valium)
dicylomine HCL (Bentyl)
didanosine (ddI)
digoxin (Lanoxin)
diltiazem (Cardizem)
dimenhydrinate (Dramamine)
diphenhydramine HCL (Benadryl)

diphenoxylate HCL plus atropine (Lomotil)
disopyramide (Norpace)
dobutamine (Dobutrex)
docusate Ca (Surfak)
dopamine (Intropin)
doxepin HCL (Sinequan)
doxorubicin (Adriamycin)
doxycycline (Vibramycin)
Ensure
Epinephrine (Adrenalin)
Erythromycin (EES)
estrogen, conjugated (Premarin)
5-fluorouracil (5-FU, Adrucil)
fluoxetine (Prozac)
flurazepam (Dalmane)
furosemide (Lasix)
gentamicin (Garamycin)
glyburide (DiaBeta, Micronase)
guaifenesin (Robitussin)
haloperidol (Haldol)
heparin sodium
hydralazine (Apresoline)
hydrochlorothiazide (Dyazide)
hydrocortisone (Cortef)
hydroxyzine HCL (Atarax, Vistaril)
ibuprofen (Motrin)
imipenem (Primaxin)
indomethacin (Indocin)
insulin, premixed 30/70
insulin, NPH, lente
insulin, regular
Isoniazid (INH)
isoproterenol (Isuprel)
isosorbide (Isordil)
lactulose (Cephulac, Chronulac)
levodopa (Dopar, Larodopa)
levothyroxine (Synthroid)
lidocaine HCL (Xylocaine)
lindane (Kwell)
lithium carbonate (Esaklith)
magnesium hydroxide (Maox, Maalox)
magnesium sulfate ($MgSO_4$)
mannitol (Osmitrol)
mebendazole (Vermox)
meperidine (Demerol)
metaproterenol (Alupent)

methyldopa (Aldomet)
methylergonovine maleate (Ergometrine)
methylphenidate (Ritalin)
methylprednisolone (Solu-Medrol)
metociopramide (Reglan)
metoprolol (Lopressor)
metronidazole (Flagyl)
morphine sulfate
nadolol (Corgard)
nitroglycerin (NTG)
nystatin (Mycostatin)
orphenadrine citrate (Norflex)
oxazepam (Serax)
oxytocin (Pitocin)
permethrin (Nix)
phenobarbital (Luminal)
phenylephrine HCL (Neo-Synephrine)
phenytoin (Dilantin)
pilocarpine HCL (Isopto Carpine)
potassium chloride (KCL, K-Tabs)
prazosin (Minipress)
prednisone (Deltasone)
primidone (Mysoline)
probenecid (Benemid)
prochlorperazine (Compazine)
promethazine HCL (Phenergan)
propranolol (Inderal)
propylthiouracil (Propacil)

protamine sulfate
psyllium (Metamucil)
Pyridoxine (vitamin B_6)
ranitidine (Zantac)
rifampin (Rifadin)
ritrodrine HCL (Yutopar)
silver sulfadiazine (Silvadine)
streptokinase (Streptase)
streptomycin
sucralfate (Carafate)
sulfadiazine
sulfamethoxazole/trimethoprim (Bactrim, Septra)
Sustical
temazepam (Restoril)
tetracycline (Achromycin)
theophylline (Aminophylline)
thiothixene (Navane)
timolol maleate (Timoptic)
tissue plasminogen activator (alteplase, t-PA)
tocainide HCL (Tonocard)
triacetin (Fungoid)
trihexphenidyl (Artane)
trimethobenzamide (Tigan)
verapamil (Calan)
vincristine (Oncovin)
Vivonex
warfarin sodium (Coumadin)
zidovudine (AZT, Retrovir)

APPENDIX D

TABLE OF MEDICATION DOSAGES, ROUTES, AND FETAL RISK CATEGORIES

Medication	Common Route	Adult Dose	Pediatric Dose	Fetal Risk Category
Acetaminophen (Tylenol)	PO	325–1000 mg 4–6 h	Depends on age and weight	B
acetazolamide Na (Diamox)	PO, IM, IV	60–250 mg q 4 h	10–15 mg/kg q 4–6 h	C
acetylcysteine (Mucomyst)	Inhal. PO	1–10 mL 20% sol 5.2 g q 4 h	1–5 mL 20% sol 70 mg/kg q 4 h	B
adenosine (Adenocard)	IV	6 mg IV bolus—repeat in 1–2 min if no results	Not approved for use	C
allopurinol (Zyloprim)	PO	100–200 mg, q 8–q 12 h	<50 mg tid	C
alprazolam (Xanax)	PO	0.25–0.5 mg q 8 to q 12 h	Not approved for use	D
aluminum hydroxide (Amphogel)	PO	30–40 mL q 6 h	50–150 mg/kg in 24 h, divided doses	Unknown
aminocaproic acid (Amicar)	PO, IV	5 g 1st h then 1 g/h	100 mg/kg 1st h then 33.3 mg/kg/h	C
amiodarone (Cordarone)	PO, IV	400 mg qd	10 mg/kg/d	D
amitriptyline (Elavil)	PO	30–100 mg qd HS	1–5 mg/kg/d	C
amoxicillin (Amoxil)	PO	200–500 mg q 8 h	6.7–13.3 mg/kg q 8 h	B
amphetamine (Dexedrine)	PO	5–20 mg qd q 8 h	5 mg q 12 h	C
ampicillin (Omnipen, et al.)	PO, IM, IV	250–300 mg q 6 h	20–50 mg/kg q 6 h	B
aspirin	PO	325–1000 mg q 6 h	60–80 mg/kg q 6 h	D
atropine	IM, IV	0.5–1 mg q 15 min	0.02 mg/kg	C
Benztropine (Cogentin)	PO	0.25–3 mg q 12 h	Not approved for use	C
bisacodyl (Dulcolax)	PO, rect.	5–15 mg qd	5–10 mg qd	Unknown
calcium carbonate (Tums)	PO	1–2 g/d	45–65 mg/kg/d	C
captopril (Capoten)	PO	12.5–25 mg q 8–12 h	0.3 mg/kg q 8 h	D
carbamazepine (Tegretol)	PO	100–200 mg q 6–12 h	10–20 mg/kg q 8–12 h	C
cefaclor (Ceclor)	PO	250–500 mg q 8 h	6.7–13.4 mg/kg q 8 h	B
cefoxitin (Mefoxin)	IM, IV	1000–2000 mg q 6–8 h	13.7–26.7 mg/kg q 4–6 h	B
ceftazidime (Fortaz)	IM, IV	500–2000 mg q 8–12 h	30–50 mg/kg q 8 h	B
cephadrine (Anspor, Velosef)	PO	250–500 mg q 6 h	6.25–25 mg/kg q 6 h	B
cephalexin (Keflex)	PO	250–500 mg q 6 h	6.25–25 mg/kg q 6 h	B
chloral hydrate (Noctec)	PO	500–1000 mg qd HS	25 mg/kg qd HS	C
chlorambucil (Leukeran)	PO	0.1–0.2 mg/kg/d	0.1–0.2 mg/kg/d	D
chloramphenicol (Chloromycetin)	PO, IV	1000 mg q 6 h	12 mg/kg q 6 h	Unknown
chlordizepoxide (Librium)	PO	5–100 mg q 4–12 h	5–10 mg q 6–12 h	D

Medication	Common Route	Adult Dose	Pediatric Dose	Fetal Risk Category
chlorothiazide (Diuril)	PO	2.5–10 mg qd q 12 h	0.4 mg/kg qd q 12 h	B
chlorpromazine (Thorazine)	PO, IM	10–25 mg q 6–12 h	0.55 mg/kg q 4–6 h	Unknown
chlorpropamide (Diabinese)	PO	125–250 mg q 8–12 h	Not approved for use	C
cimetidine (Tagamet)	PO, IV	300 mg q 6 h	20–40 mg/kg q 6 h	B
clozapine (Clozaril)	PO	300–450 mg qd	Not used	B
codeine phosphate	PO, IM	10–60 mg q 4–6 h	0.5 mg/kg q 4–6 h	C
colchicine (Novocolchine)	PO	0.5–1.2 mg q 1–2 h	Not approved for use	C
cyclophosphamide (Cytoxan)	PO, IV	750–1000 mg q 4 h × 6 d	2–8 mg/kg/day × 6 d	C
dexamethasone (Decadron)	PO, IV, top	4–25 mg q 6–12 h	0.56 mg/kg qd	B
dextromethorphan (DM)	PO	10–20 mg q 4 h	5–10 mg q 4 h	Unknown
diazepam (Valium)	PO, IV	2–10 mg q 6–12 h	1–2.5 mg q 6–8 h	D
dicylomine HCL (Bentyl)	PO	10–20 mg q 6–8 h	5–10 mg q 4–6 h	B
didanosine (ddl)	PO	125–200 mg q 12 h	75–100 mg q 8–12 h	B
digoxin (Lanoxin)	PO, IV	0.125–0.25 mg qd	20–35 μg/kg/d	C
diltiazem (Cardizem)	PO	30–120 mg q 6–8 h	Not approved for use	C
dimenhydrinate (Dramamine)	PO, IV	50–100 mg q 4 h	25–50 mg q 4 h	B
diphenhydramine HCL (Benadryl)	PO, IV	25–50 mg q 4–6 h	12.5–25 mg q 4 h	B
diphenoxylate HCL plus atropine (Lomotil)	PO	1–2 tab q 3–4 h	0.075–0.1 mg/kg q 6 h	C
disopyramide (Norpace)	PO	150 mg q 6 h	6–25 mg/kg/d	C
dobutamine (Dobutrex)	IV	2.5–10 μg/kg/min	5–20 μg/kg/min	C
docusate Ca (Surfak)	PO, rect.	240 mg qd	50–150 mg qd	D
dopamine (Intropin)	IV	0.5–10 μg/kg/min	5–20 μg/kg/min	C
doxepin HCL (Sinequan)	PO	25 mg q 8 h	Not approved for use	C
doxorubicin (Adriamycin)	IV	60–75 mg/m^2 qd	30 mg/m^2 qd	D
doxycycline (Vibramycin)	PO	50–200 mg qd q 12 h	2.2–4.4 mg/kg/d	Unknown
Ensure	PO	240 mL qd q 6 h	50–240 mL q 6 h	Unknown
Epinephrine (Adrenalin)	IV, inhal.	12.5–50 mg q 3–4 h	3 mg/kg/d	C
erythromycin (EES, Erythrocin)	PO, IV	250–500 mg q 6 h	3.75–5 mg/kg q 6 h	B
estrogen, conjugated (Premarin)	PO	0.625–7.5 mg qd	Not approved for use	X
5-fluorouracil (5-FU, Adrucil)	IV	500–1000 mg/d × 5 d	Not approved for use	D
fluoxetine (Prozac)	PO	20 mg qd in A.M.	Not approved for use	B
flurazepam (Dalmane)	PO	15–30 mg qd HS	Not approved for use	X
furosemide (Lasix)	PO, IV	20–80 mg qd q 12 h	2 mg/kg/d	C
gentamicin (Garamycin)	IV	75–200 mg q 8 h	2–2.5 mg/kg q 8 h	D
glyburide (DiaBeta, Micronase)	PO	2.5–20 mg qd	Not approved for use	C

Medication	Common Route	Adult Dose	Pediatric Dose	Fetal Risk Category
guaifenesin (Robitussin)	PO	200–400 mg q 4 h	50–100 mg q 4 h	C
haloperidol (Haldol)	PO, IM	0.5–5 mg q 8–12 h	50 μg/kg/d	C
heparin sodium	IV, SC	5000–10,000 U q 4 h; 750–1500 U/h drip	50 U/kg q 4 h	B
hydralazine (Apresoline)	PO, IV	10–25 mg q 6–12 h	0.75 mg/kg/d	C
hydrochlorothiazide (Dyazide)	PO	25–100 mg qd q 12 h	1–3 mg/kg/d	Unknown
hydrocortisone (Cortef)	PO, IV, top	20–240 mg q 4–6 h	0.56 mg/kg q 6 h	B
hydroxyzine HCL (Atarax, Vistaril)	PO, IM	25–100 mg q 6–8 h	0.6 mg q 6–8 h	C
ibuprofen (Motrin)	PO	300–800 mg q 6–8 h	20–40 mg/kg/d	B
imipenem (Primaxin)	IV, IM	250–1000 mg q 6–8 h	Not approved for use	C
indomethacin (Indocin)	PO	25–50 mg q 6–12 h	1.5–2.5 mg/kg/d	B
insulin, premixed 30/70	SC	1–35 U qd q 12 h	0.5–1 U/kg/d	B
insulin, NPH, lente	SC	1–30 U qd q 12 h	0.5–1 U/kg/d	B
insulin, regular	SC, IV	1–25 U q 6 h	0.5–1 U/kg/d	B
isoniazid (INH)	PO	300–900 mg qd × 6–12 mo	10–20 mg/kg/d	C
isoproterenol (Isuprel)	IV, inhal.	1–200 μg/5 μg/min drip	0.1 μg/kg/min	C
isosorbide (Isordil)	PO	10–40 mg q 6 h	Not approved for use	C
lactulose (Cephulac, Chronulac)	PO	15–30 mL q 6–12 h	Not approved for use	B
levodopa (Dopar)	PO	250–750 mg q 6–12 h	Not approved for use	Unknown
levothyroxine (Synthroid)	PO	75–125 μg qd	2–5 μg/kg/d	A
lidocaine HCL (Xylocaine)	IV	50–100 mg bolus/2–4 mg/min drip	1 mg/kg bolus/30 μg/kg drip	B
lindane (Kwell)	top	15–30 mL of 1% shampoo	15–30 mL of 1% shampoo	B
lithium carbonate (Eskalith)	PO	300 mg q 6–8 h	0.4–0.5 mEq/kg/d	D
magnesium hydroxide (Maox, Maalox)	PO	30–60 mL qd	15–30 mL qd	Unknown
magnesium sulfate (MgSO$_4$)	IV	4 g bolus then 1–2 g/h drip	2–10 mEq for deficiency	D
mannitol (Osmitrol)	IV	50–100 g over 30–60 min	0.25–2 g/kg over 2–6 h	C
mebendazole (Vermox)	PO	100 mg q 12 h × 3 d	100 mg q 12 h × 3 d	C
meperidine (Demerol)	PO, IM, IV	50–150 mg q 4–6 h	1–2.2 mg/kg q 4–6 h	B
metaproterenol (Alupent)	Inhal., PO	20 mg q 6–8 h	10 mg q 6–8 h	C
methyldopa (Aldomet)	PO, IV	250–500 mg q 8–12 h	10 mg/kg/d	B
methylergonovine maleate (Ergometrine)	PO, IV	200–400 μg q 6–12 h × 2–7 d	Not approved for use	C
methylphenidate (Ritalin)	PO	5–20 mg q 8–12 h	5–15 mg q 8–12 h	C

Medication	Common Route	Adult Dose	Pediatric Dose	Fetal Risk Category
methylprednisolone (Solu-Medrol)	PO, IM, IV	40–1000 mg q 6–12 h	117 µg/kg q 6–8 h	B
metoclopramide (Reglan)	PO, IM	10 mg 30 min before meal	2.5–5 mg before meal	B
metoprolol (Lopressor)	PO, IV	50–100 mg qd q 12 h	Not approved for use	B
metronidazole (Flagyl)	PO, IV	250–750 mg q 6 h	5 mg/kg q 8 h	B
morphine sulfate	PO, IV SC	2–30 mg q 4–6 h	0.025–2.6 mg/kg	C
nadolol (Corgard)	PO	40–80 mg qd	Not approved for use	C
nitroglycerin (NTG)	SL, IV	0.6 mg SL q 5 min × 3/5–20 µg/min drip	Not approved for use	C
nystatin (Mycostatin)	PO	400,000–600,000 U q 6 h	100,000–200,000 U q 6 h	B
orphenadrine citrate (Norflex)	PO	50 mg q 8 h	Not approved for use	Unknown
oxazepam (Serax)	PO	10–30 mg q 6–8 h	Not approved for use	D
oxytocin (Pitocin)	IV	0.5–20 milliunits/min	Not approved for use	Unknown
permethrin (Nix)	Top	5% cream/1% rinse for 10 min × 1	Use with caution	B
phenobarbital (Luminal)	PO, IV	30–75 mg q 8–12 h	1–6 mg/kg/d	D
phenylephrine HCL (Neo-Synephrine)	Nasal mucosa	1–2 sprays q 6 h	Not approved for use	C
phenytoin (Dilantin)	PO, IV	100–200 mg q 8 h	4–8 mg/kg/d	C
pilocarpine HCL (Isopto Carpine)	opth	1–2 drops q 6–12 h	Not approved for use	C
potassium chloride (KCL, K-Tabs)	PO, IV	20–40 mEq q 8–12 h	3 mEq/kg/d	C
prazosin (Minipress)	PO	0.5–5 mg q 8–12 h	50–400 µg/kg/d	C
prednisone (Deltasone)	PO	5–20 mg q 6–12 h	0.14–2 mg/kg/d	B
primidone (Mysoline)	PO	100–250 mg q 6–8 h	10–25 mg/kg/d	C
probenecid (Benemid)	PO	250–500 mg q 6–12 h	25 mg/kg q 6 h	B
prochlorperazine (Compazine)	PO, IV, IM	5–10 mg q 4–6 h	132 mg/kg q 4–6 h	C
promethazine HCL (Phenergan)	PO, IM	10–25 mg q 4–6 h	0.25–0.5 mg/kg q 4–6 h	C
propranolol (Inderal)	PO	20–80 mg q 6–12 h	10–100 µg/kg q 6–8 h	C
propylthiouracil (Propacil)	PO	50–600 mg qd	25–150 mg qd q 6 h	D
protamine sulfate	IV	1 mg/100 U heparin	1 mg/100 U heparin	C
psyllium (Metamucil)	PO	3–6 g q 8–12 h	1.5–3 g q 8–12 h	Unknown
pyridoxine (vitamin B$_6$)	PO, IM, IV	10–20 mg qd	2.5–10 mg qd	A
ranitidine (Zantac)	PO, IV	100–150 mg q 12 h	Not approved for use	B
rifampin (Rifadin)	PO	600 mg qd	10–20 mg/kg/d	C
ritrodrine HCL (Yutopar)	IV	50–350 µg/min	Not approved for use	Unknown

Medication	Common Route	Adult Dose	Pediatric Dose	Fetal Risk Category
silver sulfadiazine (Silvadine)	top	1% cream q 12 h	1% cream q 12 h	B
streptokinase (Streptase)	IV	250,000–1,500,000 U over 10–20 min × 1	Not approved for use	C
streptomycin	IM	500–2000 mg q 12 h	20 mg/kg/d	D
sucralfate (Carafate)	PO	1000 mg AC and HS	500–1000 mg AC and HS	B
sulfadiazine	PO	250–500 mg q 6–8 h	100–150 mg/kg q 6 h	C
sulfamethoxazole/trimethoprim (Bactrim, Septra)	PO	500–1000 mg q 8–12 h	50–60 mg/kg/d	C
Sustical	PO	240 mL q 6–12 h	No dosage recommended	Unknown
temazepam (Restoril)	PO	15–30 mg HS	Not approved for use	X
tetracycline (Achromycin)	PO	250–500 mg q 6 h	6.25–12.5 mg/kg q 6 h	Unknown
theophylline (Aminophylline)	IV, PO	100–200 mg q 6–8 h	5 mg/kg/d	B
thiothixene (Navane)	PO	2–20 mg q 8 h	Not approved for use	Unknown
timolol maleate (Timoptic)	ophth	1 gt of 0.25%–5% sol q 6–12 h	1 gt of 0.25%–5% sol q 6–12 h	C
tissue plasminogen activator (alteplase, t-PA)	IV	100 mg over 3 h	Not approved for use	C
tocainide HCL (Tonocard)	PO	400 mg q 8 h	Not approved for use	C
triacetin (Fungoid)	Top	Apply cream q 8 h	Apply cream q 8 h	C
trihexyphenidyl (Artane)	PO	1–5 mg q 6–8 h	Not approved for use	C
trimethobenzamide (Tigan)	IM	250 mg q 6–8 h	100–200 mg q 6–8 h	C
verapamil (Calan)	PO, IV	80–120 mg q 8 h	4–8 mg/kg/d	C
vincristine (Oncovin)	IV	10–30 μg/kg q wk	1.5–2 mg/m^2 q wk	D
Vivonex	PO, NGT	20–30 mL/h	10–30 mL/h	Unknown
warfarin sodium (Coumadin)	PO	2–10 mg qd	Not approved for use	Unknown
zidovudine (AZT, Retrovir)	PO	100 mg q 4 h	180 mg/m^2 q 6 h	C

APPENDIX E

MEDICATIONS GROUPED BY NCLEX-RN CONTENT AREA

MEDICATIONS COMMONLY USED IN PSYCHIATRIC NURSING

acetaminophen (Tylenol)
alprazolam (Xanax)
amitriptyline (Elavil)
amphetamine (Dexedrine)
benztropine (Cogentin)
bisacodyl (Dulcolax)
carbamazepine (Tegretol)
chloral hydrate (Noctec)
chlordizepoxide (Librium)
chlorpromazine (Thorazine)
clozapine (Clozaril)
diazepam (Valium)
dicylomine HCL (Bentyl)
docusate Ca (Surfak)
doxepin HCL (Sinequan)
fluoxetine (Prozac)
flurazepam (Dalmane)
haloperidol (Haldol)
hydroxyzine HCL (Atarax, Vistaril)
ibuprofen (Motrin)
lithium carbonate (Eskalith)
methylphenidate (Ritalin)
oxazepam (Serax)
phenobarbital (Luminal)
phenytoin (Dilantin)
prochlorperazine (Compazine)
promethazine HCL (Phenergan)
psyllium (Metamucil)
temazepam (Restoril)
thiothixene (Navane)
trihexphenidyl (Artane)

MEDICATIONS COMMONLY USED IN OBSTETRIC NURSING

acetaminophen (Tylenol)
aluminum hydroxide (Amphogel)
amoxicillin (Amoxil)
ampicillin (Omnipen, et al.)
bisacodyl (Dulcolax)
calcium carbonate (Tums)

cefaclor (Ceclor)
cefoxitin (Mefoxin)
ceftazidime (Fortaz)
cephadrine (Anspor, Velosef)
cephalexin (Keflex)
dimenhydrinate (Dramamine)
diphenhydramine HCL (Benadryl)
estrogen, conjugate (Premarin)
hydrocortisone (Cortef)
hydroxyzine HCL (Atarax, Vistaril)
ibuprofen (Motrin)
imipenem (Primaxin)
magnesium hydroxide (Maox, Maalox)
magnesium sulfate ($MgSO_4$)
meperidine (Demerol)
methyldopa (Aldomet)
methylergonovine maleate (Ergometrine)
oxytocin (Pitocin)
psyllium (Metamucil)
ritrodrine HCL (Yutopar)
sulfamethoxazole/trimethoprim (Bactrim, Septra)

MEDICATIONS COMMONLY USED IN PEDIATRIC NURSING

acetaminophen (Tylenol)
acetylcysteine (Mucomyst)
amoxicillin (Amoxil)
amphetamine (Dexedrine)
ampicillin (Omnipen, et al.)
carbamazepine (Tegretol)
cefaclor (Ceclor)
cefoxitin (Mefoxin)
ceftazidime (Fortaz)
cephadrine (Anspor, Velosef)
cephalexin (Keflex)
chlorambucil (Leukeran)
chloramphenicol (Chloromycetin)
codeine phosphate
cyclophosphamide (Cytoxin)
dexamethasone (Decadron)
dextromethorphan (DM)
didanosine (ddI)

digoxin (Lanoxin)
dimenhydrinate (Dramamine)
diphenhydramine HCL (Benadryl)
diphenoxylate HCL plus atropine (Lomotil)
doxorubicin (Adriamycin)
doxycycline (Vibramycin)
epinephrine (Adrenalin)
erythromycin (EES)
5-fluorouracil (5-FU, Adrucil)
furosemide (Lasix)
gentamicin (Garamycin)
guaifenesin (Robitussin)
hydrocortisone (Cortef)
hydroxyzine HCL (Atarax, Vistaril)
ibuprofen (Motrin)
imipenem (Primaxin)
indomethacin (Indocin)
insulin, premixed 30/70
insulin, NPH, lente
insulin, regular
isoniazid (INH)
isoproterenol (Isuprel)
lindane (Kwell)
mannitol (Osmitrol)
mebendazole (Vermox)
meperidine (Demerol)
metaproterenol (Alupent)
methylphenidate (Ritalin)
methylprednisone (Solu-Medrol)
metronidazole (Flagyl)
morphine sulfate
nystatin (Mycostatin)
permethrin (Nix)
phenobarbital (Luminal)
phenylephrine HCL (Neo-Synephrine)
phenytoin (Dilantin)
potassium chloride (KCL, K-Tabs)
primidone (Mysoline)
prochlorperazine (Compazine)
promethazine HCL (Phenergan)
rifampin (Rifadin)
silver sulfadiazine (Silvadine)
streptomycin
sulfadiazine
sulfamethoxazole/trimethoprim (Bactrim, Septra)
tetracycline
theophylline (Aminophylline)
triacetin (Fungoid)
trimethobenzamide (Tigan)
vincristine (Oncovin)

MEDICATIONS COMMONLY USED IN ADULT MEDICAL/SURGICAL NURSING

acetaminophen (Tylenol)
acetazolamide Na (Diamox)
acetylcysteine (Mucomyst)
adenosine (Adenocard)
allopurinol (Zyloprim)
alprazolam (Xanax)
aluminum hydroxide (Amphogel)
aminocaproic acid (Amicar)
amiodarone (Cordarone)
amitriptyline (Elavil)
amoxicillin (Amoxil)
ampicillin (Omnipen, et al.)
aspirin
atropine
benztropine (Cogentin)
bisacodyl (Dulcolax)
calcium carbonate (Tums)
captopril (Capoten)
carbamazepine (Tegretol)
cafaclor (Ceclor)
cefoxitin (Mefoxin)
ceftazidime (Fortaz)
cephadrine (Anspor, Velosef)
cephalexin (Keflex)
chloral hydrate (Noctec)
chlorambucil (Leukeran)
chloramphenicol (Chloromycetin)
chlordizepoxide (Librium)
chlorothiazide (Diuril)
chlorpropamide (Diabinese)
cimetidine (Tagamet)
codeine phosphate
colchicine (Novocolchine)
cyclophosphamide (Cytoxin)
dexamethasone (Decadron)
dextromethorphan (DM)
diazepam (Valium)
dicylomine HCL (Bentyl)
didanosine (ddI)
digoxin (Lanoxin)
diltiazem (Cardizem)
dimenhydrinate (Dramamine)
diphenhydramine HCL (Benadryl)
diphenoxylate HCL plus atropine (Lomotil)
disopyramide (Norpace)
dobutamine (Dobutrex)
docusate Ca (Surfak)
dopamine (Intropin)

doxorubicin (Adriamycin)
doxycycline (Vibramycin)
Ensure
epinephrine (Adrenalin)
erythromycin (EES)
estrogen, conjugated (Premarin)
5-fluorouracil (5-FU, Adrucil)
fluoxetine (Prozac)
flurazepam (Dalmane)
furosemide (Lasix)
gentamicin (Garamycin)
glyburide (DiaBeta, Micronase)
guaifenesin (Robitussin)
heparin sodium
hydralazine (Apresoline)
hydrochlorothiazide (Dyazide)
hydrocortisone (Cortef)
hydroxyzine HCL (Atarax, Vistaril)
ibuprofen (Motrin)
imipenem (Primaxin)
indomethacin (Indocin)
insulin, premixed 30/70
insulin, NPH, lente
insulin, regular
isoniazid (INH)
isoproterenol (Isuprel)
isosorbide (Isordil)
lactulose (Cephulac, Chronulac)
levodopa (Dopar, Larodopa)
levothyroxine (Synthroid)
lidocaine HCL (Xylocaine)
lithium carbonate (Eskßalith)
magnesium hydroxide (Maox, Maalox)
mannitol (Osmitrol)
meperidine (Demerol)
metaproterenol (Alupent)
methyldopa (Aldomet)
methylergonovine maleate (Ergometrine)
methylprednisone (Solu-Medrol)
metociopramide (Reglan)
metoprolol (Lopressor)
metronidazole (Flagyl)
morphine sulfate
nadolol (Corgard)

nitroglycerin (NTG)
nystatin (Mycostatin)
orphenadrine citrate (Norflex)
oxazepam (Serax)
phenobarbital (Luminal)
phenylephrine HCL (Neo-Synephrine)
phenytoin (Dilantin)
pilocarpine HCL (Isopto Carpine)
potassium chloride (KCL, K-Tabs)
prazosin (Minipress)
prednisone (Deltasone)
primidone (Mysoline)
probenecid (Benemid)
prochlorperazine (Compazine)
promethazine HCL (Phenergan)
propranolol (Inderal)
propylthiouracil (Propacil)
protamine sulfate
psyllium (Metamucil)
pyridoxine (vitamin B_6)
ranitidine (Zantac)
rifampin (Rifadin)
ritrodrine HCL (Yutopar)
silver sulfadiazine (Silvadine)
streptokinase (Streptase)
streptomycin
sucralfate (Carafate)
sulfadiazine
sulfamethoxazole/trimethoprim (Bactrim, Septra)
Sustical
temazepam (Restoril)
tetracycline
theophylline (Aminophylline)
timolol maleate (Timoptic)
tissue plasminogen activator (alteplase, t-PA)
tocainide HCL (Tonocard)
triacetin (Fungoid)
trihexphenidyl (Artane)
trimethobenzamide (Tigan)
verapamil (Calan)
vincristine (Oncovin)
Vivonex
warfarin sodium (Coumadin)
zidovudine (AZT, Retrovir)

GLOSSARY

Absorption   The process by which a medication leaves the gastrointestinal tract and enters the circulatory system or body fluids.

Acetylcholine   The neurotransmitter of the parasympathetic and somatic nervous systems.

Acidosis   A disturbance of the acid-base balance of the body with a shift toward the acid state; indicated by a low pH.

Additive interaction   A type of interaction that occurs when the end effect of two medications given at the same time is equivalent to the sum effect of each medication; lower doses of each medication can be given; decreases the side effects of each medication.

Administering medications   Any action that leads to the introduction of medication into the client's body (usual role of nurses, although most individuals who prescribe medications can also administer them).

Adrenergic   Relating to sympathetic neurons that release norepinephrine.

Adverse effect (side effect)   An unintended, unpredictable, and potentially injurious response to a medication's action. Adverse effects generally result from direct toxic medication effects, idiosyncrasies, hypersensitivity reactions, and noncompliance.

AIDS (acquired immune deficiency syndrome)   The disease syndrome caused by human immunodeficiency virus (HIV) virus.

Affinity   Tendency of a medication to attach or bind itself to a particular receptor site.

Afterload   The resistance to the blood that is being ejected by the left ventricle.

Agonist   A medication with high affinity for the receptor site and high intrinsic activity; causes a pharmacological effect by its interaction with a specific receptor site.

Agranulocytosis   A decrease in, or absence of, granulocytes (a type of white blood cell).

Alkalosis   A disturbance in the acid-base balance in the body with a shift toward the base; a high pH.

Allergy   An acquired sensitivity to medications that involves an antigen-antibody type reaction.

Alpha receptors   Adrenergic receptors that are stimulated by norepinephrine and epinephrine, with the exception of the receptors of the heart.

Amenorrhea   The absence of menstrual periods.

Analgesia   Relief of pain.

Analgesic   A medication that lessens the sensation of pain.

Anaplasia   The loss of cell differentiation found in cancer cells that allows them to reproduce cells different from the parent cells, often more primitive in structure.

Anaphylactic reaction   A sudden, severe allergic reaction that causes hypotension, shock, bronchoconstriction, and often death; constitutes a medical emergency.

Anasarca   Generalized body edema often seen in renal disease or long-term right-side congestive heart failure.

Angina pectoris   Pain in the chest caused by myocardial ischemia; usually occurs suddenly because of physical exertion or emotional stress.

Angioneurotic edema   Localized wheals or swellings occurring in subcutaneous tissue or mucous membrane probably as an allergic response to a medication or substance.

Anorexia   Loss of appetite.

Antagonist   A medication with high affinity for the receptor but minimal or no intrinsic activity; capable of preventing or reducing activity at the receptor site; may also be called a blocking agent.

Antagonist interaction   A type of interaction that occurs when the effects of two medications given at the same time cancel each other; the end result is that neither medication will produce its desired effect.

Antibacterial   Against bacteria.

Antibiotic   A medication that destroys or slows the multiplication rate of organisms.

Anticholinergic   A medication that blocks the interaction of acetylcholine with its receptor, resulting in a decrease of parasympathetic activity.

Anticoagulant   A medication that decreases the ability of the blood to clot or coagulate.

Anticonvulsant   A medication that will prevent or stop a convulsion or epileptic seizure.

Antiemetic   A medication given to relieve or prevent nausea and vomiting.

Antiepileptic   A medication that, when given prophylactically, prevents or lessens the incidence of epileptic seizures.

Antimicrobial   A medication that prevents the multiplication of microorganisms or destroys them.

Antineoplastic   A substance or medication that prevents or inhibits the growth of cancerous cells or tumors.

Antipyretic   A medication that reduces an elevated body temperature (fever).

Anxiety   A normal response to a stressful situation that may manifest itself as apprehension, fear, nervousness, emotional and physical tension, and a generalized uneasy feeling.

Aplastic anemia   A blood disorder caused by damage to the bone marrow resulting in a marked reduction in the number of red blood cells and some white cells.

Arterioles   Small arteries.

Ataxia   Loss of muscular coordination.

Axon   The longest part of the neuron; it relays the impulses to the dendrites of the next neuron.

Bacteria   Single-cell organisms without a true nucleus or functionally specific components of metabolism and that require a host to supply food and a supportive environment for reproduction.

Bacteriocidal   An antimicrobial medication that kills bacteria.

Bacteriostatic   An antimicrobial medication that arrests or inhibits the growth of bacteria.

Beta receptors   Adrenergic receptors that produce inhibition or relaxation when stimulated by epinephrine ($beta_2$ receptors) and the adrenergic receptors of the heart ($beta_1$ receptors) that produce excitation when stimulated by epinephrine.

Bioavailability   The fraction of unchanged medication that reaches the systemic circulation.

Biotransformation   Metabolic changes that occur following drug absorption and distribution; they convert the medication into products that are usually less active and that can be more readily excreted.

Bradycardia   Slow pulse rate, usually less than 60 BPM in an adult and 90 BPM in a child or infant.

Bronchospasm   A sudden, severe constriction of the bronchi resulting in airway restriction and difficulty in breathing.

Catecholamine   The neurotransmitters of the sympathetic nervous system, norepinephrine and epinephrine, and dopamine.

Carcinogen   A cancer-producing substance or drug.

Carcinoma   Cancer.

Cardiac output (CO)   The amount of blood measured in liters that is ejected from the left ventricle each minute; CO = HR (BPM) × S-V (mL/beat).

Chemotherapy   The use of medications to treat infectious diseases and cancer.

Cholinergics   Neurons of the parasympathetic and somatic nervous systems that release acetylcholine.

Chronotropic   A medication that affects the heart rate in either a positive (increased heart rate) or a negative (decreased heart rate) way.

Cinchonism A toxic condition characterized by headache, tinnitus, and deafness caused by overdose of cinchona alkaloids (quinine or quinidine).

Constipation A condition that exists when a client has decreased frequency and/or passage of hard, dry stools.

Convulsion The abnormal muscular activity that results from certain types of seizures.

Crystalluria The presence of crystals in the urine; refers especially to crystals of the sulfa medications that cause kidney damage.

Desired (expected) reaction The reason a medication is being used (therapeutic effect).

Diabetes mellitus A disease condition characterized by a lack of insulin, which results in hyperglycemia, glycosuria, and ketoacidosis.

Diarrhea A sudden increase in the number of stools that are often liquid and may be greenish.

Diplopia Double vision.

Dispensing medications The act of distributing a supply of medications to a client (usual role for a pharmacist).

Diuresis Production and passage of abnormally large amounts of urine.

Diuretic A medication that promotes the excretion of water and electrolytes.

Dyscrasia A general term used to describe an abnormal condition of the blood.

Dysmenorrhea Painful menstruation.

Dysrhythmia (arrhythmia) A general term that refers to abnormalities in the ECG pattern produced by the heart.

Dystocia (of labor) A difficult or abnormal labor.

Edema The retention of excess fluid in body tissues.

Endogenous Produced by the body.

Epilepsy A disorder of electrical activity of the brain resulting in the occurrence of periods of unconsciousness, seizures, and convulsions.

Epinephrine Also referred to as adrenaline; it is the main hormone of the adrenal medulla that stimulates the sympathetic nervous system.

Exogenous Originating outside of an organ or part; originating outside of the body.

Extrapyramidal symptoms (EPS) A group of symptoms consisting of pseudoparkinsonism (the slowing of volitional movements is also called akinesia: mask facies, rigidity, tremor at rest, and pill-rolling motions with the fingers); acute dystonia (abnormal posturing, grimacing, spastic torticollis, and oculogyric crisis); akathisia (compelling need to move without specific pattern, inability to sit still); and tardive dyskinesia (involuntary rhythmic bizarre movements of face, jaw, mouth, tongue, and sometimes extremities).

Extravasation The escape of IV fluid into surrounding tissue, causing damage to the tissue; infiltration.

First-order kinetics (kill rate) The percentage of cancer cells that are killed each time the medication is given.

Fungus (pl. fungi) Plant-type organisms that take the form of yeast, mold, or mushroom.

Fungicidal A substance or medication that kills fungi.

Fungistatic A substance or medication that inhibits the growth of fungi.

Gastritis Inflammation of the mucosal lining of the stomach caused by alcohol, salicylate, infection, oral steroid medications, or stress.

Gout A hereditary form of arthritis in which serum uric acid levels increase to a point where uric acid crystals are deposited in the joints (normal uric acid = 2.3–7 mg/dL).

Glaucoma An eye disease characterized by increased intraocular pressure associated with progressive loss of the peripheral visual fields.

Glossitis Inflammation of the tongue.

Glucocorticoids Natural or synthetic steroid hormones (adrenal cortex) which alter glucose metabolism; these steroids are also used as anti-inflammatory medications.

Glycosuria The presence of sugar in the urine.

Grand mal (tonic-clonic) A type of generalized epileptic seizure resulting in convulsions and loss of consciousness.

Granulocytopenia A reduction or decrease in the number of granulocytes (a type of white blood cell).

Half-life The time required for medication concentration in plasma or total body to decline by one half. The concept of half-life is important in time determinations of steady state and clearance of medication from the body in overdose.

Hematuria Blood in the urine.

Histamine A substance found mainly in mast cells; plays a vital role in mediating inflammatory and allergic reactions. Two types: histamine$_1$ and histamine$_2$.

Hyperglycemia A blood-glucose level that is above normal.

Hyperkalemia Serum potassium level that is above normal.

Hyperlipidemia A lipid or fat level in the blood that is above normal.

Hypernatremia A serum sodium level that is above normal.

Hypersensitivity An allergic-type reaction that is due to previous sensitization to a substance or medication.

Hyperuricemia Usually associated with gout, in which there are abnormally high levels of uric acid in the blood.

Hypnotic A medication that induces sleep.

Hypocalcemia Below normal blood calcium levels.

Hypoglycemia Below normal blood glucose level.

Hypokalemia Below normal blood potassium level.

Hyponatremia Below normal blood sodium level.

Hypotension, orthostatic A decrease in blood pressure occurring after standing in one place for an extended period of time.

Hypotension, postural A decrease in blood pressure following a sudden change in body position.

Iatrogenic reaction (effect) A reaction that occurs when a condition is produced by a medication that mimics a pathological disorder.

Idiosyncrasy An unusual and usually unpredictable response to a medication caused by a genetic variation in the client.

Incubation period The time interval between exposure to the organism and the development of the disease.

Indifferent interaction A type of interaction that occurs when two medications given at the same time do not alter the effect of each other in any way; each medication retains its effectiveness as if it were given alone.

Indigenous flora Bacteria that normally live on or in certain parts of the body (skin, respiratory tract, gastrointestinal tract) that normally do not cause infection.

Infection A general term that describes the presence and growth in the body of a foreign organism that usually produces some degree of tissue damage or inflammation.

Inflammation A nonspecific immune response that occurs in reaction to any type of tissue or organ injury no matter what the cause.

Inotropic Medications that affect the force of myocardial contraction in either a positive (increased force of contraction) or a negative (decreased force of contraction) way.

Irritant Medication that is capable of producing cell excitation, causing damage to cells—cellulitis, thrombophlebitis, and sensitivity similar to allergic reaction.

Ketonuria Ketones in the urine.

Leukopenia A decrease in the number of white blood cells.

Lipids Fat emulsion fluids that can be administered directly into the circulatory system through a central IV line.

Lipoatrophy Atrophy of subcutaneous fat caused by repeated injections of insulin in the same site over prolonged periods.

Loading dose A larger-than-normal dose of medication given at the beginning of therapy to rapidly raise the blood level to the therapeutic range.

Medication (drug) A pharmacological or chemical agent that is capable of interacting with a living organism to produce a biologic effect.

Medication incompatibility A type of interaction that can occur when IV medications are given together in the same solution, resulting in precipitation.

Medication metabolism The biochemical breakdown of medications in the body, usually in the liver.

Medication potency The relative amount of medication required to produce the desired response.

Medication therapy The use of a pharmacological agent to bring about a physiological change.

Medication tolerance A decrease in responsiveness to a medication after repeated or chronic administration; larger doses of the medication are required to produce the same effects.

Menorrhagia Excessive uterine bleeding occurring at the regular intervals of menstruation.

Metastasize The transfer or spread of cancer cells from one site (primary) to another (secondary).

Mineralocorticoid Refers to adrenal hormones, such as aldosterone, which regulate mineral (Na, K) metabolism and fluid balance.

Minimum effective concentration (MEC) The lowest level of medication in the blood that will produce the desired effects.

Minimum toxic concentration (MTC) The medication level in the blood at which the medication will begin to produce severe side effects or toxic effects.

Miosis Pinpoint pupils; constriction of the pupils.

Mode of transmission The way the infectious organism is spread from one person to another.

Myasthenia gravis A disease of the neuromuscular junction that results in muscular weakness.

Mydriasis Dilatation of the pupil of the eye.

Myocardium The muscle layer of the heart.

Necrosis Death of tissue.

Neoplastic New abnormal tissue growth, usually referring to malignant tumors.

Nephrotoxic Harmful or damaging to the kidney.

Neurosis A mental disorder involving an increased sense of fear and anxiety due to insecurity or other psychological factors.

Noncompliance The client's voluntary refusal to follow the medication regimen; a major problem in the treatment of disease.

Nonvesicant Medication that does not cause blisters on the skin nor tissue necrosis when infiltrated but that may be a mild irritant capable of producing thromboembolism.

Norepinephrine The neurotransmitter of the sympathetic nervous system.

Nosocomial infections Infections that are acquired after the person has entered the health-care system.

Nutrients Substances necessary for the promotion and maintenance of health and growth of the person.

Nystagmus An involuntary and constant movement of the eyeball.

Oligomenorrhea Light or irregular menses.

Oliguria A decrease in urinary output.

Opportunistic organisms Bacteria or fungi that are normally found in the indigenous flora that may produce infection when the host defense mechanisms are damaged or impaired.

Osteomalacia A softening of the bones.

Osteoporosis A loss of calcium from the bones, resulting in a decrease in bone density.

Ototoxic An adverse effect of some medications (diuretics, antibiotics) on the ear, resulting in deafness or vestibular disturbances.

Parasitic arthropods A number of creatures that infest humans and other mammals and often are vectors for a number of infectious diseases, including typhus, trench fever, and bubonic plague.

Parenteral Administration of a substance, such as a medication, by a route that introduces the medication below the skin.

Paresthesia An abnormal sensation such as numbness, tingling, prickling, or heightened sensitivity.

Parkinsonism A disease involving a deficiency of dopamine in the basal ganglia; symptoms usually include tremors, muscular rigidity, and ataxia.

Peak and trough A laboratory test that establishes the maximum blood level of a medication (peak) and the lowest blood level of a medication (trough) to determine whether the blood levels of the medication are within the therapeutic range.

Peak concentration The time when the level of the medication is the greatest in the blood.

Peptic ulcer disease Gastric, duodenal, and stress ulcers exist when there are ulcerations of the gastrointestinal mucosa and underlying tissue by gastric acid secretions resulting from either an increase in secretion of hydrochloric acid or from tissues that have decreased resistance to the acid itself.

Pharmacodynamics Study of the time required for medication actions to occur in the body through processes of absorption, distribution, metabolism, and elimination.

Pharmacokinetics The study of how a medication reaches its use of action and is removed from the body through processes of absorption, distribution, metabolism, and elimination.

Phlebitis Inflammation of a vein.

Photophobia An aversion to or intolerance to light.

Photosensitivity An adverse effect of some medications that causes the skin to be unusually susceptible to effects of sunlight or ultraviolet light.

Photosensitivity reaction An exaggerated sunburn reaction when the skin is exposed to sunlight.

Protozoa Modified bacteria that retain some of the properties of animals and some properties of plants.

Physical dependence The condition of being dependent on a drug (heroin, morphine, amphetamine, cocaine), which when discontinued results in withdrawal symptoms.

Pleomorphism The changes that occur in the size and shape of cancer cells, as well as in the size and shape of the nucleus.

Polydipsia Excessive thirst; symptom of diabetes.

Polyphagia Eating large amounts of food; symptom of diabetes.

Polyuria Excessive production and voiding of urine; symptom of diabetes.

Preload The amount of blood that is in the heart just prior to contraction.

Premature labor Labor between 20 and 37 weeks that produces regular contractions that are less than 10 minutes apart and cervical dilation and effacement or changes in the cervix to indicate labor progression.

Prescribing medications The process of selecting an appropriate medication to treat a client's problem based upon an assessment and diagnosis of the disease process (usual role of physicians, dentists, nurse practitioners, veterinarians, physician's assistants).

Prodromal symptoms The first symptom that indicates the onset of a particular disease. It is not always the most typical symptom.

Prophylaxis Using a medication or method to prevent a disease from developing or spreading.

Prostaglandins Chemical substances that are released whenever there is trauma or injury to tissues.

Pruritus An itching sensation on the skin that may be the first indication of an allergic reaction to a medication.

Psychosis A serious mental disorder involving a breakdown of personality and a loss of the sense of reality.

Resistant organisms Bacteria, viruses, or parasites that are no longer able to be destroyed by the usual amounts and types of anti-infective medications.

Salicylism A toxic condition characterized by nausea, vomiting, and tinnitus caused by an overdose of salicylates (aspirin).

Shock An abnormal physiological state in which there is widespread serious reduction of tissue perfusion.

Secondary reaction A type of reaction that occurs when medications have more than one primary action and use.

Sedative A medication that reduces activity and produces relaxation.

Seizure A physiological condition caused by abnormal electrical activity in the brain. This abnormal activity involves organized and repetitive discharges from some area in the brain and may or may not produce a convulsion.

Serum sickness Symptoms of chills, fever, edema, joint and muscle pain, malaise.

Side effects Effects produced by a drug that are in addition to the therapeutic effect (adverse reactions).

Status epilepticus A continuing series of grand mal seizures that may result in death without immediate medical treatment.

Stomatitis Inflammation of the mouth.

Sublingual Under the tongue.

Superinfection An infection that results when the balance of the body's normal flora is disrupted by use of antibiotics or other antimicrobial medications.

Sympatholytic A medication that inhibits or blocks the sympathetic nervous system.

Sympathomimetic A medication that mimics medications that stimulate the sympathetic nervous system.

Synapse The point at which the axon of one neuron communicates with the dendrites of another neuron.

Synergistic interaction A type of interaction that occurs when two medications taken at the same time have an end effect greater than would be expected from the sum of the effects; sometimes stated as, "Medication X potentiates medication Y." Results of a synergistic interaction are often difficult to predict; some side effects may be increased because of this interaction.

Synthetic Manufactured or produced by artificial methods, usually in a scientific laboratory.

Teratogen Anything that can damage the rapidly growing cells in a fetus, often leading to birth defects.

Therapeutic range The concentration of medication in the blood when the desired effects are produced without severe side effects; that is, the level between the minimum effective concentration and the minimum toxic concentration.

Thrombocytopenia A decrease in the number of platelets.

Thrombosis Development of a thrombus.

Thrombus A blood clot (pl. thrombi).

Tinnitus Ringing in the ears.

Titrate The adjustment of the dosage of a medication based on a predetermined, specific physiological response.

Tolerance Reduced responsiveness during repeated administration of a medication, requiring increasingly larger doses.

Toxicity Refers to the poisonous or toxic effects produced by medications when the blood levels exceed the therapeutic range.

Toxic reaction (effect) A serious and potentially lethal type of adverse reaction that occurs when the blood level of the medication reaches toxic levels, producing permanent damage to organ systems.

Unpredictable reactions Less frequent reactions to medications that are not dose-related and that are usually due to a unique or individual response by a client to a medication.

Uricosuric Any agent or medication that increases the urinary excretion of uric acid.

Urticaria Eruption of itching wheals, usually of systemic origin; early sign of an allergic reaction to a medication.

Vasodilation Dilation of a vessel.

Vasopressor A constriction of the blood vessels that when widespread results in a rise in blood pressure.

Venous Pertaining to the vein(s).

Venules Small veins.

Vertigo A sensation of moving or of objects moving, usually accompanied by difficulty in walking and maintaining balance.

Vestibular Pertaining to the structures of the inner ear.

Vesicant Medication capable of producing blisters on the skin and tissue necrosis if it becomes infiltrated.

Virus Obligate intracellular parasites that cannot live outside of cells because of their inability to obtain food or replicate DNA without a host.

Vitamins Several types of substances that are required in small amounts for normal development and functioning of the body.

Vomiting A condition that occurs when the chemoreceptor trigger zone (CTZ) in the medulla of the brain is stimulated, in turn stimulating the vomiting center (VC), also located in the medulla.

BIBLIOGRAPHY

Drug Facts and Comparisons. JB Lippincott, St Louis, 1998.

Kee, JL, and Marshall, SM: Clinical Calculations, ed 3. WB Saunders, Philadelphia, 1996.

Kee, JL, and Hayes, ER: Pharmacology. WB Saunders, Philadelphia, 1997.

Kuhn, M: Pharmacotherapeutics: A Nursing Process Approach, ed 4. FA Davis, Philadelphia, 1998.

McEvoy, GK (ed): AHFS '95 Drug Information. American Society of Health-System Pharmacists, New York, 1995.

Medical Center of Delaware: Formulary and Drug Therapy Guide. Lexi-Comp, Hudson, Ohio, 1996.

Physician's Desk Reference, ed 52. Medical Economics, Montvale, N.J., 1998.

Pinnell, NL: Nursing Pharmacology. WB Saunders, Philadelphia, 1996.

Shannon, MT, Wilson, BA, and Stang, CL: Govoni & Hayes Drugs and Nursing Implications. Appleton & Lange, Norwalk, Conn., 1995.

Taber's Cyclopedic Medical Dictionary, ed 18. FA Davis, Philadelphia, 1997.

United States Pharmacopeia Drug Information (USP-DI) for the Health Care Professional, ed 16. US Pharmacopeial Convention, Rockville, Md., 1997.

INDEX

Note: Page numbers followed by "f" indicate figures; those followed by "t" indicate tables.

Pituitary gland, 75, 78t
Pleomorphism, 103
Pleural space, 69
PMS. *See* Premenstrual syndrome
Poison control, 29
Positive attitude, 16
Post-myocardial infarction, 19
Potassium, 120–121
Potency, medication, 21
Practice effect, 11
Practice questions/tests, 11, 125–326
Preeclampsia, 88–89
Pregnancy
    fetal risk, 333–337
    hypertension and preeclampsia, 88–89
    labor, 87–88, 89
    medications during, 23
Preload, 48
Premature ventricular contractions (PVCs), 54
Premenstrual syndrome (PMS), 89–90
Primary hypertension, 50
Prinzmetal angina. *See* Variant angina
Probenecid, 100
Process of elimination, 12
Prodromal symptom, 107
Prostaglandins, 39, 98
Protamine sulfate, 61
Protein, 27, 30
Protozoa, 106
PSVT. *See* Paroxysmal supraventricular tachycardia
Psychiatric conditions, 40–45, 338
Psychosis, 44–45
Psychosocial Integrity Needs, 4, 5
Purified protein derivative, 24
Purines, 100
PVCs. *See* Premature ventricular contractions
Pyridoxine, 120

Qualifying words, 13

Refractory period, 48
Relative refractory period, 48
Renal system, 25–26, 63–67
Renin, 51f
Resistant organism, 107
Respiratory system, 69–73
Review books, 10, 11
Rhythmicity, 47
Ribonucleic acid. *See* RNA

Ringworm, 111
RNA (ribonucleic acid), 103
Roundworms, 112

Safe and Effective Care Environment, 4
Scabies, 107, 113
Schizophrenia, 44
Secondary hypertension, 50
Sedatives, 40–41
Seizure, 38
Seizure disorder. *See* Epilepsy
Sella turcica, 75
Sensory system, 97–101
Septic shock, 56
Sequence of actions, 16
Serotonin, 42
Serum albumin, 27
Sexual contact route, 107
Shock, 55–56
Skeletal muscle relaxants, 40
Small intestine, 91
Sociocultural theory, 44
Sodium, 120
Somatotropin, 78t
Specific binding medications, 32
Stable angina, 49
Stimulators. *See* Agonist medications
Stomach, 91
Streptokinase, 60, 61
Study strategies, 10–11
Subcutaneous fat, 29
Subcutaneous injection, 24
Sublingual route. *See* Oral mucosa route
Sucralfate, 93
Sulfonamide, 109
Superinfection, 107
Suppositories, 25
Sylvan Learning Centers, 9–10
Sympathetic system, 32, 33, 34–35
Sympatholytic agents, 34
Sympathomimetic agents, 33
Synapses, 31
Synergistic interaction, 22
Systemic infections, 111

Teratogen, 23
Terminology, 21
Tetracycline, 108–109
Therapeutic range, 25, 26f